W9-CDY-599

Nurses' Guide to Clinical Procedures

Second Edition

Jean Smith-Temple, MSN, RN
Clinical Assistant Professor of Nursing
Baccalaureate Nursing Program
Adult Health
The University of South Alabama
Mobile, Alabama

Joyce Young Johnson, PhD, RN, CCRN
Assistant Professor
Adult Health Nursing
College of Health Science
Georgia State University
Atlanta, Georgia

J. B. Lippincott Company
Philadelphia

Sponsoring Editor: Donna L. Hilton
Coordinating Editorial Assistant: Susan M. Keneally
Project Editors: Mary Kinsella and Barbara Ryalls
Indexer: David Ammundson
Design Coordinator: Kathy Kelley-Luedtke
Interior Designer: Holly Reid McLaughlin
Cover Designer: Lou Fuiano
Production Manager: Helen Ewan
Production Coordinator: Nannette Winski
Compositor: Graphic Sciences Corporation
Printer/Binder: R. R. Donnelly & Sons, Crawfordsville
Cover Printer: R. R. Donnelly & Sons, Crawfordsville

Second Edition

Copyright © 1994, by J. B. Lippincott Company.
Copyright © 1990, by J. B. Lippincott Company. All rights reserved.
No part of this book may be used or reproduced in any manner what-
soever without written permission except for brief quotations embodied
in critical articles and reviews. Printed in the United States of America.
For information write J. B. Lippincott Company, 227 East Washington
Square, Philadelphia, Pennsylvania 19106.

6 5 4 3

Library of Congress Cataloging-in-Publication Data
Smith-Temple, Jean.
    Nurses' guide to clinical procedures / Jean Smith-Temple
Joyce Young Johnson : 2nd ed.
        p.   cm.
    Includes bibliographical references and index.
    ISBN 0–397–54987–3
    1. Nursing—Handbooks, manuals, etc.   I. Smith-Temple, Jean.
II. Title.   III. Title: Clinical procedures.
    [DNLM: 1. Nursing Assessment—handbooks.   2. Nursing Process-
–handbooks.   WY 39 S6425n   1994]
RT51.S65   1994
610.73—dc20
DNLM/DLC
for Library of Congress   94–10211
                                                                                    CIP

Any procedure or practice described in this book should be applied by
the health-care practitioner under appropriate supervision in accordance
with professional standards of care used with regard to the unique circumstances that apply in each practice situation. Care has been taken to
confirm the accuracy of information presented and to describe generally
accepted practices. However, the authors, editors, and publisher cannot
accept any responsibility for errors or omissions or for any consequences
from application of the information in this book and make no warranty
express or implied, with respect to the contents of the book.

Every effort has been made to ensure that drug selections and dosages
are in accordance with current recommendations and practice. Because of
ongoing research, changes in government regulations and the constant
flow of information on drug therapy, reactions and interactions, the read-
er is cautioned to check the package insert for each drug for indications,
dosages, warnings and precautions, particularly if the drug is new or in-
frequently used.

To my husband, Richard . . . as we expand our future.
To my family and friends . . . thanks.

Jean

To my husband, Larry, who has helped me make miracles
with his patience, encouragement, assistance, and love.

To my family, who are always there for me
when I need them.

To my best friends, who always believe in me.

Joyce

To our students and colleagues
for contributing to our professional growth
and development.

Jean and Joyce

CONTRIBUTORS

Second Edition
Rosie Calvin, RN, MSN
> *Clinical Specialist*
> *University of Mississippi Medical Center*
> *Jackson, Mississippi*

Phyllis Prather Hicks, RN, BSN
> *Instructor*
> *Harrisburg Area Community College*
> *Harrisburg, Pennsylvania*

Richard Temple, Jr., LPTA, BS
> *Licensed Physical Therapist Assistant*
> *Mobile Infirmary Medical Center*
> *Mobile, Alabama*

First Edition
Louise Gore Grose, RN, PhD
> *Nurse Consultant*
> *Board of Nurse Examiners*
> *for the State of Texas*
> *Staff Nurse*
> *Home Health Care Department*
> *Holy Cross Hospital*
> *Austin, Texas*

LaDonna Powell, RN, MSN
> *Pediatric Clinical Nurse Specialist*
> *University Medical Center*
> *Children's Hospital*
> *Jackson, Mississippi*

Nurses' Guide to Clinical Procedures is a quick-reference clinical support tool designed to serve students in all types of educational programs and practicing nurses in any clinical setting. It explains the key steps necessary to perform nursing skills and provides cues to the critical thinking needed for client care.

This guide contains information about nearly 200 skills. A detailed table of contents and index are provided for easy reference to procedures. The procedures within the 12 chapters of *Nurses' Guide to Clinical Procedures* are organized in a nursing process format, with procedures listed at the beginning of each chapter for convenience. Chapter overviews review basic principles and concepts. A list of potential nursing diagnoses accompanies each procedure. Nursing procedures are organized as follows:

Equipment
Purpose(s)
Assessment
Nursing Diagnoses
Planning (includes client-centered goals and highlighted special considerations with general, pediatric, geriatric, home health, and transcultural aspects)
Implementation (actions with rationales)
Evaluation (includes examples of desired outcomes)
Documentation (includes examples of charting)

Actions are presented concisely with clear illustrations to assist the user. Universal blood and body fluid precautions are considered whenever applicable. A pictogram next to the procedure title indicates that gloves should be worn.

Nursing procedures have been organized to facilitate safe, expedient performance. *Nurses' Guide to Clinical Procedures* should be used as a clinical reference; it is *not* intended for initial instruction of nursing procedures. The user should review principles in the chapter overview before proceeding to the nursing procedures. Procedures should be read in their entirety to ensure that all relevant health-care matters are considered during performance. Narrative documentation format will be used for charting examples, although many other forms of documentation may be used in the clinical setting. Illustrations, tables, and appendices provide further support. Users should refer to these aids, as well as to related nursing procedures, as needed.

Jean Smith-Temple, RN, MSN
Joyce Young Johnson, RN, PhD, CCRN

ACKNOWLEDGMENTS

We would like to thank Donna Hilton for her support; Phyllis Prather-Hicks and Rosie Calvin for their contributions; Clemmie L. Riggins and Dorothy Young for their invaluable assistance; and the following people for their support during writing the first edition of Nurses' Guide to Clinical Procedures: *Dr. Frances Henderson; Patricia Cleary; Louise Grose; LaDonna Powell; Gwendolyn J. Johnson; Kim Golmon; Cynthia Henderson; Jo Tina Johnson; and Myra Young.*

CONTENTS

11 *Medication Administration* 579

Nurses' Guide to Clinical Procedures

Second Edition

CHAPTER 7

Verbal Communication Skills

OVERVIEW

- Verbal communication involves a sender, a receiver, a message, and the environment in which the interaction takes place.
- Communication includes the attitude projected—gestures, voice tone, rhythm, volume, and pitch—in addition to words spoken.
- Effective communication is
  - *simple*—briefly and comprehensively relates data using commonly known and understood terms
  - *clear*—states exactly what is meant covering the who, what, when, where, why, and how of the matter
  - *pertinent*—contains data that are important to the current situation and ties data to an apparent need to show significance
  - *sensitive*—considers readiness of the receiver and adapts depth and breadth of data to meet receiver's needs
  - *accurate*—includes factual information related with confidence and credibility

Jean Smith-Temple and Joyce Young Johnson:
Nurses' Guide to Clinical Procedures, Second Edition.© 1994
J. B. Lippincott Company

- Building effective communication skills requires a constant awareness of one's self as a sender and a receiver of messages.
- Communication approaches should be modified to meet the cultural needs of the client.

Shift Report

☒ Equipment

- Client Kardex or plan of care
- Client summary notes (kept throughout shift)
- Tape recorder, if warranted by facility protocol

Purpose

Facilitates continuity of client care through accurate and comprehensive communication of relevant client data from off-going to oncoming care-givers

Assessment

Assessment should focus on the following:

Current status of client (comfort, medications/fluid infusions, treatments pending) 30 to 60 minutes before nurse begins to write report (prior to end of shift)

Planning

Key Goals and Sample Goal Criterion

The client will

Receive appropriate treatments, medications, and other care measures consistent with plan of care

Special Considerations

When "walking rounds" are employed, visual verification of the client's condition should supplement reported data.

When reporting to care-givers with little previous exposure to the client, more background may be needed or desired. Care-givers with extensive previous exposure to the client may require only a brief update of pertinent changes.

Remember to report data or occurrences from previous shifts, when pertinent.

Include concerns of the client, family members, or significant others.

Home Health

The assessment and report of a homebound client should include the client's status at the time of the last home health visit, the client's response to interventions, any restrictions present in the environment (such as no running water or no electricity), and any adaptations that have been made in client-care procedures (such as irrigating a wound while in the bathtub).

The visit report should also include the client's address (with directions if it is difficult to locate), any special supplies or equipment to be taken on the next visit, and client-teaching needs.

 Transcultural

Pertinent data about the client's sociocultural background should be included if the data are significant to some aspect of the client's care.

Implementation

Action	Rationale
1. Gather equipment.	Facilitates organizing report
2. Report client identification data:	Ensures association of reported data with correct client
- Name	
- Room number	
- Age	
- Sex	
- Medical diagnosis (primary and secondary)	
- Doctor's name (Display 1.1)	
3. Record special circumstances of client:	Promotes client safety and psychosocial well-being
- Sight or hearing deficits	
- Language or cultural barriers	Recognizes ethical and legal concerns
- Safety needs (*e.g.*, client at high risk for falls)	

Action	Rationale

- Support needs
   - Family concerns
   - Religious concerns	

4. Summarize client's status using nursing diagnoses to indicate active emotional or physical problems (Display 1.1).	Validates established nursing diagnoses and need for continued intervention
BEGIN WITH DIAGNOSES OF HIGHEST PRIORITY AND PROCEED TO THOSE OF LEAST PRIORITY.	Establishes priority of client's needs
5. For each diagnosis addressed, record the following: - Actual or potential diagnosis	
- Assessment data (complaints, wound/dressing status, IVs, drains, O₂, etc.)	Summarizes current status of treatments
- Interventions used (medications, IV, treatments, monitoring, teaching) - Evaluation (intake and output, client response to treatments, teaching, etc.)	
6. Report recent results of diagnostic procedures and lab tests.	Provides status update
7. Report new medical/nursing orders (diagnostic tests, medications, treatments, surgery, dietary or activity restrictions, or discharge planning).	Provides update on planned medical and nursing interventions
8. Summarize general environmental concerns (tubes; drains; infusions, with fluid counts; and mechanical supports [include settings]).	Facilitates maintenance of support equipment

Action	Rationale

Display 1.1   Report Format—Summary

Client identification data
Special circumstances
Client status—physical/emotional
   Priority nursing diagnoses
   Assessment data
   Interventions (treatments, teaching, monitoring needs)
   Evaluation (client response to interventions)
Recent diagnostic test results
New orders medical/nursing
Environmental concerns
   Tubes
   Infusions (fluid count)
   Drains
Immediately pending treatments

Action	Rationale
9. Summarize treatments, fluid replacements, medication needs, tests, and so forth required during first hour of oncoming shift.	Facilitates punctuality and continuity in execution of treatment regimen

Evaluation

Goals met, partially met, or unmet?

Desired Outcomes (sample)

Appropriate treatments and medications are received as scheduled.

Sample Report

Mr. Homes, room 102, is a 75-year-old client of Dr. Smith admitted with diverticulitis; he has a history of hypertension and diabetes.

He is slightly hard-of-hearing in his left ear.

Priority nursing diagnosis: altered comfort related to abdominal cramps. Mr. Homes complained of pain at 9:00 A.M. and 2:00 P.M., was medicated with meperidine (50 mg IM each time), and experienced relief within ½ hour.

His potassium level was 3.7 this A.M. and the last fingerstick glucose level was 140.

He is scheduled for a barium enema this P.M. at 5:00 and has received enemas till clear. Food and fluids are restricted (NPO).

He has dextrose 5% in water (D_5W) infusing at 50 ml/hr with 400 ml left to count.

He is scheduled for a fingerstick glucose level test at 4:00 P.M.

Client Education

Equipment

- Selected teaching tools (booklets, pamphlets, audiovisual materials, games, and so forth)

Purpose

Assists client in learning information necessary for participation in self-care

Reduces anxiety

Assessment

Assessment should focus on the following:

Client's or family's readiness to learn and ability to comprehend
Client's age and educational level
Amount and accuracy of client's prior knowledge about content
Community resources for referral
Prior knowledge of significant others, if they are to be included
Presence of any communication barriers such as visual, hearing, or speech problems
Presence of any physical or emotional barriers (conditions or medications that alter mental state or cause pain or stress)

Nursing Diagnoses

The nursing diagnoses may include the following:

Knowledge deficit related to unfamiliarity with new illness
Anxiety related to knowledge deficit

Planning

Key Goals and Sample Goal Criteria

The client will

Demonstrate procedure using correct technique with 100% accuracy by discharge

State the purpose prior to beginning the procedure

State solutions to potential complications of the procedure by discharge

Special Considerations

Individuals with similar problems are frequently helpful in facilitating client learning.

A list of support or referral groups may be available through an agency.

Geriatric

Because of delayed reaction times that occur with normal aging, elderly clients may require more response time during actual teaching and evaluation.

Consider response time when planning time frame.

Pediatric

Visual aids and demonstrations are often effective when teaching children.

Always include parents or family (for reinforcement), if available.

Same-age-group teaching can be used.

Home Health

Incorporate adaptations or modifications of procedures that are likely to occur in the home setting.

Transcultural

- Examples used for clarification or explanation of information may in some instances be understood more easily if they relate to some aspect of the client's culture. Pictures may be useful if a different language is spoken. Many facilities have access to interpreters of various languages if needed.
- It is important to find out how the client views health. Many clients of various cultures view illness as a curse or bad luck. This may affect the nurse's ability to engage the client successfully in active learning.

Implementation

Action	Rationale
1. Establish verbal contract with client regarding teaching plans.	Provides mutual goals for client and nurse
2. Eliminate environmental distractions such as excess noise, poor lighting, uncomfortable room temperatures, cluttered rooms, excess visitor and staff traffic, and clinical treatments and procedures.	Facilitates environment for communication and learning
3. During assessment and along with client, determine exactly what information client needs and is able to retain.	Provides teaching focus Involves client Teaching is most effective when it occurs in response to specific needs expressed by the learner

---

Display 1.2   Preparation Guide for Development of a Teaching Plan

---

Objectives to be met by end of session
Content
    What content will be taught to meet objectives?
    Will complex content need to be taught in divided stages?
Teaching methods
    What reading materials are needed?
    What audiovisual aids are needed?
    Will games or role-playing be used?
    Will support groups or group sessions be used?
    What equipment/supplies are needed?
    Will tours or visits to related agencies be helpful?
    How much time is needed to cover each section of material?
    Will practice time be needed?
    How much time is realistic for this client?
Evaluation methods
    How much time will be needed to evaluate learning?
    Will evaluation be:
        verbal?
        written?
        return demonstration?

Action	Rationale
4. Determine nursing diagnoses based on assessment findings.	Provides focus for goal-setting
5. Set realistic, measurable goals with client and significant others.	Allows client participation Provides focus for implementing teaching
6. Develop teaching plan (Display 1.2) that specifically addresses: - Objectives to be met by the end of teaching session - Content to be taught - Methods of teaching - Methods of evaluation	Facilitates optimal learning Provides questions to guide teaching plan preparation
7. Obtain all necessary equipment.	
8. Implement teaching plan.	
9. Evaluate plan and implementation.	

Evaluation

Goals met, partially met, or unmet?

Desired Outcomes (sample)

Client states purpose of procedure before beginning procedure.
Client demonstrates procedure correctly with 100% accuracy by discharge.
Client states solutions to potential complications of procedure by discharge.

Documentation

The following should be noted on the client's chart:

- Extent to which each objective was met (fully, partially, not met)
- Nature of material taught
- Persons other than client included in session
- Client response to teaching

- Client concerns expressed during teaching
- Need for additional teaching or alternate method of teaching
- Need for revision of plans with client input

Sample Documentation

DATE	TIME	
6/11/94	0900	Client teaching done regarding importance of low-sodium diet in relation to managing hypertension. Client demonstrated selection of low-sodium foods with 80% accuracy from list. Participated actively in learning. Denies concerns in relation to topic at this time.

Therapeutic Communication

⊠ Equipment

- Calendars
- Clocks
- Picture or word boards
- Any items needed to add clarity to message

Purpose

Facilitates client's sense of well-being and control
Promotes beneficial nurse–client interaction

Assessment

Assessment should focus on the following:

Client's age, developmental level, cultural or ethnic background, educational level
Physical and mental barriers to communication, such as poor sight or hearing, speech impediment, pain, and so forth
Client's use of nonverbal gesturing
Client's perceptions of people and situations
Sources of stress for client
Client's use of defense and coping mechanisms
Immediate environment (*e.g.*, noise, lighting, visitors)
Support systems (family, friends, community agencies)

Nursing Diagnoses

The nursing diagnoses may include the following:

Anxiety related to inability to communicate needs
Noncompliance related to feelings of lack of control
Individual ineffective coping related to multiple stressors

Planning

Key Goals and Sample Goal Criteria

The client will

Communicate needs and their satisfactions effectively
Comply with diet and activity regimen
Verbalize feelings about recent occurrences

Special Considerations

The nurse should anticipate questions and concerns when explaining factual information.

Plan interaction times to ensure privacy and avoid interruptions.

When planning interactions consider the phase of the nurse-client relationship:

- *Orientation phase:* initial meeting of client and nurse; verbal contract is made
- *Working phase:* basic nurse–client trust established and relationship solidified through meeting of objectives
- *Termination phase:* preparation for discharge and ending of relationship

When interacting with clients consider their stage of coping or possible grief: denial, anger, bargaining, depression, and acceptance (see Display 1.3.1).

Avoid statements or behaviors that might result in barriers to communication (Display 1.3.2).

Geriatric

Elderly clients may have one or more communication barriers that may readily be removed once discovered; necessary dentures, hearings aids, and glasses should be acquired, if possible.

With increasing age, a client's speech and comprehension may be slowed, requiring more time for communication.

Pediatric

A child may perceive sudden body movements by an adult as threatening; approach slowly, after informing the child of your intentions.

When communicating with a child, consider developmental stage.

Home Health

Encourage the client and family to prepare a list of questions or concerns during the time between the nurse's visits.

Display 1.3.1   Considerations for Interactions with Special Clients/Families

When interacting with an anxious client, recognize client's decreased ability to focus on and respond to multiple stimuli:
- maintain quiet, calm environment
- keep messages simple, concrete, and brief
- repeat messages often
- minimize need for extensive decision making
- monitor anxiety level, using verbal and nonverbal cues

When interacting with an angry client:
- use careful, unhurried, deliberate body movements
- provide an open, nonthreatening environment
- clear area of anger-provoking stimuli (persons, objects, etc.)
- maintain a nonthreatening demeanor, using open body language, soft voice tones and so forth

When interacting with a depressed client:
- allow additional time for interactions
- emphasize use of physical attending
- avoid giving client time-limited tasks due to slowed reflexes
- monitor closely for cues of self-destructive tendencies
- keep messages simple, concrete, and brief
- minimize need for extensive decision making

When interacting with a client exhibiting denial:
- use direct questions to determine the situation triggering use of coping mechanism
- do not avoid the reality of the situation, but allow client to maintain denial defense; it often serves a protective function
- recognize that denial may be the first of a series of crisis phases, to be followed by phases of: increased tension, disorganization, attempts to reorganize, attempts to escape the problem, local reorganization, general reorganization, and possibly resolution
- be alert for cues that the phase is ending (*i.e.,* questions from client regarding the disturbing situation)

 Transcultural
- Use of an interpreter for clients whose native language is not English may reduce chances of miscommunication by client and nurse.
- Clients of some cultures may view direct eye contact as offensive and intrusive. It is best to follow the cues of the client in developing a rapport.

- Sociocultural differences should be considered when inter-preting a client's nonverbal behavior (*i.e.,* lack of eye contact may signify respect, not insecurity, and a shuffling gait may signify "cool" use of body language, not physical debilitation).

Implementation

Action	Rationale
1. Approach the client in a purposeful but unhurried manner.	Facilitates controlled but nonthreatening interaction
2. Identify self and relation-ship to client.	Initiates orientation phase of nurse–client relationship
3. Arrange environment so that it is conducive to type of interaction needed.	Eliminates environmental distractions
4. Use physical attending skills throughout the inter-action process:	Exhibits nonverbal body language consistent with verbalizations
- Face directly and lean to-ward client	Conveys interest, attentive-ness, sincerity, and nonde-fensiveness
- Maintain eye contact and an open posture (do not cross legs or arms)	
5. Begin interaction using therapeutic techniques when eliciting or sharing information or responses:	Facilitates purposeful and mutually beneficial interac-tion for nurse and client
- Use open-ended state-ments and questions	Allows ventilation of those feelings and concerns most important to client at the time
- Restate or paraphrase client statements when indicated	Confirms significance of client's comments
- Clarify unclear com-ments	Ensures intended message
- Focus the statement when client tends to ramble or is vague	Promotes concreteness of message
- Explore further when additional information is needed.	Promotes more complete information gathering
- Provide rationale why more information is	Maintains professional integrity of interaction

Action	Rationale
needed, when appropriate	
- Use touch and silence, when appropriate	Conveys compassion and allows time for client composure
6. Use active listening techniques:	
- Do not interrupt client in the middle of comments	Prevents distraction
- Use verbal indicators of acceptance and understanding ("um-hmm," "yes")	Expresses interest
- Focus on verbal and nonverbal message	Facilitates receipt of complete message
7. When client communicates, note use of gestures as well as facial expression and elements of speech—tone, pitch, emphasis of words, etc.	Facilitates receipt of complete message
8. Note client's nonverbal gestures as you are speaking (facial grimacing, smiling, crossing arms or legs).	Facilitates detection of cues indicating acceptance or nonacceptance of message
9. Toward end of the interaction, summarize important aspects of the conversation.	Avoids abrupt and incomplete closure

Display 1.3.2   Blocks to Therapeutic Communication

Giving advice
Using responses that imply approval or disapproval
Agreeing or disagreeing
Not listening attentively
Appearing distracted
Imposing judgment
Stereotyping
Providing false reassurance
Using clichés
Excessive probing
Questioning without basis
Responding defensively

Evaluation

Goals met, partially met, or unmet?

Desired Outcomes (sample)

Client evidences no sign of anxiety and communicates needs effectively.
Client complies with dietary and activity regimen.
Client discusses major stressors in current life.

Documentation

The following should be noted on the client's chart:

- Date, time, and place of interaction
- Nature and significant highlights of the discussion
- Communication barriers (if any) and interventions used
- Significant nonverbal gestures

Sample Documentation

DATE	TIME	
2/29/94	1400	Client in bed and tearful; upset because husband has not visited in 3 days. States concern about husband's feelings regarding loss of her breast. Reach to Recovery support group discussed. Nurse will contact husband this P.M.

CHAPTER **2**

Written Communication Skills

2.1 Nursing Process/Plan of Care Preparation
2.2 Nurses' Progress Notes

OVERVIEW

- Written communication is often the major and occasionally the only medium for data exchange between health care team members.
- Communication that is client oriented and reflects the nursing process will be more focused and organized than disjointed, task-oriented communication.
- Written communication often provides proof of practice or malpractice. **Legally speaking, if it wasn't documented, it wasn't done.** Focus charting or charting by exception may be used to minimize lengthy narrative charting through the use of check lists. Clear documentation is best proof that responsible, well-planned nursing care was given.
- Written communication should follow the guidelines of good communication and should be simple, clear, pertinent, sensitive, and above all, accurate.
- Nurse's notes and plans of care often will be the only proof in future years that clients were monitored and cared for.
- Well-written plans of care, completed flow sheets and

notes lay a strong foundation for continuity of client care.
- Standardized care plans may be used in some settings; however, some individualization of the plan of care should be possible, and basic knowledge of plan of care preparation remains beneficial.
- Patient-outcome or critical-path time line plans may guide patient care. Documentation of patient outcomes remains important for evaluation.
- Although nursing diagnoses accepted by the North American Nursing Diagnosis Association (NANDA) are available as a reference, additional clinically useful diagnoses such as collaborative problems (Carpenito, 1992) may be used if institutionally acceptable.

Nursing Process/Plan of Care Preparation

☒ Equipment

- Pencil or pen (if care plan is permanent part of chart)
- Client Kardex or care plan
- Appropriate reference books

Purpose

Provides a guiding foundation for individualized client care
Facilitates continuity of nursing care

Assessment

Assessment should focus on the following:

Data gathered from client environment, client history, physical and mental status, and social supports

Nursing Diagnoses

Will vary related to client circumstances (see individual procedures)

Planning

Key Goals and Sample Goal Criterion

The client will

Receive consistent, continuous care as designed in the plan of care

Special Considerations

When planning and implementing care, always consider safety and privacy needs of the client.

Involve client/family as much as possible in all stages of the nursing process.

Implementation

Action	Rationale
Assessment includes gathering and analyzing client data and involves appraising areas in which client might require nursing care or assistance to meet basic or higher level needs.	

Data Gathering

Action	Rationale
1. Systematically gather data: assess client status from admission history, physical examination, and diagnostic tests (may use body systems or basic needs areas).	Organizes data
2. Underline any abnormal data or note on separate pad.	Designates areas of concern and probable causes
3. Interview client regarding perceptions of condition and need priorities.	Determines what needs client feels are of highest priority and how those needs might be met

Data Analysis

Action	Rationale
4. Organize and group areas of concern.	Facilitates clear definition of needs or problems
5. Determine client abilities and inabilities to meet identified needs; match client strengths and supports to needs.	Determines level of nursing care needed—teaching, guidance, or direct nursing intervention

Action	**Rationale**

Developing Nursing Diagnoses

6. Determine nursing diagnoses centering on needs requiring nursing intervention or teaching. Write diagnoses with two parts and a connector:

Part One–actual or potential client problem (Example: noncompliance to diet therapy)

Part Two–probable cause of problem (Example: knowledge deficit)

Connector–connecting phrase such as **related to** or *associated with* (Example: impaired skin integrity related to immobility)

Serves as guide for individualizing plan of care

Clearly communicates problems

7. Prioritize diagnoses according to critical nature of problem and client's perceptions of need priority; life-threatening needs take first priority. Potential problems can often be addressed under a major actual concern (see goals).

Determines priorities for plan of care

Planning involves the establishment of key goals of care with criteria for evaluating if goals have been met. A goal is a statement of behavior that would reflect measurable progress toward resolution of the problem.

8. Develop goals using these key elements:
   - Statement of what client is expected to accomplish (Example: demonstrates adequate tissue perfusion)

Expresses goals in concrete terms.

Action	Rationale

- Goal criteria, in terms of measurable behaviors (Example: evidenced by capillary refill of 5–10 sec, 2+ or greater pulses, and warm skin)
  - Specific date at which expectation should be met
  - Conditions or special circumstances associated with meeting goal (Example: with the assistance of vasodilator therapy)	

9. Use the following guidelines when writing goals:
  - Goals should be client-centered (Example: "The client will . . . .")
  - Goals should be written in active and measurable terms (Example: "The client will walk. . . .")
  - Establish realistic goals of health care and or maintenance
  - Set realistic time limits, including short- and long-term goals
  - Set one goal at a time
	Develops clear, concise, realistic goals

- Avoid terms like *understand, realize,* and so forth	Decreases measurability of goal

Sample goal: By discharge, the client will demonstrate knowledge of diabetic self-care by giving own insulin and planning a 1500-calorie ADA diet without assistance or coaching.

Implementation involves carrying out actions/nursing orders designed to help client meet goals.

Action	Rationale
10. Determine who will perform actions to resolve problem.	Designates locus of control as: - **client-centered**—actions performed by client - **shared**—client and nurse jointly perform actions - **nurse-centered**—actions performed by nurse
11. List actions needed to reach goals. Nursing actions may include supervising, teaching, assisting, monitoring, or direct intervention.	Identifies actions to meet goals
12. State actions clearly, including the following elements: - **Who** will perform the action (*i.e.*, client, nurse, assistant) - **How often** or to what extent the action will be performed (Examples: three times daily; three out of four foods will be named) - **Under what conditions** action will be performed (*i.e.*, with assistance, after instruction, with supervision)	Clearly communicates planned interventions
13. State actions singularly. Explain or clarify as needed.	
14. Perform action (nurse or designated health team member).	

Evaluation is an ongoing step of reassessment and interpretation of new data to determine if goals are being met fully, partially, or not at all.

15. Assess client in view of goals and criteria.	Identifies extent of progress toward goal
16. If some behaviors are noted, determine if goal	

Action	Rationale

has been fully met or partially met.
17. Review behaviors and criteria.
18. Revise plan as needed:
    - Continue effective actions.
    - Determine factors hindering the meeting of goal and remove or minimize them.
    - Modify goal, if needed, by expanding time limits or lowering expectations.
    - Modify actions and eliminate those no longer indicated.
    - Add new actions, if needed.
    - If indicated, shift locus of control.
    - Continuously assess client status using data-gathering process.

Maintains goal behaviors, or progress toward goal
Makes goal more reachable

Makes goal more realistic for the client

Documentation
19. Documentation should be placed on appropriate temporary or permanent forms.
20. For samples of documentation, see examples in text.

Nurses' Progress Notes

☒ Equipment

- Small pad and pencil (for client summary notes)
- Client Kardex or care plan
- Pen (of appropriate color for shift)
- Client-specific progress note or nurses' note sheets

Purpose

Facilitates comprehensive communication of relevant client data from one nursing care-giver to other nurses or members of health care team

Assessment

Assessment should focus on the following:

Previous shift notes from nurses, physicians, and other team members for an update on client status

Current status, as indicated by:
- Vital signs
- Intake (infusion rates and amount remaining in tube feedings, IVs, and other infusions)
- Output (drainage amounts); indicate locations of tubes and drains
- Dressings (degree and type of soiling, frequency of changes, and status of underlying skin/wound)
- Treatments (number of times performed, duration, and client response)

Planning

Key Goals and Sample Goal Criterion

The client will

Receive continuity of care through dissemination of information in an accurate, comprehensive, and brief form.

Special Considerations

Assessment data should be obtained at beginning of and throughout shift and should be recorded in small notebook until needed.

Health care agencies may require that client data be recorded in a specialized format using the following categories: Subjective, Objective, Assessment, Planning, Implementation, and Evaluation. These categories may be used in whole (SOAPIE), in part (SOAP, APIE), or in other variations. You may organize data into this format in your notebook as they are collected by indicating the type with an initial (*e.g., A* for Assessment or *Pl* for Planning).

If routine client care flow sheets or checklists are used, do not duplicate data. Use nurses' notes to record data not covered on flow sheets and to elaborate, if needed.

Home Health

Notations should be made for each care visit regarding homebound status of client.

Content of notes should address how "sick" client is. Report findings in objective and specific terminology.

Implementation

Action	Rationale
1. Designate body systems requiring detailed assessment and documentation.	Provides framework for concise charting addressing only pertinent areas in great detail
2. Assess client in an orderly manner (see Procedure 3.1) and record findings in small notebook.	Organizes notes and facilitates accuracy through minimum dependence on memory
3. When time allows, record initial client assessment in	Provides other health care team members with an update on pertinent client data

Action	Rationale
chart (Table 2.1 lists guidelines).	
4. As day progresses, record in small notebook or bedside activity flowchart, if available, time of, precise details of, and client response to treatments or teaching. Also record occurrences pertinent to client's physical or mental state.	Indicates possible changes in client's status requiring update in documentation Facilitates prompt and accurate recording of client data

TABLE 2.1   Guidelines for Initial Assessment Notes

Assessment Area	Criteria
Neurological	Level of consciousness, orientation, verbal response, pupil size and reaction, incisions or head dressings, intracranial pressure monitor, sensory or mobility deficits (if applicable expand musculoskeletal–mobility limitations, cast or traction, and extremity status) **Safety measures**—side rails, restraints (skin status and care)
Respiratory	Rate, depth, character, dyspnea, symmetry of chest movement, breath sounds, secretions, cough, incisions, dressings, oxygen therapy, and chest tubes
Circulatory	Skin color, temperature, capillary refill, heart sounds, pulse rate, rhythm, EKG pattern (if available), heart sounds, pulse assessment (absent to 4+), skin turgor, edema, neck vein distension, hemodynamic pressures (if available), intravenous therapy (with counts), and incisions/dressings
Gastrointestinal	Bowel sounds, shape and feel of abdomen, tenderness, nausea, emesis, diet and intake, dysphagia, bowel movements, nasogastric tube/tube feeding, ostomy site, stoma, drainage and care, and incision/dressings
Genitourinary	Urinary output, continence, appearance of urine, and Foley catheter status
Support therapy	Wound drains, irrigations, invasive lines, pain-control measure (transelectrical nerve stimulation unit, patient-controlled analgesia pump)

Action	Rationale
5. Record pertinent observations in chart in an organized manner. USE ACTIVITY FLOW SHEETS IF AVAILABLE. Or use SOAPIE categories (in whole or in part) or other formats. - **S**ubjective and **O**bjective data with **A**ssessment (interpretation of data in reference to identified client problems) - **P**lan with goals to address noted client problems - **I**mplementation of actions - **E**valuation of implementation to determine degree to which goals were met	Promotes problem-oriented charting and organized, thorough documentation Eliminates repetition and shortens notes
6. Document any changes from initial assessment, or the absence of any changes, at least every 4 hours.	Indicates ongoing nursing assessment and care
7. Use final note to highlight major shift events or progress toward goals.	Emphasizes priority shift occurrences and facilitates rapid review of notes
8. Document p.r.n. medication (medication given as necessary) in nurses' notes as per hospital policy.	Demonstrates adherence to established policy
9. Adhere to the following legalities in documentation: - Never erase or scratch out errors in charting. Draw a line through the sentence(s) and indicate the error. - Check for and correct small errors (*e.g.*, wrong time or date) - When recording events not witnessed or performed by you, use fol-	Decreases indications of falsification or deception Minimizes errors in charting that may decrease total credibility Clarifies that recorder did not personally perform or view action

Action	Rationale
lowing form: "_____ reported administering or witnessing. . . ."	
- Draw a line through space at end of completed notes	Prevents addition of information by someone else
- Sign notes before chart leaves your possession	Avoids confusion of authorship should other persons write on same form
- Chart actions on completion and not prior to performing	Avoids charting error due to delays in or cancellation of action
- Use complete words or acceptable abbreviations only (see Appendix C)	Eliminates miscommunication

Evaluation

Goals met, unmet, or partially met?

Desired Outcomes (sample)

Client receives continuity of care through dissemination of information to members of health care team in an accurate, comprehensive, and brief form.

Documentation

Sample Documentation

DATE	TIME	NARRATIVE CHARTING
1/23/94	1330	Alert, oriented ×3. Family at bedside. Skin warm and dry with capillary refill of less than 5 seconds. Respirations even and nonlabored with faint expiratory wheezes noted. Cough strong with scant, thin, yellow secretions produced. Pillow pressed to chest by client to splint incision site during cough. Abdomen soft with active bowel sounds. Voiding without difficulty. Chest tubes intact on right chest wall, with dressing clean and dry. Drainage serous and moderate—

(continued)

		NARRATIVE CHARTING (*continued*)
		30 to 40 ml/hr. TENS unit intact at settings of 45 and 30. No complaints of severe pain.

DATE	**TIME**	**CHARTING BY EXCEPTION**
1/23/94	1330	(Graphic sheet and assessment flow sheet or checklist is used to validate normal findings.) Faint expiratory wheezes noted bilaterally in lower lobes. Thin yellow secretions produced with coughing. Moderate serous drainage—30 to 40 ml/hr noted from chest tubes. TENS unit in place at settings of 45 and 30.

DATE	**TIME**	**SOAPIE CHARTING**
1/23/94	1330	S — "I don't have any pain." O — Skin warm and dry with capillary refill less than 5 seconds, respirations even with expiratory wheezes, cough strong with scant, thin, yellow secretions produced, chest tubes intact with clean, dry dressing. Drainage is serous and moderate—30 to 40 ml/hr. TENS unit intact at settings of 45 and 30. A — Pain free P — Continue supportive care with TENS unit. Encourage use of pillow to splint chest incision site when coughing. I — Pillow pressed to chest by client during deep breathing and cough exercise. E — Verbalized lack of pain after coughing.

(*continued*)

DATE	TIME	FOCUS CHARTING	(continued)
1/23/94	1330		
Incisional pain		D (Data)	Grimacing during and 15 minutes after deep breathing and cough exercises. In-
or		A (Action)	structed to hold pillow to
Pain related to chest incision		R (Response)	chest to splint incision when coughing, return demonstration from patient received. Verbalized decrease in discomfort when coughing.

CHAPTER 3

Basic Health Assessment

OVERVIEW

- In most situations, the TREND of vital sign readings is more relevant than any individual reading.
- To obtain a TRUE assessment of client status when using mechanical equipment, correlation of data with clinical findings is essential.
- A thorough clinical assessment provides the foundation for competent and complete follow-up care.
- Assessment consists of objective and subjective data related to the client's present or past mental and physical status.
- Assessment performed in a systematic manner helps eliminate errors and oversights in data collection.
- Measuring the client's weight provides data about health state and cues for direction of treatment.
- Blood pressure and pulse may be obtained by a variety of methods to determine cardiac or vascular status. One method may be more appropriate in certain clinical situations than in others; however, each method requires precision.

Jean Smith-Temple and Joyce Young Johnson:
Nurses' Guide to Clinical Procedures, Second Edition.© 1994
J. B. Lippincott Company

Basic Assessment

☒ Equipment

- Pen
- Appropriate assessment form
- Gown
- Drape or sheet
- Blood pressure cuff
- Stethoscope
- Penlight
- Sphygmomanometer
- Thermometer
- Scales
- Watch with second hand
- Measurement tape
- Cotton balls
- Nonsterile gloves

Purpose

Determines strengths and weaknesses of physical and mental health status

Assessment

Assessment should focus on the following:

Medical diagnosis
Source of information
Information obtained on health history
Need for partial versus in-depth assessment

Nursing Diagnoses

The nursing diagnoses may include the following:

Altered physiologic and mental status related to drug overdose
Decreased tissue perfusion related to low blood cell level

Planning

Key Goals and Sample Goal Criterion

The client will

Have no undetected signs and symptoms of altered physiologic or mental status

Special Considerations

Acute clients may require a more in-depth assessment of certain systems.

Assessment in acute situations should be prioritized to address life-threatening areas immediately, with assessment of other areas undertaken as soon as possible thereafter.

After initial detailed assessment is obtained for baseline data, an abbreviated assessment of problem areas noted from initial assessment may be performed each shift. A detailed assessment may then be performed periodically (every 24 to 72 hours depending on agency policy and client state of health).

Geriatric and Pediatric

Normal developmental stage and physiologic changes must be taken into consideration when assessing the client.

Although most of the information in the history may be obtained from the parent(s), the child's perspective regarding illness and care will be valuable throughout treatment plan.

Home Health

A complete assessment must be completed on the client initially with abbreviated updates on each visit.

Transcultural

- When interviewing clients for whom English is not their native language, secure an interpreter to reduce the potential for mistaken interpretations of client responses.
- Biocultural norms should be determined before judging whether findings are pathologic (*i.e.*, mongolian spots are a normal skin variation in children of African, Asian, or Latin cultural background, but may be pathologic in Caucasian children).
- Color changes in persons of color may be best observed in areas of minimal pigmentation—sclera, conjunctiva, nail beds, palms and soles, and the mucosal areas. Consider, however, that a bluish hue may be normal for persons of Mediterranean or African descent.

Implementation

Action	Rationale
1. Wash hands and organize equipment.	Reduces microorganism transfer Promotes efficiency
2. Explain procedure to client, emphasizing importance of accuracy of data.	Decreases anxiety Increases compliance
3. Provide for privacy.	Decreases embarrassment

Health History

Action	Rationale
4. Obtain health history by interviewing client using therapeutic communication techniques (see Procedure 1.3).	Provides baseline data for future reference when providing care
Include the following areas:	
- Biographical information (name, age, sex, race, marital status, informant)	Identifies client
- Chief complaint (as stated in client's own words)	Explains why client sought health care and what problem means to client
- History of present problem (date of onset, detailed description of problem: nature, location, severity, and duration as well as associating, contributing, and precipitating factors)	Defines details of manifestations of problems Helps define diagnosis
- Past medical and surgical history (date and description of problems, previous hospitalizations, doctor's name, allergies as well as current medications and time of last dose)	Serves as baseline and guide for treatment decisions Identifies potential problems related to present complaints
- Family history of mental and physical conditions	Identifies hereditary factors that may affect health status
- Psychosocial history (occupation; educational	Identifies psychosocial, spiritual, and educational factors

Action	Rationale
level; abuse of alcohol and other drug substances; tobacco use; religious preference; cultural practices)	that may contribute to state of health
- Nutritional information (diet, food likes and dislikes, special requirements, and compliance to diets)	Identifies nutritional factors related to present state of health
- Review of body systems (client's self-report of conditions or problems)	Detects subjective cues that may further define problem

Physical Assessment

Action	Rationale
5. Assess general appearance.	Provides objective cues about overall health state
6. Obtain vital signs, height, and weight.	Provides objective data about health state
7. Assess the following in relation to neuromuscular status:	Detects cues to abnormalities of neurologic or muscular status

Level of Consciousness
- Awake, alert, drowsy, lethargic, stuporous, or comatose

Orientation
- Oriented to person, time, and place or disoriented

Sensory Function
- Able to distinguish various sensations on skin surface (*i.e.*, hot/cold, sharp/dull) and aware of when and where sensation occurred

Motor Function
- Muscle tone (as determined by strength of extremities against resistance), gait, coordination of hands and feet, and reflex responses

Action	**Rationale**
Range of Motion - Structural abnormalities such as burns, scarring, spinal curvatures, bone spurs, contractures	

8. While proceeding from head to toe, inspect skin of head, neck, and extremities:
  - Note color, lesions, tears, abrasions, ulcerations, scars, degree of moistness, edema, vascularity
  - Measure size of all abnormal lesions and scars with tape measure
	Detects skin abnormalities
	
	Provides baseline data for comparison

9. Palpate skin, lymph nodes, pulses, capillary refill, and joints of head, neck, and extremities. Note temperature, turgor, raised skin lesions, or lumps:
  - Lymph node tenderness and enlargement (Fig. 3.1.1 identifies lymph nodes areas)
  - Pulse quality, rhythm, and strength (Fig. 3.1.2 identifies pulse sites)
  - Crepitus, nodules, and mobility
	Detects skin abnormalities and lymph enlargement
	
	Determines quality and character of pulses

10. Complete assessment of head and neck including eye, ear, nose, mouth, and throat:
 	
Eye
  - Pupillary status (size, shape, and response to light and accommodation)
  - Visual acuity
  - Condition of cornea, conjunctival sac
	Detects cues to pathophysiologic abnormalities of eye, ear, nose, mouth, and throat

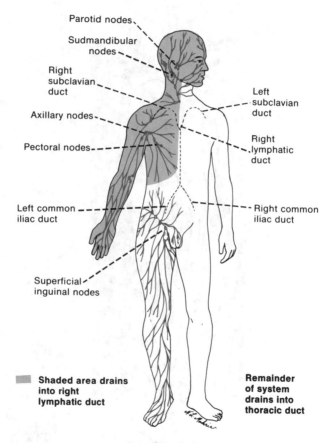

Figure 3.1.1

Action   **Rationale**

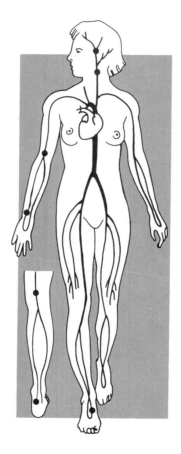

Figure 3.1.2

Action	**Rationale**

  - Abrasions, discharge, discoloration

Ear
- External ear structure (shape, presence of abnormalities on inspection and palpation)
- Hearing acuity (ability of client to respond to normal sounds)
- Presence of ear discharge and degree of wax buildup

Nose
- External and internal structure
- Presence of unusual or excessive discharge
- Ability to inhale and exhale through each nostril
- Ability to identify common odors correctly

Mouth
- Presence of lesions internally or externally
- Color of mucous membranes
- Abnormalities of teeth
- Unusual odor

Throat
- Presence of swelling, inflammation, or abnormal lesions
- Ability to swallow without difficulty

11. Inspect skin status of anterior and posterior trunk and extremities, including the feet.

    Detects skin abnormalities

12. Palpate chest, breasts, and back, noting:

    Detects abnormal masses and lesions

Action	**Rationale**
- Raised lesions on any area, tenderness on palpation - Symmetry of breasts and nipples; skin status; lymph nodes; presence of discharge, lumps, or nodules	

13. Assess cardiac status for the following:
  - Unusual pulsations at precordium
  - Character of first (S1) and second (S2) heart sounds
  - Presence or absence of third (S3) or fourth (S4) heart sounds
  - Presence of murmurs or rubs
	Detects cues related to pathologic cardiac abnormalities

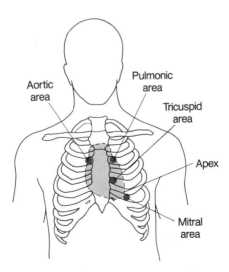

Figure 3.1.3

Action	Rationale
- Auscultate heart sounds in the following areas (Fig. 3.1.3): *Aortic*—at second or third intercostal space just to the right of sternum *Pulmonic*—at second or third intercostal space just to left of sternum *Tricuspid*—at fourth intercostal space just to left of sternum *Mitral*—in left midclavicular line at fifth intercostal space	
14. Assess respiratory status: Note character of respirations and of anterior and posterior breath sounds in the following areas: *Bronchial*—over trachea *Bronchovesicular*—on each side of sternum between	Determines if adventitious breath sounds (rales, rhonchi, or wheezes) are present, indicating abnormal pathophysiologic alterations Side-to-side comparison approach increases possibility

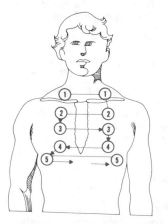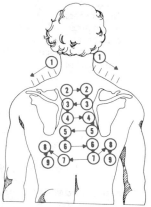

Figure 3.1.4

Action	Rationale
first and second inter-costal space *Vesicular*—peripheral areas of chest Note: When auscultating breath sounds, use side-to-side sequence to compare breath sounds on each side (Fig. 3.1.4). Avoid auscultating over bone or breast tissue.	of detecting abnormalities in a given client
15. Assess abdomen. PERFORM AUSCULTA-TION BEFORE PALPA-TION AND PERCUS-SION OF ABDOMEN. - Inspect size and contour. - Auscultate for bowel sounds in all quadrants. - Palpate tone of ab-domen and check for underlying abnormali-ties (masses, pain, ten-derness) and bladder distension.	Detects masses, abnormal fluid retention, or decrease or absence of peristalsis Palpation and percussion set underlying structures in mo-tion, possibly interfering with character of bowel sounds
16. Assess genitalia and urethra. - Inspect for abnormali-ties in structure, dis-coloration, edema, abnormal discharge, or foul odor	Detects abnormalities of geni-talia and urethral opening
17. Restore or discard equip-ment properly.	Removes microorganisms
18. Wash hands.	Prevents spread of micro-organisms

Evaluation

Goals met, partially met, or unmet?

Desired Outcomes (sample)

Signs and symptoms of underlying mental or physical alter-ations do not go undetected.

Documentation

The following should be noted on the client's chart:

- Time of assessment
- Informant
- Chief complaint
- Information from client history
- Detailed description of assessment area related to chief complaint
- Detailed description of abnormalities
- Reports of abnormal subjective data (pain, nausea, and so forth)
- Priority areas of assessment
- Assessment procedures deferred to a later time
- Ability of client to assist with assessment

Sample Documentation

DATE	TIME	
4/29/94	0830	A 44-year-old black male presented with nagging chest pain in center of chest that started 24 hours ago. Denies nausea, headache, or radiation of pain to arms or back. No abnormal heart sounds detected. Vital signs: blood pressure, 130/90; pulse, 82; temperature, 98.8°F; respirations, 22. Bedside oscilloscope displays normal sinus rhythm. No jugular vein distention. Pulses in upper and lower extremities weak (1+). Skin slightly moist but warm. No jugular vein distention or lower extremity edema noted.

Electronic Vital Signs Measurement

☒ Equipment

- Electronic blood pressure monitor with appropriate-sized cuff for size and age
- Noninvasive blood pressure printer (optional)
- Flow sheet for frequent reading (if printer is not used)
- Watch with second hand

Purpose

Provides objective data for determining client's blood pressure status

Allows frequent monitoring of blood pressure electronically through noninvasive means

Assessment

Assessment should focus on the following:

Ordered frequency of readings, if any

Conditions that might indicate need for frequent readings (*e.g.,* head injury, trauma, surgery)

Skin integrity of arm (or extremity being used)

Initial and previous blood pressure recordings

Circulation in extremity in which readings are obtained (skin color and temperature, pulse volume, capillary refill)

Presence of shunt, fistula, or graft in extremity

History of mastectomy or lymph node removal from extremity

Choice of extremity to use to obtain blood pressure (*e.g.,* if arm cannot be used for brachial blood pressure, use leg for popliteal pressure)

Nursing Diagnoses

The nursing diagnoses may include the following:

Decreased peripheral tissue perfusion related to hypotension or dehydration

Altered cardiopulmonary perfusion related to dehydration or decreased venous return

Planning

Key Goals and Sample Goal Criteria

The client will

Experience no undetected blood pressure changes

Show signs of adequate tissue perfusion (brisk capillary refill; warm, pink, and dry skin; normal heart rate)

Special Considerations

Readings reflecting a 20-mm Hg change in blood pressure, or pulse below 60 or above 100 beats per minute, should be reported. Assess frequently clients who show such a change.

Assess frequently clients in immediate postoperative or post-trauma states, or clients with acute neurologic deficits.

If client has had a mastectomy, do not take pressure in affected extremity.

Avoid placing cuff on extremity in which hemodialysis shunt, fistula, graft, or IV infusion is being maintained.

Ensure that blood pressure cuff falls within range parameters when wrapped around extremity to verify adequacy of cuff size. Small cuff will result in elevation of blood pressure; large cuff will excessively decrease blood pressure (Fig. 3.2.1).

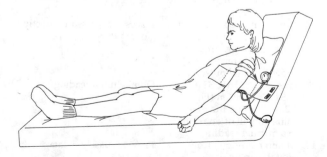

Figure 3.2.1

Pediatric
Use game to encourage cooperation and decrease anxiety.

Implementation

Action	Rationale
1. Explain procedure to client.	Reduces anxiety
2. Wash hands and organize equipment.	Reduces microorganism transfer
3. Check the cuff and tubing of automated vital signs machine for air leaks and kinks.	Facilitates accurate readings
4. Attach noninvasive blood pressure printer to blood pressure module, if available, and turn both machines on.	Activates equipment Allows continuous recording of vital signs
5. Place arm at level of heart in straight position (Figure 3.2.1)	Facilitates correct reading—if arm is below the level of the heart, the blood pressure will be elevated; if above, the blood pressure will be decreased
6. Palpate brachial pulse.	Determines most accurate position for cuff placement
7. Assess client's pulse and blood pressure manually using the arm you will use for automated vital signs readings.	Provides baseline vital signs for comparison to determine the accuracy of automated readings
8. Remove manual cuff and place cuff of automated machine snugly around extremity (artery arrow) above brachial pulse.	Places cuff pressure directly over artery
9. Press MANUAL, STAT, or START button (Fig. 3.2.2). Turning the machine on will often result in a manual reading.	Obtain initial reading
10. Obtain reading(s) from digital display panel:	Provides baseline data

Action	Rationale

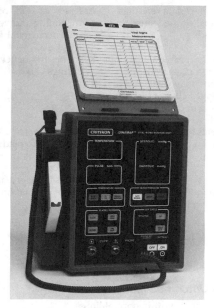

Figure 3.2.2

- Systolic pressure
- Diastolic pressure
- Arterial mean pressure
- Heart rate

Action	Rationale
11. Compare manual blood pressure and pulse readings to those obtained from the automated vital signs machine.	Assesses accuracy of monitor function
12. Check cuff for full deflation.	Prevents prolonged obstruction of blood flow in extremity
13. Set timer for recheck of readings in 1 to 2 minutes and check time interval with a reliable watch.	Assesses accuracy of timing device

Action	Rationale
14. Check new data readings and time elapsed since last reading.	Assesses accuracy of machine functioning and verifies range of current blood pressure
15. Set timer for frequency of readings as desired. (Method may vary, but time is usually set by increasing or decreasing minutes until desired time intervals are obtained.)	Regulates frequency of readings
16. Set alarm limits with appropriate controls.	Alerts nurse to readings which require immediate attention
17. Reassess circulation status of extremity and cuff deflation with each reading.	Prevents inadvertent compromise of circulation

Evaluation

Goals met, partially met, or unmet?

Desired Outcomes (sample)

Blood pressure is within normal limits.
Skin is warm and dry, mucous membranes pink, capillary refill brisk.

Documentation

The following should be noted on the client's chart:

- Blood pressure readings (record in nurses' notes only if reading is significantly different from previous readings)
- Summary of trends of readings
- Condition of extremity from which pressure was taken
- Need for increase or decrease of frequency of readings

Sample Documentation

DATE	TIME	
2/24/94	1500	Left arm BP 120/80. Left hand remains pink with brisk capillary refill.

Blood Pressure by Palpation

☒ Equipment

- Blood pressure cuff
- Sphygmomanometer
- Flow sheet for reading of frequent assessments

Purpose

Obtains blood pressure measurement by palpation for pulse return (systolic pressure) when blood pressure cannot be obtained by auscultation

Assessment

Assessment should focus on the following:

Ordered frequency of readings, if any, or conditions that might indicate need for frequent readings (*e.g.*, cardiac failure, trauma, postoperative hemorrhage)

Extremity being used to obtain blood pressure (if arm cannot be used for brachial blood pressure, use leg for popliteal pressure)

Skin integrity of extremity being used

Initial and previous blood pressure recordings

Circulation in extremity in which readings are being obtained (skin color and temperature, color of mucous membranes, pulse volume, capillary refill)

Nursing Diagnoses

The nursing diagnoses may include the following:

Decreased tissue perfusion related to fluid volume deficit

Altered cardiopulmonary perfusion related to dehydration, decreased venous return

Planning

Key Goals and Sample Goal Criteria

The client will

Have no undetected significant changes in blood pressure
Show signs of adequate tissue perfusion (brisk capillary refill;
 heart rate normal; skin warm, pink, and dry)

Special Considerations

If blood pressure was audible previously and becomes palpable
 only, notify the physician and continue to monitor the client
 closely with blood pressure, pulse, and respirations every 5 to
 10 minutes.
Readings reflecting a 20-mm Hg change in blood pressure
 should be reported.
Systolic readings in popliteal area are usually 10 to 40 mm Hg
 above brachial readings.
Although a diastolic pressure can be obtained by palpation, frequent errors occur in obtaining results.
If you are unable to palpate blood pressure, try using Doppler
 (see Procedure 3.4).
If client has had a mastectomy or has a hemodialysis shunt or IV
 infusion, avoid taking blood pressure in the affected extremity.

Geriatric
Avoid leaving blood pressure cuff on elderly clients, because
 skin may be thin and fragile.

Pediatric
In the young pediatric client, the flush method frequently is
 used to obtain blood pressures rather than the palpation
 method. Consult a nursing fundamentals text or agency policy
 manual for instructions.

Implementation

Action	Rationale
1. Explain procedure to client and family.	Decreases anxiety Promotes cooperation
2. Wash hands and organize equipment.	Reduces microorganism transfer Promotes efficiency

Action	Rationale
3. Palpate for brachial or radial pulse.	Finds pulse offering best palpable volume for procedure
4. Place cuff on arm selected for blood pressure.	Positions cuff for inflation
5. Palpate again for pulse. Once pulse is obtained, continue to palpate.	Relocates pulse for procedure
6. Inflate cuff until unable to palpate pulse.	Occludes arterial blood flow
7. Inflate cuff until measurement gauge is 20 mm Hg past the point at which pulse was lost on palpation.	Clearly identifies point of pulse return
8. Slowly deflate cuff at 2 to 3 mm Hg per second.	Prevents missing first palpable beat
9. Note reading on measurement gauge when pulse returns.	Identifies systolic blood pressure reading
10. Repeat steps 5 through 9.	Confirms readings
11. Remove cuff (or leave on if readings are being obtained at frequent intervals).	Promotes comfort
12. Restore equipment.	Prepares for next use
13. Wash hands.	Reduces microorganisms

Evaluation

Goals met, partially met, or unmet?

Desired Outcomes (sample)

Significant changes in blood pressure are detected at early stages.
Client shows signs of adequate tissue perfusion (brisk capillary refill; normal heart rate; warm, pink, and dry skin).

Documentation

The following should be noted on the client's chart:

- Systolic blood pressure measurement upon palpation
- Extremity from which blood pressure was obtained

- Circulatory indicators (capillary refill, color of skin and mucous membranes, skin temperature, quality of pulses)
- Level of consciousness

Sample Documentation

DATE	TIME	
3/4/94	0830	Blood pressure by palpation, 80 mm Hg systolic from right arm. Client slightly lethargic at times. Skin cool to touch. Nailbeds and mucous membranes slightly blanched in color. Capillary refill, 5 seconds.

Doppler Pulse Assessment

⊠ Equipment

- Doppler
- Coupling gel
- Washcloth
- Small basin of warm water
- Soap
- Towel

Purpose

Determines presence of arterial blood flow when pulse is not
palpable

Assessment

Assessment should focus on the following:

Medical diagnosis
History of medical problems related to cardiovascular deficits
Quality of pulses in extremities
Circulatory indicators of extremities (color, temperature, sensa-
tion, and capillary refill)
Pulse rate and blood pressure

Nursing Diagnoses

The nursing diagnoses may include the following:

Decreased tissue perfusion related to occlusion of blood flow to
lower extremities.

Planning

Key Goals and Sample Goal Criterion

The client will

Experience no undetected loss of pulses in extremities during postoperative period

Implementation

Action	Rationale
1. Explain procedure to client and family.	Decreases anxiety Promotes cooperation
2. Wash hands and organize equipment.	Reduces microorganism transfer Promotes efficiency
3. Squirt coupling gel over pulse area. (Inform client that gel will be cold.)	Enhances transmission of vascular and pulse sounds
4. If using portable manual Doppler, place eartips of Doppler scope in ears (similar to positioning stethoscope).	Enables sound to be detected by nurse
5. Place Doppler transducer over identified pulse area (Fig. 3.4).	Places transducer over area that will transmit pulse sound
6. Turn Doppler on until faint static sound is audible. Adjust volume with control knob.	Activates system Sets volume to suit listener's hearing range
7. Identify pulse by listening for a hollow, rushing, *pulsatile* sound (a "swooshing" sound).	Confirms presence of pulse
8. If pulse is not audible within 4 to 5 seconds, slowly slide Doppler over a ½-inch radius within same pulse area. If pulse still is not audible, continue this step increasing radius by ½ inch until pulse	Locates pulse

Action   **Rationale**

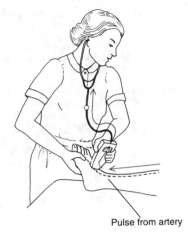

Pulse from artery

Figure 3.4

is audible *or* until convinced that pulse is not present.	
9. Wash gel from skin, rinse, and pat dry.	Prevents skin irritation
10. If pulse was difficult to obtain, draw circle around pulse site.	Outlines location of pulse for next assessment
11. Restore equipment.	Prepares for next use
12. Wash hands.	Promotes cleanliness

Evaluation

Goals met, partially met, or unmet?

Desired Outcomes (sample)

Adequate circulation to extremities is maintained, as evidenced by pulse detection by Doppler.

Documentation

The following should be noted on the client's chart:

- Area in which pulse was obtained
- Circulatory indicators in all extremities (capillary refill, color and temperature of skin, quality of pulses)
- Pulse rate and blood pressure

Sample Documentation

DATE	TIME	
3/3/94	0600	Right foot cool, nailbeds and sole of foot slightly bluish. Pedal pulse detectable only by Doppler. Left foot cool, with faint palpable pulse. Capillary refill, 6 seconds in right foot and 3 seconds in left foot.

Apical–Radial Pulse Measurement

☒ Equipment

- Stethoscope
- Watch with second hand

Purpose

Detects presence of pulse deficit that is related to poor ventricular contractions or dysrhythmias

Assessment

Assessment should focus on the following:

Ordered frequency of readings with follow-up orders
History of dysrhythmias, cardiac conditions
Pulse characteristics
Previous pulse recordings
Medication regimen for cardiac drugs

Nursing Diagnoses

The nursing diagnoses may include the following:

Decreased tissue perfusion related to irregular pulse

Planning

Key Goals and Sample Goal Criterion

The client will

Experience no undetected pulse irregularities or pulse deficit during immediate postoperative period

Special Considerations

Clients with ventricular (pump) pathologies and cardiac dysrhythmias are particularly prone to pulse deficits.

Geriatric

Clients with such chronic conditions as diabetes and atherosclerosis are particularly prone to pulse deficits and should be checked every 24 hours for apical–radial pulse deficit.

Pediatric

Some infants and children experience occasional nonpathologic dysrhythmias, such as premature ventricular contractions (PVCs).

Obtain a baseline of pulse deficit occurrence and note client response.

Monitor for change in frequency of occurrence or response.

Home Health

Since procedure requires two persons, enlist and train a family member to assist. Teach family member(s) to perform the procedure between nurse visits.

Implementation

Action	Rationale
1. Explain procedure to client.	Decreases anxiety
2. Wash hands and organize equipment.	Reduces contamination Promotes efficiency
3. Have one nurse position herself to take radial pulse (at radial artery).	
4. Have second nurse place stethoscope under gown at apex (fifth intercostal space at midclavicular line) to obtain apical pulse. Maintain privacy.	Locates apical pulse
5. Place watch so that both nurses can see second hand.	Facilitates accuracy in beginning and ending
6. State "begin" when ready to start (nurse counting apical pulse will state when to begin and end counting).	Prevents error in count, because nurse with stethoscope in ear cannot hear count call

7. Both nurses should count pulse for 1 full minute AT THE SAME TIME.	Ensures accuracy of reading
8. Call out "stop" when minute has passed.	Ends 1-minute count
9. Compare rates obtained. If a difference is noted between apical and radial rates, subtract the radial rate from the apical rate.	Determines if pulse deficit exists. Pulse deficit will be the number obtained by deducting radial from apical
10. Repeat steps 6 through 9.	Verifies results
11. Lower gown and adjust for comfort.	Restores privacy
12. Wash hands.	Reduces microorganisms
13. Notify doctor if pulse deficit was noted.	Initiates prompt medical intervention

Evaluation

Goals met, partially met, or unmet?

Desired Outcomes (sample)

No undetected pulse irregularities or pulse deficit is experienced during immediate postoperative period.

Documentation

The following should be noted on the client's chart:

- Apical–radial pulse rate
- Quality of pulse
- Irregularities of pulse rhythm (if present)
- Calculated pulse deficit, if present
- Response to deficit
- Current cardiac drugs

Sample Documentation

DATE	TIME	
1/6/94	0830	Apical–radial pulse, 94 apical and 74 radial with pulse deficit of 20. Pulse irregular. Client states no dizziness, faintness, or chest discomfort. Dr. Britt notified.

Obtaining Weight With a Sling Scale

☒ Equipment

- Sling scale with sling (mat)
- Disposable cover for sling (or disinfectant and cleaning supplies)
- Washcloth
- Pen
- Graphic sheet or weight record

Purpose

Obtains body weight when client is unable to stand or tolerate sitting position

Assessment

Assessment should focus on the following:

Doctor's orders regarding frequency and specified time of weighing
Medical diagnosis
Previous body weight
Rationale for bedscales (*e.g.*, client's weakness or inability to stand; standing contraindicated)
Type and amount of clothing being worn (should always be weighed in same type and amount of clothing)
Adequacy of bedscale function

Nursing Diagnoses

The nursing diagnoses may include the following:

Altered nutrition: more than body requirements related to poor dietary habits
Weight gain related to fluid volume excess

Planning

Key Goals and Sample Goal Criteria

The client will

Lose 3 kg per week on a 1100-calorie diet
Lose 1 kg during next three series of dialysis exchanges

Special Considerations

If the client is unable to turn independently or has drainage tubes that could become dislodged, obtain assistance to move client.

If client's weight possibly exceeds weight capacity of sling scale, seek alternative means for weighing client.

See Figure 3.6 for identification of parts of the sling scale.

Pediatric

Infants and small toddlers should be weighed on pediatric scales for exactness.

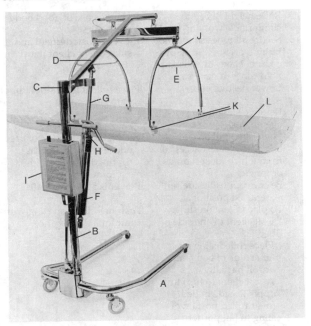

Figure 3.6

Implementation

Action	Rationale
1. Explain procedure to client.	Decreases anxiety
2. Wash hands and organize equipment.	Reduces microorganism transfer Promotes efficiency
3. Calibrate (zero balance) scales (with sling across stretcher frame) according to manufacturer's directions.	Ensures accuracy of results
4. Remove sling from stretcher frame and cover with disposable cover. Roll sling into tube and place in storage holder. Leave scale close to bed.	Reduces transfer of microorganisms between clients
5. Raise height of bed to comfortable working level.	Promotes use of good body mechanics
6. Secure all tubes so that no pulling occurs during procedure. Have an assistant hold tubes, if necessary.	Prevents dislodgment and subsequent client injury
7. Lower head of bed.	Places client in position to roll onto sling
8. Remove sling from storage holder.	
9. Lower bed rail on side of bed with clearest access or from which most tubings originate. Be sure opposite side rail is in raised position.	Facilitates placement of base under bed without disrupting tubings or other equipment Prevents accidental falls
10. To place client on sling: - Roll client to one side of bed - Place rolled sling on other side of bed and unroll partially - Assist client to turn to opposite side of bed (over rolled portion of sling to flat portion) - Unroll entire sling until flat	Positions client on sling with minimal disturbance

Action	Rationale
- Turn client supine on sling	
- Position top sheet over client	Maintains privacy
BE SURE BED RAILS ARE UP ON UNAT-TENDED SIDE OF BED.	Prevents accidental falls
11. Roll scale to bedside, lower bed rail, and roll caster base under bed.	
12. Center stretcher frame over client.	Ensures centering of body
13. Widen stance of base with shifter handle of caster base.	Provides support base for weight
14. Slowly release control valve and lower stretcher frame. Tighten valve when frame reaches mat-tress level.	Enables proper placement of hooks in holes
15. Place rings (hooks) on end of stretcher frame into sling holes.	Attaches sling to weighing portion of scale
16. Have client fold arms across chest.	Prevents injury to arms
17. Raise client up with hy-draulic pump handle until body is clear of bed.	Places weight of body and attached tubing on scale
18. Hold all tubing, wires and equipment above client's body.	Removes weight from equipment
19. Press button on readout console.	Obtains weight (in pounds or kilograms)
20. Lower client onto bed by slowly releasing control valve.	Returns client to bed gently
21. Remove client from sling, rolling from side to side as in step 10. Remove sling cover, roll sling, and place in storage holder (or place sling in holder for cleaning of sling cover at later point).	
22. Remove caster base from under bed.	

Action	Rationale
23. Lift side rails.	Ensures safety
24. Raise head of bed and lower height of bed. Place client in comfortable position.	Restores bed to position of safety and comfort
25. Replace covers.	Ensures privacy
26. Restore or discard all equipment appropriately.	Reduces transfer of microorganisms between patients and prepares equipment for future use
27. Wash hands.	Reduces microorganisms
28. Record weight immediately.	Avoids loss of data and reweighing of client

Evaluation

Goals met, partially met, or unmet?

Desired Outcomes (sample)

Daily sling scale readings indicate weight loss of 3 kg per week.
A 1-kg weight loss per sling scale weight is noted after three series of dialysis exchanges.

Documentation

The following should be noted on the client's chart:

- Weight obtained in pounds or kilograms
- Type (and number or location) of scale used for weighing (*e.g.*, "sling bedscale on unit 41")
- Client's tolerance of procedure

Sample Documentation

DATE	TIME	
3/9/94	0600	Weight after third dialysis exchange: 82 kg on sling scale. Weight loss of 1 kg from predialysis weight. Client reported slight shortness of breath in flat position, although respirations were smooth and nonlabored during weighing process. Client resting quietly in semi-Fowler's position.

Oxygenation

OVERVIEW

- One key to successful chest drainage and oxygen therapy is tube patency. Tubing must remain free of clots, kinks, or other obstructions to ensure proper equipment function.
- Agency policy and physician protocols vary regarding milking or stripping of chest tubes. Consult policy prior to intervening.
- Increasing restlessness or decreased level of consciousness are characteristic signs of hypoxia. Note

Jean Smith-Temple and Joyce Young Johnson:
Nurses' Guide to Clinical Procedures, Second Edition.© 1994
J. B. Lippincott Company

associated signs or symptoms: elevated respiratory rate, tachycardia, or dysrhythmia.

- Improperly maintained artificial airway or tube cuff can cause trauma to mucous membranes, edema, and obstruction.
- High oxygen levels can be LETHAL to certain clients.
- **Remember "NO SMOKING" signs—OXYGEN IS HIGHLY COMBUSTIBLE.**

 Transcultural

- The assessment of skin color is subjective and dependent on the sensitivity of the observer to color.
- For clients of African, Mediterranean, American Indian, Spanish, or Indian descent:
  - When caring for patients with highly pigmented skin, the nurse must first establish the baseline skin color.
  - Daylight is the best source for this assessment, but when not available, a lamp with at least a 60-watt bulb should be used.
  - Observation of skin surfaces with the least amount of pigmentation may be helpful. These include palms of hands, soles of feet, the abdomen and buttocks, and the volar (flexor surface) of the forearm.
  - The nurse should look for an underlying red tone, which is typical of all skin, regardless of how dark or light its pigment. An absence of this red tone may indicate pallor.
  - Nailbeds may be highly pigmented, thick, or lined and may contain melanin deposits. Nonetheless, for baseline assessment, it is important to evaluate how rapidly the color returns to the nailbed after pressure has been released from the nail.

🖐 Chest Drainage System Preparation (4.1)

🖐 Chest Tube Maintenance (4.2)

❌ Equipment

- Chest drainage system (bottles or disposable system)
- Suction source and set-up (wall cannister or portable)
- Nonsterile gloves
- Sterile irrigation saline or sterile water (500-ml bottle)
- Funnel
- 2-inch tape
- Sterile gauze sponges

Purpose

Removes fluid or air from chest cavity
Restores negative pressure facilitating lung re-expansion

Assessment

Assessment should focus on the following:

Doctor's orders for type of drainage system (water-seal or suction) and amount of suction
Purpose and location of chest tube(s)
Type of drainage systems available
Agency policy regarding use of saline or water in drainage system
Baseline data: breath sounds; respiratory rate, depth, and character; pulse rate and rhythm; temperature; blood gases; and chest drainage type and amount

Nursing Diagnoses

The nursing diagnoses may include the following:

Ineffective breathing pattern related to decreased lung expansion

Planning

Key Goals and Sample Goal Criteria

The client will

Ventilate effectively, as evidenced by smooth, nonlabored respirations and a respiratory rate within client's normal limits

Show lung re-expansion by breath sounds audible in all lobes

Special Considerations

Rules regarding clamping or not clamping chest tubes vary greatly among facilities and doctors. Investigate agency's policy BEFORE an emergency occurs.

Geriatric and Pediatric

Prolonged immobility can result in joint stiffening in geriatric clients and in increased frustration for hospitalized pediatric clients. Obtain rolling cart for drainage system and encourage ambulation as soon as it is allowed.

Implementation

Action	Rationale

PROCEDURE 4.1 CHEST DRAINAGE SYSTEM PREPARATION

Action	Rationale
1. Wash hands and organize equipment.	Decreases microorganism transfer Promotes efficiency
2. Open saline or water container.	
3. Unwrap drainage system and stand it upright.	
4. Fill bottle(s) or chambers to appropriate level: *One-bottle System* Place funnel in port or tubing leading to long rod (straw) and fill bottle with	Establishes proper amount of water-seal pressure

Action	Rationale

solution until end of rod is
2 cm below fluid level or
until marked fluid line is
reached (Fig. 4.1.1).

Two- or Three-bottle/chamber System
– Place funnel in tubing or
  port leading to suction-
  control chamber or
  bottle.
– Pour fluid into suction-   Level of water controls
  control port until des-   amount of suction pressure
  ignated amount is
  reached—per doctor's
  orders, or to specific line
  marked on bottle—usu-
  ally indicating the 20-cm
  water pressure level.

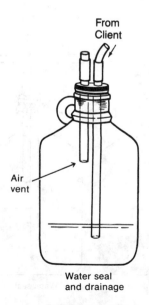

From
Client

Air
vent

Water seal
and drainage

Figure 4.1.1

Action	Rationale
	The suction-control bottle in a two-bottle system is the bottle with the long rod (Fig. 4.1.2). The closed-chamber drainage system (Fig. 4.1.3) is more commonly used than the three-bottle system (Fig. 4.1.4). The bottles and chambers of the systems are similarly aligned. The three-bottle systems have a suction control bottle with two short rods and one long rod (Fig. 4.1.4). Chamber systems have marked ports that corre-

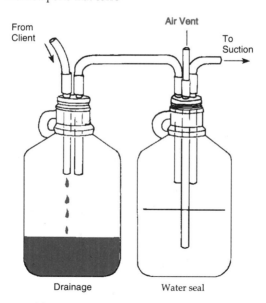

From Client

Air Vent

To Suction

Drainage

Water seal

Figure 4.1.2

Action	Rationale
late with the bottles of the three-bottle system (Fig. 4.1.3).	
– Fill water-seal chamber or bottle of drainage system to the 2-cm level. (Tip of long rod should be 2 cm below fluid level. Rod may require adjustment in some two-bottle systems.)	Allows air to escape chest while preventing air reflux into chest Stabilizes suction control altered by chest drainage
5. Don gloves and connect drainage system to chest tube and suction source, if suction is indicated.	
– Connect tubing from client to tubing entering drainage collection bottle or chamber. MAINTAIN STERILITY OF CONNECTOR ENDS.	
– If changing drainage systems, ask client to take a deep breath, hold it, and bear down slightly while tubing is being changed quickly.	Prevents air influx into chest while water seal is broken
– If indicated, connect tubing from suction-control chamber to the suction source. (MOST ONE-BOTTLE SYSTEMS SHOULD NOT BE CONNECTED TO SUCTION.)	Provides gravity drainage and water seal only
6. Adjust suction-flow regulator until quiet bubbling is noted in suction control chamber.	Regulates flow of suction, not pressure; vigorous flow is unnecessary unless large air leak is present
7. Discard gloves and disposable materials.	
8. Position client for comfort with call button within reach.	

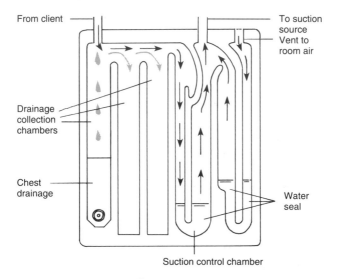

From client

To suction source

Vent to room air

Drainage collection chambers

Chest drainage

Water seal

Suction control chamber

Figure 4.1.3

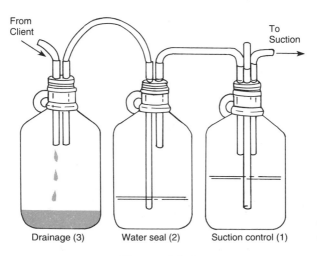

From Client

To Suction

Drainage (3)   Water seal (2)   Suction control (1)

Figure 4.1.4

Action	Rationale

PROCEDURE 4.2 CHEST TUBE MAINTENANCE

1. Observe water-seal chamber for bubbling. Suspect air leak if bubbling is present and client has no known pneumothorax. Also suspect air leak if bubbling is noted and chest tube is clamped, or if bubbling is excessive. Check security of tube connections.

   Indicates air entering system (from client or air leak)
   Determines if air is entering system through loose tube connections

2. Every 1 to 2 hours (depending on amount of drainage):
   – Mark drainage in collection chamber/bottle.

   Detects hemorrhage or increased or decreased drainage
   Indicates suction is intact

   – Monitor the drainage system for bubbling in suction-control chamber.

   – Check for fluctuation in water-seal chamber with respirations.

   Indicates patent tubing (may not fluctuate if lung re-expanded)

3. If drainage slows or stops, consult agency policy and, if allowed, gently milk chest tube (or strip as last resort):

   Stripping tubes causes extreme pain and can cause hemorrhage

   Milking
   – Grasp tube close to chest and squeeze tube between fingers and palm of hand (Fig. 4.2A).

   Pushes clotted blood toward drainage system

   – Move other hand to next lower portion of tube and squeeze.

   Exerts gentle increased suction to facilitate drainage

   – Release first hand and move to next portion of tube.

   – Continue toward drainage bottle.

Action	Rationale

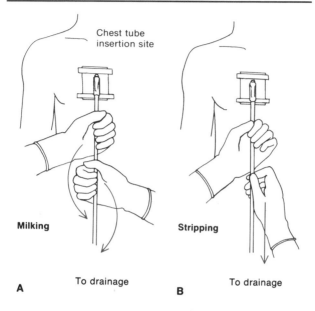

Figure 4.2

Stripping
- Place lubricant on fingers of one hand and pinch chest tube with fingers of other hand (Fig. 4.2*B*).
- Squeeze tubing below pinched portion with lubricated fingers and slide fingers down tube toward drainage system.
- Slowly release pinch of nonlubricated fingers, then release lubricated fingers.
- Repeat one to two times
  Notify doctor if unable to clear clots from tubing.

Decreases pulling on tube while stripping
Stabilizes tube to prevent dislodging
Exerts increased suction to facilitate drainage (may disrupt tissue healing and cause hemorrhage, so perform with caution)

Facilitates prompt tube replacement and avoids development of hemothorax

Action	Rationale
Monitor for tension hemo/pneumothorax.	
4. Every 2 hours (more frequently if changes are noted) monitor: – chest tube dressing for adequacy of tape seal and amount and type of soiling	Determines possible source of air leak, hemorrhage, or tube obstruction, and leakage at tube insertion site
– breath sounds	Indicates progress toward lung reinflation
5. Every 2 to 4 hours, monitor vital signs and temperature. Use the following troubleshooting tips in maintaining chest tube drainage.	Facilitates detection of such complications as hemorrhage, tension pneumo/hemothorax and infection

Troubleshooting Tips

If:

– *Drainage system is turned over and water seal is disrupted,* re-establish water seal and assess client.	Prevents additional air reflux and determines presence of pneumothorax
– *Drainage decreases suddenly,* assess for tube obstructions (*i.e.,* clots or kinks) and milk tubing.	Determines if drainage has been blocked and re-establishes tube patency
– Check that gravity drainage systems and suction systems are below level of client's chest.	Ensures proper gravitational pull and negative water seal
WATCH FOR TENSION HEMO/PNEUMO-THORAX.	Indicates air or blood is entering chest cavity, increasing pressure on structures in chest cavity
– *Drainage increases suddenly or becomes bright red,* take vital signs, observe respiratory status, and notify doctor	Indicates possible hemorrhage
– *Dressing becomes saturated,* reinforce with gauze, and tape securely. If per-	Retains original seal around chest tube

Action	Rationale
mitted, remove soiled dressings without disturbing petroleum jelly gauze seal, and apply new gauze pads.	
– *Drainage system is broken*, clamp tube with Kelly clamp or hemostat and replace system immediately, OR place end of tube in sterile saline bottle, place bottle below level of chest, and replace drainage system immediately.	Prevents entrance of air into chest Establishes temporary water seal
CLAMP CHEST TUBES FOR NO MORE THAN A FEW MINUTES (SUCH AS DURING SYSTEM CHANGE).	Air can enter pleural cavity with inspiration and, if not able to escape, will cause tension hemo/pneumo-thorax

Evaluation

Goals met, partially met, or unmet

Desired Outcomes (sample)

Respirations are nonlabored with breath sounds in all lobes.

Documentation

The following should be noted on the client's chart:

System function (type and amount of drainage)
Time suction was initiated or system changed
Client status (respiratory rate, breath sounds, pulse, blood pressure, skin color and temperature, mental status, and core body temperature)
Chest dressing status and care done

Sample Documentation

DATE	TIME	
6/8/94	1100	Client alert and oriented; skin warm and dry. Chest tubes intact with dressing dry and intact. Disposable drainage system changed with no signs of air leak noted. Suction maintained at 20 cm. Drainage scant with 10 ml serous fluid this hour. Respirations, 12; nonlabored with breath sounds in all lobes. Pulse and blood pressure within client's normal range.

✋ Postural Drainage (4.3)

✋ Chest Percussion (4.4)

✋ Chest Vibration (4.5)

✖ Equipment

- Large towel (optional)
- Suctioning equipment
- Emesis basin or tissues and paper bag

Purpose

This three-part regimen, often referred to as *chest physiotherapy*, achieves the following:

Loosens secretions in airways
Uses gravity to drain and remove excessive secretions
Decreases accumulation of secretions in unconscious or weakened clients

Assessment

Assessment should focus on the following:

Bilateral breath sounds
Respiratory rate and character
Doctor's orders regarding activity/position restrictions

Tolerance of previous physiotherapy
Current chest radiographs

Nursing Diagnoses

The nursing diagnoses may include the following:

Ineffective airway clearance related to excessive secretions

Planning

Key Goals and Sample Goal Criterion

The client will

Ventilate with clear airways, evidenced by a respiratory rate within client's normal limits and clear breath sounds in all lobes

Special Considerations

Postural drainage should be omitted in clients with poor tolerance to lying flat (*i.e.*, clients with increased intracranial pressure or those with extreme respiratory distress)

Length of time of therapy or degree of head elevation should be altered for client tolerance.

Therapy should not be initiated until 2 or more hours after solid food intake (1 hour after liquid diet intake).

Performance of therapy prior to meals and at bedtime opens airways for easier breathing during meals and at night.

Do not percuss or vibrate over areas of skin irritation or breakdown, soft tissue, the spine, or wherever there is pain.

Always have suction equipment available (particularly with pediatric clients) in case of aspiration.

Geriatric and Pediatric

Pressure used in percussion or vibration must be modified to prevent fracture of the brittle bones of elderly or pediatric clients.

Home Health

Pillows and rolled linens may be used to achieve positions.

Implementation

Action	Rationale

PROCEDURE 4.3 POSTURAL DRAINAGE

Action	Rationale
1. Explain and demonstrate procedure to client and family.	Facilitates relaxation and cooperation
2. Wash hands and organize equipment.	Reduces microorganism transfer Promotes efficiency
3. Administer broncho-dilators, expectorants, or warm liquids, if ordered or desired.	Loosens and liquifies secretions
4. Encourage client to void.	Prevents interruption of therapy
5. Position client to drain specific lung area (Fig. 4.3). To drain *upper lung segments/lobes,* position client:	
– Sitting upright in bed or chair; perform therapy to right and left chest (Fig. 4.3*A*)	Drains anterior right and left apical segments
– Leaning forward in sitting position; perform therapy to back (Fig. 4.3*B*)	Drains posterior right and left apical segments
– Lying flat on back; perform therapy to right and left chest (Fig. 4.3*C*)	Drains anterior segments
– Lying on abdomen, tilted to right or left side; perform therapy to right or left back (Fig. 4.3*D*)	Drains posterior segments
To drain *middle lobe,* position client:	
– Lying on back, tilted to left side in Trendelenburg's position; therapy to right chest (Fig. 4.3*E*)	Drains middle anterior lobe
– Lying on abdomen, tilted to left side, with hips ele-	Drains middle posterior lobe

Action	Rationale
vated; therapy to right back (Fig. 4.3F)	
To drain *basal/lower lobes*, position client:	
– Lying in Trendelenburg's position on back; perform therapy to right and left chest (Fig. 4.3G)	Drains anterior basal lobes
– Lying in Trendelenburg's position on abdomen; perform therapy to right and left back (Fig. 4.3H)	Drains posterior basal lobes
– On right or left side, in Trendelenburg's position; perform therapy to back (Fig. 4.3I)	Drains lateral basal lobes

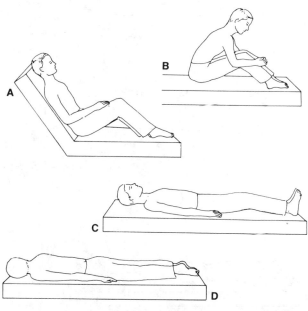

Figure 4.3

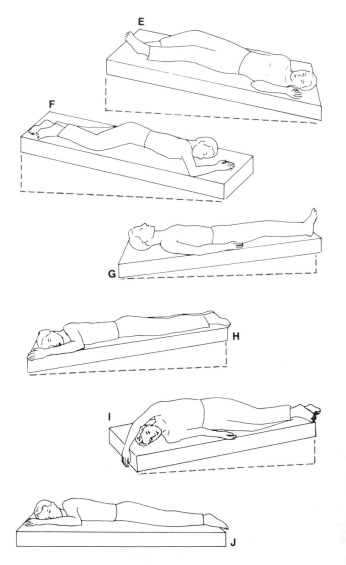

Figure 4.3 (cont.)

Action	**Rationale**
– Lying on abdomen with therapy to right and left back (Fig. 4.3*J*)	Drains superior basal lobes
6. Maintain client in position until chest percussion and vibration are completed (approximately 5 minutes).	Loosens secretions in target area
7. Assist client into position for coughing, or position client for suctioning of trachea.	Removes secretions from lungs accumulating in trachea
8. Position client to drain next target area and repeat percussion and vibration.	
9. Continue sequence until identified target areas have been drained.	Completes drainage of congested lung fields

PROCEDURE 4.4 CHEST PERCUSSION

1. Place client in position to drain target lung field and place towel over skin if desired (see Procedure 4.3).	Decreases friction against skin
2. Close fingers and thumb together and flex them slightly, making shallow cups of your palms (Fig. 4.4).	Allows palms to be used to trap air and cushion blows to chest
3. Strike target area using palm cups, holding wrists stiff, and alternating hands (a hollow sound should be produced).	Delivers cushioned blows and prevents "slapping" of skin with flat palm or fingertips

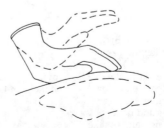

Figure 4.4

Action	Rationale
4. Percuss entire target area using a systematic pattern and rhythmic hand alternation.	Ensures loosening of secretions in entire target area
5. Continue percussion 1 to 2 minutes per target area, if tolerated.	Facilitates maximum loosening of secretions from airway
6. Perform chest vibration to site (see Procedure 4.5), assist client to clear secretions, and position client for new target area (see Procedure 4.3).	
7. Repeat percussion, vibration, and cough/suction sequence until identified lung fields have been drained.	

PROCEDURE 4.5 CHEST VIBRATION

1. Prepare and position client to drain target area.	
2. Perform chest percussion to target area (Procedures 4.3 and 4.4).	Facilitates the loosening of secretions
3. Instruct client to breathe in deeply and exhale slowly (may use pursed lip breathing).	Uses air movement to push secretions from airways
4. With each respiration, perform vibration techniques as follows: – Place your hands on top of one another over target area (Fig. 4.5). – Instruct client to take deep breath. – As client exhales slowly, deliver a gentle tremor or shaking by tensing your arms and hands and making hands shake slightly.	Provides gentle vibration to shake secretions loose

Action	Rationale

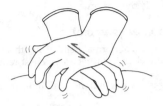

Figure 4.5

Action	Rationale
– Continue tremor throughout exhalation phase. – Relax arms and hands as client inhales.	Moves secretions from lobes of lungs and bronchi into trachea
5. Repeat vibration process for five to eight breaths, moving hands to different sections of target area.	Facilitates loosening secretions over entire target area
6. Assist client in clearing secretions (through coughing or suction).	Removes secretions drained into trachea and pharynx from lungs
7. Position client for drainage of next target area.	
8. Repeat steps 2 to 7 until all targeted lung fields have been drained.	Clears secretions from obstructed lung fields and prevents obstruction of airways
9. Assess breath sounds in targeted lung fields.	Evaluates effectiveness of therapy and need for additional treatment
10. Assist client with mouth care.	Removes residual secretions from oral cavity and freshens mouth
11. Position client in bed with head of bed elevated 45 degrees or more.	Facilitates lung expansion and deep breathing
12. Turn client to side with pillow at back.	Facilitates movement of secretions
13. Raise side rails and place call light within reach.	Facilitates client safety and communication with nurse
14. Wash hands and chart procedure.	

Evaluation

Goals met, partially met, or unmet?

Desired Outcomes (sample)

Respirations, 14 to 20, of normal depth, smooth, and symmetrical.
Breath sounds are clear in target areas; chest radiograph reveals
clear lung fields.
Arterial blood gases are within normal limits for client.

Documentation

The following should be noted on the client's chart:

- Breath sounds before and after procedure
- Character of respirations
- Significant changes in vital signs
- Color, amount, and consistency of secretions
- Tolerance to treatment (*e.g.,* state of incisions, drains)
- Replacement of oxygen source, if applicable

Sample Documentation		
DATE	**TIME**	
1/12/94	1200	Postural drainage with chest percussion and vibration performed to right upper, middle, and lower lobes of lungs. Cough productive with thick, yellow sputum. Positioned on left side with O_2 at 2 liters per cannula.

🖐 Nasal Cannula/Face Mask Application

❎ Equipment

- Oxygen humidifier (and distilled water if needed for humidifier)
- Oxygen source (wall or cylinder)
- Oxygen flow meter
- Nasal cannula or appropriate facemask
- Nonsterile gloves
- "NO SMOKING" signs
- Cotton balls
- Wash cloth
- Petroleum jelly

Purpose

Provides client with additional concentration of oxygen to facilitate adequate tissue oxygenation

Assessment

Assessment should focus on the following:

Doctor's order for oxygen concentration, method of delivery, and parameters for regulation (blood gas levels)
Baseline data: level of consciousness, respiratory status (rate, depth, signs of distress), blood pressure, and pulse

Nursing Diagnoses

The nursing diagnoses may include the following:

Ineffective breathing pattern related to neuromuscular impairment
Anxiety related to inability to breathe

Planning

Key Goals and Sample Goal Criterion

The client will

Demonstrate adequate oxygenation as evidenced by alertness, full orientation, blood gases within acceptable level for client, and pink mucous membranes

Special Considerations

In most *acute* situations, placing client on oxygen is a nursing decision and does not require a doctor's order prior to initiation of therapy; check agency policy. Once oxygen is applied, notify doctor for further orders.

A face mask provides better control of inspired oxygen concentration than the nasal cannula.

The nasal cannula may be unsuitable for emergency oxygen delivery if high oxygen percentages are desired.

If client has history of chronic lung disease or extensive tobacco abuse, DO NOT PLACE ON MORE THAN 2 TO 3 LITERS OF NASAL OXYGEN (30% FACE MASK) WITHOUT A DOCTOR'S ORDER.

Geriatric

Monitor for signs of chronic lung disease and take appropriate precautions.

Pediatric

An oxygen tent or canopy is the most suitable oxygen delivery method for infants and very young children.

Young children are very sensitive to high levels of oxygen. Be careful not to expose to high percentage of oxygen for extended periods unless ordered.

Home Health

If problems are noted in oxygen equipment, contact medical equipment supplier for assistance.

"NO SMOKING" signs should be placed on door of client's home if oxygen is in use.

Clients may require extra-long tubing to permit movement from room to room without moving oxygen cylinder.

Oximeter may be used to assess oxygenation instead of requiring blood samples for blood gases.

Transcultural

- Prior to touching the client's head, note ethnic/cultural background. Acknowledge related cultural taboos, and discuss alternatives (*e.g.*, have client or family member apply cannula/mask).

- With clients of African or Mediterranean descent, exercise caution when assessing for cyanosis, particularly around the mouth, as this area may be dark blue normally. Coloration varies from client to client and should be carefully evaluated on an individual basis.*

*Boyle and Andrews. Transcultural Concepts in Nursing Care. p 80. Scott, Foresman/Little, Brown, 1989.

Implementation

Action	Rationale
1. Wash hands and organize equipment.	Decreases microorganism transfer
	Promotes efficiency
2. Explain equipment and procedure to client.	Decreases anxiety and facilitates cooperation
3. Insert flow meter into outlet on wall, or place oxygen cylinder near client.	
4. Prepare humidifier: Add distilled water if needed, or remove prefilled bottle from package and screw enclosed spiked cap to bottle (Fig. 4.6.1*A*).	Delivers moistened oxygen to mucous membranes of airway
5. Connect humidifier to flow meter (Fig. 4.6.1*B*).	Controls flow of oxygen
6. Connect humidifier to tubing attached to cannula or mask (Fig. 4.6.1*C*).	Connects humidification to delivery mechanism
7. Turn on oxygen flow meter until bubbling is noted in humidifier. If no bubbling is noted, check that flow meter is securely inserted, ports of humidifier are patent, and connections are tight. Contact respiratory therapist or supervisor if unable to correct problem.	Determines if oxygen flow is adequate and connections are intact
8. Regulate flow meter as ordered (with Venturi	Regulates oxygen delivery

A:ction	Rationale

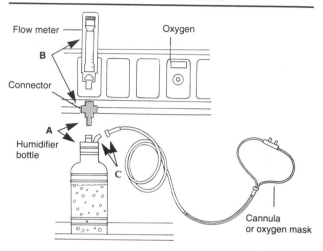

Figure 4.6.1

masks, attach oxygen per-
centage regulator to oxy-
gen mask). Regulate flow
as indicated.

9. Check oxygen flow rate
and doctor's orders every
8 hours.

Assures correct level of
oxygen administration

10. Don gloves.
11. Place oxygen cannula or
mask on client.

Cannula

– Clear nares of secretions
with moist cotton balls.

Removes secretions

– Place cannula prongs
into client's nares.

– Slip attached tubing
around client's ears and
under chin (Fig. 4.6.2).
Cotton between tubing
and ear may add
comfort.

Holds tubing in place

Action	Rationale

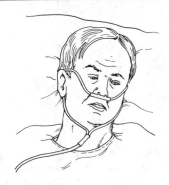

Figure 4.6.2

- Tighten tubing to secure cannula, but make sure client is comfortable.

Mask
- Place mask over nose, mouth, and chin.

Places mask correctly

- Adjust metal strip at nose bridge of mask to fit securely over bridge of client's nose.

Individualizes fit

- Pull elastic band around back of head or neck.

Secures mask

- Pull band at sides of mask to tighten (Fig. 4.6.3). Cotton under bridge of face mask may decrease pressure on nose.

Ensures secure fit

12. Remove cannula each shift or every 4 hours to assess skin, apply petroleum jelly to nares, and clean away accumulated secretions. Remove mask every 2 to 4 hours, wipe away accumulated mist, and assess underlying skin.

Provides opportunity to assess skin condition
Promotes comfort
Prevents infection

Action   **Rationale**

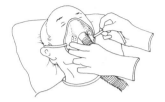

Figure 4.6.3

Action	Rationale
13. Position client for comfort with head of bed elevated.	Facilitates lung expansion for gas exchange
14. Dispose of or store equipment appropriately.	Decreases spread of microorganisms
15. Place "NO SMOKING" signs on door and over bed.	Prevents contact of fire with combustible oxygen

Evaluation

Goals met, partially met, or unmet?

Desired Outcomes (sample)

Respirations are 14 to 20, of normal depth, smooth, and symmetrical; lung fields are clear; no cyanosis.

Documentation

The following should be noted on the client's chart:

- Time of initiation of oxygen therapy
- Amount of oxygen and delivery method
- Respiratory status prior to and after initiation
- Color of skin and mucous membranes
- Client teaching performed regarding therapy and client understanding of teaching
- Blood gas results

Sample Documentation

DATE	TIME	
1/12/94	1200	Client complained of chest pain and shortness of breath. Three liters of O_2 begun per nasal cannula. Respiratory rate, 32/minute prior to oxygen administration, decreased to 24/minute within 10 minutes. Resting comfortably, states pain decreased.

🖐 Oral Airway Insertion

☒ Equipment

- Oral airway
- Equipment for suctioning
- Tape strips—one approximately 20 inches, one 16 inches (may use commercially manufactured airway holder)
- Tongue depressor
- Petroleum jelly
- Mouth moistener or swabs with mouthwash
- Nonsterile gloves

Purpose

Holds tongue forward and maintains open airway
Facilitates easy removal of secretions

Assessment

Assessment should focus on the following:

Level of consciousness, agitation, and ability to push airway from mouth
Respiratory status (respiratory rate, congestion in upper airways), blood pressure, pulse
Color, amount, and consistency of secretions
Alternative methods of maintaining airway

Nursing Diagnoses

The nursing diagnoses may include the following:

Ineffective breathing pattern related to airway blockage by tongue

Planning

Key Goals and Sample Goal Criteria

The client will

Attain and maintain clear airway passage, evidenced by non-labored respirations and clear breath sounds

Maintain skin integrity of lips and moist, intact oral mucous membranes

Special Considerations

If client is alert and agitated enough to push airway out or resist it, DO NOT INSERT. Airway could stimulate gag reflex and cause client to aspirate. Use another method of maintaining airway, if needed.

If goal is to prevent client from biting on endotracheal tube, use a bite block, preferably a dental bite block, and secure well to prevent block from sliding to back of throat.

Implementation

Action	Rationale
1. Explain procedure to client and family.	Decreases anxiety and facilitates cooperation
2. Wash hands and organize equipment.	Reduces microorganism transfer
	Promotes efficiency
3. Lay long strip of tape down with sticky side up, and place short strip of tape over it with sticky side down, leaving equal length of sticky tape exposed on each end of long strip. Split each end of tape 2 inches (See Fig. 4.12.1 and Procedure 4.12) May substitute commercial holder.	Prepares tape as holder for oral airway
4. Don gloves.	Avoids contact with secretions
5. Rinse airway in cool water.	Facilitates insertion
6. Open mouth and place tongue blade on front half of tongue.	Flattens tongue and opens mouth, facilitating airway insertion

Action	Rationale
7. Turn airway on side and insert tip on top of tongue (Fig. 4.7.1).	Promotes deeper insertion of airway without stimulating gag
8. Slide airway in until tip is at lower half of tongue.	Assures accurate placement
9. Remove tongue blade.	
10. Turn airway so that tip points toward tongue, (outer ends of airway should be vertical).	Places tongue under curve of airway, thus holding tongue forward and away from pharynx
11. Place tape under client's neck with ends lying on either side.	Places nonsticky portion under neck
12. Pull one end of tape across client's mouth with splits taped across upper and lower ends of airway (Fig. 4.7.2).	Secures airway in mouth
13. Repeat with other end of tape.	
14. Suction mouth and throat, if needed.	Removes pooled secretions
15. Swab mouth with moisturizer and mouthwash.	Freshens mouth and removes microorganisms
16. Apply petroleum jelly to lips.	Decreases dryness of lips

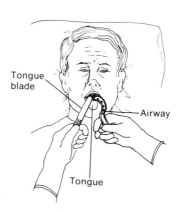

Tongue blade

Airway

Tongue

Figure 4.7.1

Action	Rationale

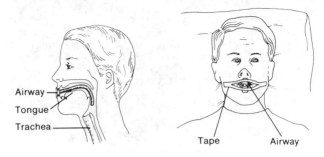

Airway
Tongue
Trachea

Tape   Airway

Figure 4.7.2

17. Position client in good alignment and for comfort.	
18. Raise side rails and place call light within reach.	Ensures safety Permits communication
19. Remove gloves and wash hands.	Removes microorganisms

Evaluation

Goals met, partially met, or unmet?

Desired Outcomes (sample)

Airway is patent and free of secretions.
Skin and mucous membranes of lips and oral area are intact without dryness or irritation.

Documentation

The following should be noted on the client's chart:

- Respiratory rate, quality, degree of congestion
- Status of lips and mucous membranes
- Time of airway insertion
- Suctioning and mouth care performed
- Tolerance of procedure

Sample Documentation

DATE	TIME	
3/4/94	0830	Client semicomatose, moves arms to painful stimuli. Upper airway congestion noted with tongue at back of throat. Oral airway inserted with no resistance. Suctioned clear secretions from mouth. Lemon-glycerin swabs to oral area, petroleum jelly to lips. No broken skin noted on lips or in oral area.

✋ Nasal Airway Insertion

☒ Equipment

- Nasal airway
- Equipment for suctioning
- Petroleum jelly
- Moist tissue/cotton balls
- Cotton-tip swabs
- Nonsterile gloves
- Washcloth

Purpose

Facilitates easy removal of secretions

Assessment

Assessment should focus on the following:

Level of consciousness, agitation, and inability to tolerate oral airway

Available alternative methods of maintaining airway

Respiratory status (respiratory rate, congestion in upper airways)

Blood pressure, pulse

Color, amount, and consistency of secretions

Nursing Diagnoses

The nursing diagnoses may include the following:

Ineffective airway clearance related to excessive secretions

Planning

Key Goals and Sample Goal Criteria

The client will

Attain and maintain clear airway passage, evidenced by smooth, nonlabored respirations, and clear breath sounds

Maintain good skin integrity of nose and intact nasal mucous membranes

Special Considerations

The decision to use continuous or intermittent nasal airway should be based on client's needs and the status of circulation to the underlying tissue. If circulation is poor, the nasal airway may need to be alternated between nares frequently or an alternate method of airway maintenance should be considered.

If airway is difficult to insert, it may be maintained continuously, but it will require frequent checks and care.

Geriatric

Tissue is often thin and fragile, requiring frequent checks and skin care.

Pediatric

The small airway diameter of pediatric clients can easily become obstructed by blood, mucus, vomitus, or the soft tissue of the pharynx; therefore, inspect airway every 1 to 2 hours.

Home Health

Teach family to insert airway and perform maintenance for care between nurse's visits.

Implementation

Action	Rationale
1. Explain procedure to client and family.	Decreases anxiety Facilitates cooperation
2. Wash hands and organize equipment.	Reduces microorganism transfer Promotes efficiency
3. Don gloves.	Avoids contact with secretions
4. Ask client to breathe through one naris while the other is occluded.	Determines patency of nasal passage

Action	Rationale
5. Repeat step 4 with other naris.	Determines patency of nasal passage
6. Have client blow nose with both nares open (if client is comatose proceed to next step).	Facilitates removal of excess mucus and dried secretions
7. Clean mucus and dried secretions from nares with wet tissue or cotton-tip swab.	Clears nasal passage
8. Lubricate airway.	Facilitates insertion
9. Insert airway into naris in a smooth downward arch (Fig. 4.8).	Decreases trauma to nasal tissue
10. Roll airway side to side while gently pushing downward.	Promotes deeper insertion of airway without tissue damage
11. Slide airway in until horn of airway fits against outer naris.	Ensures accurate placement
12. Remove excess lubricant.	
13. Suction pharynx and mouth, if needed (see Procedure 4.9).	Removes pooled secretions

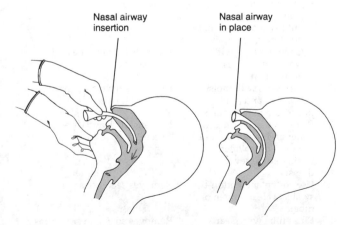

Nasal airway insertion

Nasal airway in place

Figure 4.8

Action	Rationale
14. Apply petroleum jelly to nares.	Decreases dryness of nares
15. Reposition client.	
16. Discard gloves.	Decreases spread of organisms
17. Raise side rails and place call light within reach.	Facilitates client safety and permits communication

Maintenance Techniques

18. At least once each shift, don gloves, slide airway slightly outward and inspect underlying tissue.	
19. Lubricate naris with petroleum jelly and massage gently.	Keeps tissue moist Promotes skin circulation
20. Alternate nares (if both are unobstructed) if airway is to be maintained for extended periods or inserted and removed for each suctioning episode.	

Cleaning and Storage

21. Remove tube by:	
– Donning gloves	
– Gently pulling airway out using a side-to-side twisting motion	
– Covering tube with washcloth as it is withdrawn	Prevents client witness of dirty tube
22. Clean nares with moist cotton ball and apply petroleum jelly to nares.	Decreases dryness of nares
23. Place tube in warm, soapy water and soak for 5 to 10 minutes; pass water through tube several times.	Loosens thick and dried secretions
24. Use cotton and cotton-tip swabs to clean lumen of tube.	Removes secretions
25. Rinse tube with clear water.	Removes soap and secretions

Action	Rationale
26. Dry lumen with cotton-tip swabs.	Removes remaining water
27. Cover in clean, dry cloth and store at bedside.	Keeps airway clean and dry for future use
28. Remove gloves and discard soiled equipment appropriately.	Removes microorganisms

Evaluation

Goals met, partially met, or unmet?

Desired Outcomes (sample)

Client's airway is patent and free of secretions.
Skin and mucous membranes of nasal area are intact, without dryness or irritation.

Documentation

The following should be noted on the client's chart:

- Time of airway insertion
- Client's tolerance of procedure
- Suctioning and skin care performed
- Respiratory rate, quality, degree of congestion
- Status of nares

Sample Documentation

DATE	TIME	
3/4/94	0830	Client alert, restless, moves arms to painful stimuli. Upper airway congestion noted with tongue at back of throat. Nasal airway inserted with no resistance. Suctioned clear secretions from pharynx. Lemon-glycerin swabs to oral area, petroleum jelly to nasal entrance. No broken skin on nares.

✋ Oral Airway Suctioning

☒ Equipment

- Suction source (wall suction or portable suction machine)
- Large towel
- Nonsterile gloves
- Irrigation saline or sterile water
- Oral moisturizer swabs
- Mouthwash (optional)
- Petroleum jelly
- Suction catheter (adult, size 14 to 16 French; pediatric, 8 to 12), or oral suction (Yankauer)

Purpose

Clears oral airway of secretions
Facilitates breathing
Decreases halitosis and anorexia

Assessment

Assessment should focus on the following:

Respiratory status (respirations, breath sounds)
Lips and mucous membranes (dryness, color, amount and consistency of secretions)
Ability or desire of client to perform own suctioning

Nursing Diagnoses

The nursing diagnoses may include the following:

Ineffective airway clearance related to weak cough
Anorexia related to excess oral secretions

Planning

Key Goals and Sample Goal Criterion

The client will

Attain and maintain a patent upper airway, evidenced by respiratory rate of 14 to 20 breaths per minute (or within normal limits for client), with clear upper airway and no pooling of oral secretions

Special Considerations

If a client, adult or pediatric, is capable and wishes to manage suctioning independently, provide instruction in the use of the suction catheter or Yankauer.

Pediatric
Suctioning of infants may require two people. Parents may be particularly helpful in assisting and in allaying the infant's fears.

Home Health
A bulb syringe may be purchased at pharmacy and used.

Implementation

Action	Rationale
1. Explain procedure to client.	Reduces anxiety
2. Wash hands and organize equipment.	Reduces microorganism transfer
	Promotes efficiency
3. Check suction apparatus for appropriate functioning.	Maintains safety
4. Position client in semi-Fowler's or Fowler's position.	Facilitates forward draining of secretions in mouth
5. Turn suction source on and place finger over end of attached tubing.	Tests suction apparatus (use 50 to 120 mm Hg pressure)
6. Open sterile irrigation solution and pour into sterile cup.	Allows for sterile rinsing of catheter

Action	Rationale
7. Open mouthwash and dilute with water (optional).	Freshens mouth and decreases oral microorganisms
8. Don gloves.	Prevents contact with secretions
9. Open suction catheter package.	Facilitates organization
10. Place towel under client's chin.	Prevents soiling of clothing
11. Attach suction control port of suction catheter to tubing of suction source.	Ensures correct attachment of catheter to suction source
12. Lubricate 3 to 4 inches of catheter tip with irrigating solution.	Prevents mucosal trauma when catheter is inserted
13. Ask client to push secretions to front of mouth.	Facilitates secretion removal
14. Insert catheter into mouth along jawline and slide to oropharynx until client coughs or resistance is felt. BE SURE FINGER IS NOT COVERING OPENING OF SUCTION PORT.	Promotes removal of pooled secretions Prevents application of suction as catheter is inserted
15. Withdraw catheter slowly while applying suction and rotating catheter between fingers. AVOID DIRECT CONTACT OF CATHETER WITH IRRITATED OR TORN MUCOUS MEMBRANES.	Facilitates removal of secretions from oropharynx Prevents additional trauma to oral tissue
16. Place tip of suction catheter in sterile solution and apply suction for 1 to 2 seconds.	Clears secretions from tubing
17. Ask client to take three to four breaths while you auscultate for bronchial breath sounds and assess status of secretions.	Permits reoxygenation Determines need for repeat suctioning
18. Repeat steps 13 to 17 once or twice if secretions are still present.	Promotes adequate clearing of airway

Action	Rationale
19. When secretions are adequately removed, irrigate mouth with 5 to 10 ml of mouthwash and ask client to rinse out mouth.	Removes microorganisms and thick secretions, Freshens breath and improves taste sensation
20. Suction mouth; repeat irrigation and suctioning.	Removes secretions and residual mouthwash
21. Disconnect suction catheter from machine tubing, turn off suction source and discard catheter.	
22. Apply petroleum jelly to lips, and mouth moistener to inner lips and tongue, if desired.	Prevents cracking of lips and maintains moist membranes
23. Dispose of or store equipment properly.	Decreases spread of microorganisms
24. Position client for comfort with head of bed elevated 45 degrees.	Lowers diaphragm and promotes lung expansion
25. Raise side rails and leave call light within reach.	Promotes safety Permits communication

Evaluation

Goals met, partially met, or unmet?

Desired Outcomes (sample)

Respirations are 14 to 20 breaths per minute, the oral airway is clear, and oral intake is adequate.

Documentation

The following should be noted on the client's chart:

- Breath sounds after suctioning
- Character of respirations after suctioning
- Color, amount, and consistency of secretions
- Tolerance to treatment
- Replacement of oxygen equipment on client after treatment

Sample Documentation

DATE	TIME	
2/30/94	1400	Suctioned moderate amount of thick cream-colored secretions from mouth and oropharynx. Mouth care given. Upper airway clear; respirations non-labored. Ventimask reapplied at 40% FIO_2.

✋ Nasopharyngeal/Nasotracheal Suctioning

❎ Equipment

- Suction machine or wall suction setup
- Large towel or linen saver
- Sterile irrigation saline or water
- Suction catheter (adults, size 14 to 16 French; pediatrics, 8 to 12 French)
- Sterile gloves
- Cotton-tip swabs
- Moist tissue/cotton swabs

Purpose

Clears airway of secretions
Facilitates breathing

Assessment

Assessment should focus on the following:

Chart for doctor's order
Respiratory status (respiratory character, breath sounds)
Circulatory indicators (skin color and temperature, capillary refill, blood pressure, pulse)
Nasal skin and mucous membranes
Color, amount, and consistency of secretions

Nursing Diagnoses

The nursing diagnoses may include the following:

Ineffective airway clearance related to weak cough
Anxiety related to inability to breathe effectively

Planning

Key Goals and Sample Goal Criterion

The client will

Attain or maintain a patent upper airway, indicated by respiratory rate of 14 to 20 breaths per minute, normal depth, smooth symmetrical, lungs clear, no cyanosis

Special Considerations

Clients sensitive to decreased oxygen levels should be suctioned for shorter durations, but more frequently, to ensure adequate airway clearance without hypoxia.

Whenever possible, an assistant should be secured to minimize unnecessary tube manipulation and to facilitate bagging with less risk of contamination.

Pediatric

Two people may be required to suction infants and children in order to minimize trauma.

Proper length for insertion of suction catheter should be determined by measuring from the tip of the child's nose to the ear lobe, then to midsternum. The premeasured length should be used, *not* the stimulated cough, to prevent tracheal trauma.

Implementation

Action	Rationale
1. Explain procedure to client.	Reduces anxiety
2. Wash hands and organize equipment.	Reduces microorganism transfer
	Promotes efficiency
3. Apply nonsterile gloves.	Prevents contact with secretions
4. Position client in semi-Fowler's position.	Facilitates maximal breathing during procedure
5. Turn suction machine on and place finger over end of tubing attached to suction machine.	Tests suction pressure (use 60 mm Hg for children and up to 120 mm Hg for adults for normal secretions)
7. Open sterile irrigation solution and pour into sterile cup.	Allows for sterile rinsing of catheter
8. Open sterile gloves and suction catheter package.	Maintains aseptic procedure

Action	Rationale
9. Place towel under client's chin.	Prevents soiling of clothing
10. Ask client to breathe through one naris while the other is occluded.	Determines patency of nasal passage
11. Repeat step 10 with other naris.	Determines patency of nasal passage
12. Have client blow nose with both nares open.	Clears nasal passage without pushing microorganisms into inner ear
13. Clean mucous and dried secretions from nares with moist tissues or cotton-tip swabs.	Clears nasal passage
14. Don sterile glove on dominant hand.	Maintains sterile technique
15. Holding suction catheter in sterile hand, attach suction control port to tubing of suction source (held in nonsterile hand).	Maintains sterility while establishing suction
16. Slide sterile hand from control port to suction catheter tubing (wrap tubing partially around hand).	Facilitates control of tubing
17. Lubricate 3 to 4 inches of catheter tip with irrigating solution.	Prevents mucosal trauma when catheter is inserted
18. Ask client to take several deep breaths—with oxygen source near.	Provides additional oxygen to body tissues before suctioning
19. Insert catheter into an unobstructed naris, using a slanted, downward motion. BE SURE FINGER IS NOT COVERING OPENING OF SUCTION PORT.	Facilitates unrestricted insertion of catheter Prevents trauma to membranes due to suction from catheter
20. As catheter is being inserted, ask client to open mouth.	Allows for visibility of tip of catheter once inserted
21. Proceed to step 22 for pharyngeal suctioning or to step 27 for nasotracheal suctioning.	

Action	Rationale

Nasopharyngeal Suctioning

22. Once catheter is visible in back of throat or resistance is felt, place thumb over suction port (Fig. 4.10). — Applies suction

23. Withdraw catheter in a circular motion, rotating it between thumb and finger. — Promotes cleaning of large area and sides of lumen

    SUCTION SHOULD NOT BE APPLIED FOR MORE THAN 10 to 12 SECONDS. — Prevents unnecessary hypoxia

24. Place tip of suction catheter in sterile solution and apply suction for 1 to 2 seconds. — Clears secretions from tubing

25. Allow client to take about five breaths while you listen to bronchial breath sounds and assess status of secretions. — Determines if repeat suctioning is needed

26. Repeat steps 22 to 25 once or twice if assessment indicates that secretions have not cleared well. Proceed to step 35 for completion of procedure. — Promotes adequate clearing of airway

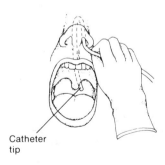

Catheter
tip

Figure 4.10

Action	Rationale

Nasotracheal Suctioning

27. Once catheter is visible in back of throat or resistance is felt, ask client to pant or cough.

Opens trachea and facilitates entrance into trachea

28. With each pant or cough, attempt to insert the catheter deeper.

Decreases resistance to catheter insertion

29. Place thumb over suction port.

Initiates suction of secretions

30. Encourage client to cough.

Facilitates loosening and removal of secretions

31. Withdraw catheter in a circular motion, rotating it between thumb and finger.
SUCTION SHOULD NOT BE APPLIED FOR MORE THAN 10 to 12 SECONDS.

Minimizes adherence of catheter to the sides of the airway

Prevents unnecessary hypoxia

32. Place tip of suction catheter in sterile solution and apply suction for 1 to 2 seconds.

Clears clogged tubing

33. Allow client to take about five breaths while you listen to bronchial breath sounds and assess status of secretions.

Determines if repeat suctioning is needed

34. Repeat steps 27 to 33 once or twice if assessment indicates that secretions have not cleared well.

Promotes adequate clearing of airway

35. To complete the suctioning procedure:
    – Perform oral airway suctioning

Clears secretions from oral airway

    – Disconnect suction catheter from suction tubing and turn off suction machine
    – Properly dispose of or store all equipment

Prevents spread of microorganisms

Action	Rationale
36. Assess incisions and wounds for drainage and approximation.	Detects complications, such as bleeding or weakened incisions, from coughing and straining
37. Position client for comfort.	Facilitates slow, deep breathing
38. Raise side rails and leave call light within reach.	Promotes safety Permits communication
39. Wash hands.	Removes microorganisms

Evaluation

Goals met, partially met, or unmet?

Desired Outcomes (sample)

Respirations are 14 to 20 breaths per minute, of normal depth, smooth, and symmetrical.
Upper lung fields are clear; no cyanosis.

Documentation

The following should be noted on the client's chart:

- Breath sounds after suctioning
- Character of respirations
- Significant changes in vital signs
- Color, amount, and consistency of secretions
- Tolerance to treatment (*e.g.*, state of incisions, drains)
- Replacement of oxygen equipment on patient after treatment

Sample Documentation

DATE	TIME	
12/3/94	0400	Suctioned moderate amount of thick, cream-colored secretions via nasopharynx (nasotrachea). Lungs clear in all fields after suctioning. Client slightly short of breath after procedure. Deep breaths with 100% O_2 taken. Respirations are 22, smooth and nonlabored. O_2 per nasal cannula reapplied at 3 liters/minute. Chest dressing dry and intact.

✋ Endotracheal Tube Suctioning (4.11)

✋ Endotracheal Tube Maintenance (4.12)

❎ Equipment

- 5-ml syringe
- Nonsterile gloves
- Suction machine or wall suction setup
- Sterile gloves (in kit)
- Large towel (or linen saver, possibly in kit)
- Sterile irrigation saline in sterile container
- Suction catheter or kit (adult, 14 to 16 French; pediatric, 6½ to 12 French)
- Irrigation saline (prefilled tubes or a filled 3- to 10-ml syringe)
- Wrist restraints (optional)
- Goggles or protective glasses
- Gown or protective apron
- Endotracheal tube holder, 1-inch tape, or Elastoplast
- Benzoin or skin preparation (optional)
- Face mask (optional)
- Nasal/oral care items (*e.g.,* oral swabs or moistener, cotton swabs)
- Petroleum jelly
- Sphygmomanometer

Purpose

Maintains open airway for breathing assistance and continuous positive airway pressure

Facilitates maximum clearance of secretions

Assessment

Assessment should focus on the following:

Doctor's orders

Airway patency (clear inspiratory and expiratory breath sounds, absence of mucous plugs in tubing, consistency of secretions, absence of triggering of ventilator pressure alarm)

Ventilation adequacy (respiratory rate of 12 to 16 breaths per minute or within range of baseline rate; respirations even and nonlabored; mucous membranes and nailbeds pink)

Endotracheal (ET) tube stability (tube placed securely; cuff properly inflated with minimum or no leak audible; pressure in cuff at 14 to 18 mm Hg or 20 to 25 cm H_2O)

Functioning of oxygen apparatus (chest rises with ventilator cycle, excursion symmetrical, breath sounds audible bilaterally to bases, and respiratory rate not less than ventilator rate setting [with mandatory ventilation setting—IMV])

Apparatus settings: Oxygen level (FIO_2), type of setting (assist-control or mandatory ventilations), tidal volume, and positive end expiratory pressure (PEEP or CPAP)

Orientation of client (tendency to pull or disconnect tubing, resist ventilation, or resist suctioning)

Nursing Diagnoses

The nursing diagnoses may include the following:

Inadequate respiratory pattern related to muscle paralysis
Ineffective airway clearance related to weak cough
Anxiety related to inability to breathe effectively

Planning

Key Goals and Sample Goal Criteria

The client will

Attain and maintain a patent airway, evidenced by a respiratory rate of 14 to 20 breaths/minute, clear breath sounds, and an absence of cyanosis

Demonstrate adequate oxygenation, indicated by alertness, full orientation, blood gases within acceptable level for client, and pink mucous membranes

Special Considerations

Clients sensitive to decreased oxygen levels (*e.g.*, with head injury or with possible increased intracranial pressure) must be well ventilated and oxygenated prior to beginning suctioning to prevent carbon dioxide buildup. Suction these clients briefly and increase frequency of suctioning.

For maximum client safety and oxygenation during suctioning and tracheostomy care, an assistant should be secured before beginning the procedure.

Confused clients or pediatric clients may need to be restrained. Place them in soft wrist restraints to prevent ET tube dislodgment.

Geriatric

The skin is often thin and sensitive to pressure in the elderly; therefore, special care should be taken to avoid breakdown.

Pediatric

The head may need to be stabilized with sandbags to prevent extubation.

Use two persons when performing suctioning or ET tube care.

Home Health

May substitute oxygen saturation per oximeter for blood gases.

An emergency power source must be available for ventilator-dependent clients.

Implementation

Action	Rationale
PROCEDURE 4.11 ENDOTRACHEAL TUBE SUCTIONING	
1. Explain procedure to client.	Reduces anxiety
2. Wash hands and organize equipment.	Reduces microorganism transfer Promotes efficiency
3. Perform any procedures that loosen secretions (*e.g.*, postural drainage, percussion, nebulization).	Facilitates removal of secretions from all lobes
4. If changing ET tube, prepare tape (see Procedure 4.12). To determine length of catheter to be inserted:	Maintains proper tube placement

Action	Rationale
– Nasal tracheal—measure distance from tip of nose to earlobe and along side of neck to thyroid cartilage (Adam's apple).	
– Oral tracheal—measure from mouth to midsternum.	
5. Don gloves, goggles, gown, and mask.	Protects nurse from contact with secretions
6. Position client on side or back with head of bed elevated.	Facilitates maximal breathing during procedure
7. Turn suction machine on and place finger over end of tubing attached to suction machine.	Tests suction pressure (should range from 50 mm Hg in infants to 120 mm Hg in adults)
8. Open sterile irrigation solution and pour into sterile cup.	Allows for sterile rinsing of catheter
9. Open sterile gloves and suction catheter package.	Maintains sterility of procedure
10. Place towel under client's chin.	Prevents soiling of clothing
11. Don sterile glove on dominant hand.	Maintains sterile technique
12. Pick up suction catheter with sterile hand and attach suction control port to tubing of suction source (held with non-sterile hand).	Maintains sterility Ensures correct attachment of catheter
13. Slide sterile hand from control port to suction catheter tubing (may wrap tubing around hand).	Facilitates control of tubing
14. Lubricate 3 to 4 inches of catheter tip with irrigating solution.	Facilitates passage of suction catheter into endotracheal tube
15. Set oxygen on Ambu breathing bag to 100% and turn on full flow.	
16. Have assistant deliver ventilations (Fig. 4.11.1):	Provides additional oxygen to body tissues before suctioning

Action	Rationale

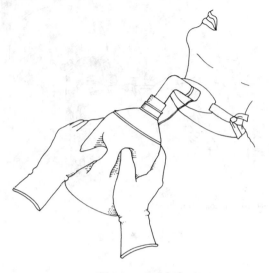

Figure 4.11.1

- Disconnect oxygen supply tubing and attach Ambu bag.
- Administer 3 to 5 deep ventilations, or allow client to take 3 to 5 deep breaths, if able.
- Remove Ambu bag.
17. Perform suction maneuvers:
    - Insert catheter into endotracheal tube using a slanted, downward motion (Fig. 4.11.2). BE SURE FINGER IS NOT COVERING OPENING OF SUCTION PORT. Continue insertion until resistance is met or coughing is stimulated.

Prevents trauma to membranes due to suction from catheter

Action	Rationale

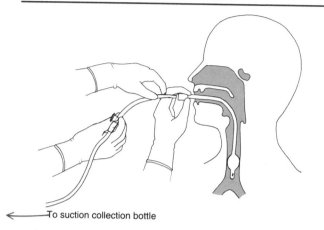

To suction collection bottle

Figure 4.11.2

If catheter meets resistance after being inserted the expected distance, it may be on the carina. If so, pull back 1 cm before advancing further or suctioning.

– Place thumb over suction port.

Applies suction

– Encourage client to cough.

Facilitates loosening and removal of secretions

– Withdraw catheter in a circular motion rotating between thumb and finger.

Promotes cleaning of sides of lumen of endotracheal tube

SUCTION SHOULD NOT BE APPLIED FOR MORE THAN 10 TO 12 SECONDS.

Prevents unnecessary hypoxia and mucosal trauma from suction

18. Place tip of suction catheter in sterile solution and apply suction for 1 to 2 seconds.

Clears clogged suction catheter and tubing

Action	Rationale
19. If secretions are thick, place 2 or 3 ml saline into ET tube and administer deep ventilations with Ambu bag.	Loosens thick secretions for removal
20. Repeat steps 17 through 18 once.	Removes loosened secretions
21. Allow client to take about 5 breaths while you auscultate bronchial breath sounds and assess status of secretions.	Determines if repeat suctioning is needed
22. Repeat steps 17 to 21 once or twice if assessment indicates that secretions are not well cleared.	Promotes adequate clearing of airway
23. Deflate ET tube cuff and repeat suctioning (steps 17 and 18).	Removes secretions pooled above tube cuff
24. Reinflate cuff to appropriate pressure.	Prevents trauma to tracheal tissue from excessive pressure
25. Suction oral airway and perform oral care (see Procedure 4.9).	Removes pooled secretions
26. Disconnect suction catheter from suction tubing and turn off suction machine.	
27. Assess incisions and wounds for approximation and drainage.	Promotes early detection of complications or bleeding
28. Position client with head of bed at 45 degrees, side rails up, and call light within reach (restraints on, if ordered and required).	Maximizes lung expansion Facilitates communication and client safety Prevents tube dislodgment
29. Discard equipment appropriately.	Promotes clean environment
30. Proceed to Procedure 4.12 to perform routine maintenance or to change tube holder.	

Action	Rationale

Closed Tracheal or In-Line Suctioning

1–3. Follow steps 1, 2, and 3 of Procedure 4.11, Endotracheal Tube Suctioning.

4. Attach 10-cc unit dose saline to the lavage/rinse port. — Prepares for lavage and rinse

5. Attach suction connecting tube, if not already attached. — Prepares for the suctioning and removal of secretions from the client

6. Turn on suction 15% to 20% higher than usual (120 mm Hg). — Adjusts for the extra length of the tracheal care catheter

7. Advance catheter 1 to 2 inches down tracheal tube or 4 to 5 inches down endotracheal (ET) tube. — Begins to move catheter into position for secretion removal

8. Instill 3 to 5 cc saline solution. — Lubricates and loosens secretions

9. Turn on thumb port. — Allows suction

10. Stabilize the endotracheal tube with nondominant hand while advancing the catheter 2 inches at a time until the carina is reached (at premeasured point for child). — Avoids movement of the ET tube while advancing the catheter

11. Pull back 1 cm and begin withdrawing slowly, using continuous suction. — Prevents trauma to membranes due to suction from catheter

12. Repeat as necessary.

13. Withdraw the catheter until the black line can be seen through the bag. — Ensures that catheter is out of airway

14. Depress the thumb port and hold it down while gently squeezing in the remaining saline from the unit dose syringe. — Allows for the rinsing of the catheter

15. Lock thumb port. — Prevents the inadvertent application of suction

16. Close lavage/rinse port. — Closes potential entry port into catheter

17. Position catheter in secure area. — Prevents the inadvertent displacement of catheter

Action	Rationale

18. Then follow steps 21 to 30 of Procedure 4.11, Endotracheal Tube Suctioning.

PROCEDURE 4.12 ENDOTRACHEAL TUBE MAINTENANCE

1. Don nonsterile gloves.
2. Every 2 hours assess client for:
   - Level of consciousness, respiratory status, vital signs, and temperature IF CLIENT IS CONFUSED, USE SOFT WRIST RESTRAINTS (obtain doctor's order, if required).

   Determines client is adequately oxygenated

   Prevents client dislodging of endotracheal tube

   - Symmetry of chest excursion with inspiration and presence of breath sounds bilaterally

   Determines correct tube placement (main stem bronchus)

3. Inspect ET tube every 2 to 4 hours to determine if obstructed by kinks, mucous plugs, secretions, or client's bite. Check ventilator, if applicable, for high or increasing ventilation pressures.

   Indicates need for suctioning, tube repositioning, or bite block to maintain patency
   Indicates resistance to flow of air

4. Check tube holder or tape for severe odor, soiling, and stability. IF ET TUBE HOLDER/TAPE REQUIRES REPLACEMENT, ENLIST AN ASSISTANT TO HOLD TUBE STABLE.

   Indicates need for adjustment or replacement of holder/tape
   Maintains placement of tube during manipulation

5. Replace tape/holder only when needed. To replace holder, see vendor instructions.
   To prepare tape to secure tube:
   - Tear two long strips of tape (one 14 inches, the other 24 inches).

Action	Rationale
– Lay 24-inch strip of tape down with sticky side up.	Prepares nonsticky area of tape for neck
– Place short strip of tape (sticky side down) on center of 24-inch strip.	Facilitates secure taping of ET tube
– Split each end of 24-inch strip 4 inches (Fig. 4.12.1).	
– Place nonsticky tape under client's neck.	
– For oral tube, position tube in corner of mouth, grasp one sticky tape end, press half of split tape end across upper lip, and wrap other half around the tube (Fig. 4.12.2). Repeat steps with other end of tape.	
– For nasal tube, press half of split tape end across upper lip and wrap other half around tube. DO NOT OCCLUDE NARIS. Repeat steps with other end of tape.	

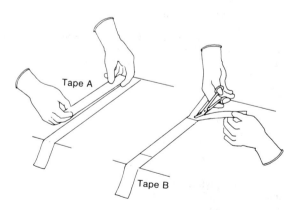

Tape A

Tape B

Figure 4.12.1

Action **Rationale**

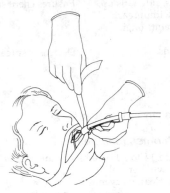

Figure 4.12.2

Action	Rationale
(Use of Elastoplast or application of benzoin may provide a secure holder.)	Resists perspiration and skin oils
6. With nasal ET tube, inspect naris for redness, drainage, ulcer, or pressure area around tube.	Constant pressure to tissue due to immobility of nasal tube compromises blood flow
With oral ET tube, inspect oral cavity and lips for irritation, ulcer, or pressure areas. Rotate tube position to opposite side of mouth every 24 to 48 hours.	Detects development of skin breakdown Prevents continuous pressure on one area of lips
7. Perform oral care every 2 to 4 hours (suctioning, swabs, petroleum jelly to lips).	Removes pooled secretions and moistens lips and mucous membranes
8. Assess cuff status (see Procedure 4.16).	Prevents tracheal tissue damage from cuff overinflation
9. Properly dispose of or store supplies or equipment.	Prevents spread of microorganisms
10. Position client for comfort with head of bed at	Facilitates lung expansion Permits communication

Action	Rationale
45 degrees, side rails up, call light within reach (and restraints on, if needed).	Ensures client safety
11. Wash hands.	Decreases spread of organisms

Evaluation

Goals met, partially met, or unmet?

Desired Outcomes (sample)

Respirations are 14 to 20 breaths per minute, of normal depth, smooth, and symmetrical.
Lung fields are clear; no cyanosis.
Nasal or oral passage is free of skin breakdown.

Documentation

The following should be noted on the client's chart:

- Breath sounds after suctioning
- Character of respirations
- Significant changes in vital signs
- Color, amount, and consistency of secretions
- Status of oral or nasal passage
- Tolerance to treatment (*e.g.*, state of incisions, drains)
- Replacement of oxygen equipment after treatment

Sample Documentation

DATE	TIME	
12/3/94	0400	Suctioned moderate amount of thick, cream-colored secretions via endotracheal tube. Lungs clear in all fields after suctioning. Respirations smooth and nonlabored. Ventilator resumed with IMV 6, FIO_2 40%; spontaneous respirations 10 to 14/minute. Lips and mucous membranes pink and without irritation. Right chest incision line dry and intact.

✋ Tracheostomy Suctioning (4.13)

✋ Tracheostomy Cleaning (4.14)

✋ Tracheostomy Dressing and Tie Change (4.15)

☒ Equipment

- Tracheostomy care kit:
  - sterile bowls or trays (two)
  - cotton-tip swabs
  - pipe cleaners
  - nonabrasive cleaning brush
  - tracheostomy ties
  - gauze pads
- Normal saline (500-ml bottle)
- Hydrogen peroxide
- Equipment for suctioning:
  - suction machine or wall suction setup
  - suction catheter (size should be ½ lumen of trachea; adult, 14 to 16 French)
- Pair of nonsterile gloves
- Pair of sterile gloves (often in suction catheter kit)
- Towel or waterproof drape
- Goggles or protective glasses
- Face mask (optional)
- Gown or protective apron (optional)
- Irrigation saline (prefilled tubes or filled 3-, 5-, or 10-ml syringe)
- Hemostat

Purpose

Clears airway of secretions
Facilitates tracheostomy healing
Minimizes tracheal trauma or necrosis

Assessment

Assessment should focus on the following:

Agency policy regarding tracheostomy care
Status of tracheostomy (*i.e.*, time since immediate postoperative
    period)
Type of tracheostomy tube (*i.e.*, metal, plastic, cuffed)
Respiratory status (respiratory character, breath sounds)
Color, amount, and consistency of secretions
Skin around tracheostomy site

Nursing Diagnoses

The nursing diagnoses may include the following:

Ineffective airway clearance related to weak cough
Potential for infection related to impaired skin integrity

Planning

Key Goals and Sample Goal Criterion

The client will

Attain and maintain a patent airway, indicated by respiratory
    rate of 14 to 20 breaths/minute, smooth, symmetrical, normal
    depth; breath sounds clear, and no cyanosis

Special Considerations

For maximum client safety and oxygenation during suctioning
    and tracheostomy care, an assistant should be secured before
    beginning procedure.
Clients sensitive to decreased oxygen levels should be suctioned
    for shorter durations but more frequently to ensure adequate
    airway clearance without hypoxia or carbon dioxide buildup.
If client has nasogastric (NG) tube and cuffed tracheostomy,
    monitor closely for signs of pharyngeal trauma.

Client participation in tracheostomy care provides opportunity to teach home care.

Home Health

Clean technique may be substituted for sterile technique in home health care, extended care, and care in other facilities.

Family members should be taught to perform care and assist nurse in care.

Tape hemostat to head of bed or wall above bed for emergency use if tracheostomy tube becomes dislodged.

Implementation

Action	Rationale
1. Explain procedure to client.	Reduces anxiety
2. Wash hands and organize equipment.	Reduces microorganism transfer
	Promotes efficiency
3. Perform any procedure that loosens secretions (*e.g.,* postural drainage, percussion, nebulization)	Facilitates removal of secretions from all lobes of lungs

PROCEDURE 4.13 TRACHEOSTOMY SUCTIONING

4. Don nonsterile gloves, goggles, gown, and mask.	Protects nurse from contact with secretions
5. Position client on side or back with head of bed elevated.	Facilitates maximal breathing during procedure
6. Turn suction machine on and place finger over end of tubing attached to suction machine.	Tests suction pressure (should not exceed 120 mm Hg)
7. Open sterile irrigation solution and pour into sterile cup.	Allows for sterile rinsing of catheter
8. Draw 10 ml sterile saline into syringe and place back into sterile holder (or place 3-ml saline containers on table).	Provides fluid for irrigation of lungs to loosen secretions during suctioning
9. If performing tracheostomy care, set up tracheostomy	

Action	Rationale
care equipment (see Fig. 4.14.1 and Procedure 4.14). If not, proceed to step 10.	
10. Increase oxygen concentration to tracheostomy collar or Ambu bag to 100%.	Increases oxygen level inspired before suctioning
11. Open sterile gloves and suction catheter package.	Ensures aseptic procedure
12. Place towel or drape on client's chest under tracheostomy.	Prevents soiling of clothing
13. Don sterile glove on dominant hand.	Maintains sterile technique
14. Pick up suction catheter with sterile hand and attach suction control port to tubing of suction source (held with nonsterile hand).	Maintains sterility Ensures correct attachment of catheter
15. Slide sterile hand from control port to suction catheter tubing (may wrap tubing around hand).	Facilitates control of tubing
16. Lubricate 3 to 4 inches of catheter tip with irrigating solution.	Prevents mucosal trauma when catheter is inserted
17. Ask client to take several deep breaths with tracheostomy collar intact (Fig. 4.13) or Ambu bag at tracheostomy tube entrance. If necessary, have assistant deliver 4 to 5 deep breaths with Ambu bag.	Provides additional oxygen to body tissues before suctioning
18. Remove tracheostomy collar or Ambu bag.	Allows entrance into tracheostomy
19. Insert catheter approximately 6 inches into inner cannula (or until resistance is met or cough reflex is stimulated). BE SURE FINGER IS NOT	Places catheter in upper airway and facilitates clearance Prevents trauma to membranes due to suction from catheter

Action	Rationale

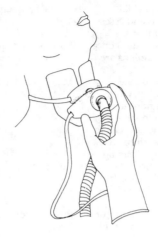

Figure 4.13

COVERING OPENING
OF SUCTION PORT.

Action	Rationale
20. Encourage client to cough.	Facilitates loosening and removal of secretions
21. Place thumb over suction port.	Initiates suction of secretions (often catheter stimulates cough)
22. Withdraw catheter in a circular motion, rotating catheter between thumb and finger. Intermittent release and application of suction during withdrawal is recommended.	Facilitates removal of secretions from sides of the airway
APPLY SUCTION FOR NO MORE THAN 10 TO 15 SECONDS.	Prevents unnecessary hypoxia Minimizes trauma to mucosa
23. Place tip of suction catheter in sterile solution and apply suction for 1 to 2 seconds.	Clears clogged tubing
24. Allow client to take about five breaths while you	Assesses if repeat suctioning is needed

Action	Rationale
auscultate bronchial breath sounds and assess status of secretions.	Permits reoxygenation
25. Repeat steps 19 to 24 once or twice if secretions are still present.	Promotes adequate clearing of airway
26. If performing tracheostomy cleaning, wrap catheter around sterile hand (do not touch suction port), and proceed to step 4 of Procedure 4.14, Tracheostomy Cleaning.	Maintains sterility and control
27. If not performing tracheostomy cleaning or dressing/tie change, discard materials.	Completes procedure
28. Position client for comfort and place call light within reach.	Provides for client safety and communication
29. Wash hands.	Prevents spread of microorganisms

PROCEDURE 4.14 TRACHEOSTOMY CLEANING

1. If tracheostomy cleaning is to follow tracheostomy suctioning, leave suction catheter around sterile hand (see Procedure 4.13), and proceed to step 4.	Clears secretions Maintains sterility
2. If suctioning is not required, set up tracheostomy care equipment (Fig. 4.14.1):	
– Open tracheostomy care kit and spread package on bedside table.	Provides sterile field
– Maintaining sterility, place bowls and tray with supplies in separate locations on paper.	Arranges equipment for easy access without contamination
– Open sterile saline and peroxide bottles and fill first bowl with equal parts of peroxide and	Provides ½ strength peroxide mixture for tracheostomy cannula cleaning Maintains sterility of supplies

Action	**Rationale**

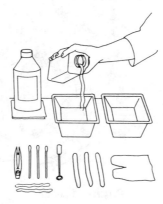

Figure 4.14.1

saline (do not touch container to bowl).	
– Fill second bowl with saline.	Provides rinse for cannula
– Don sterile gloves.	
3. Place four cotton-tip swabs in peroxide mixture, then place across tracheal care tray.	Provides moist swabs for cleaning skin
4. Pick up one sterile gauze with fingers of sterile hand.	Allows nurse to touch nonsterile items while maintaining sterility
5. Stabilize neck plate with nonsterile hand (or have assistant do so).	Decreases discomfort and trauma during removal of cannula
6. With sterile hand, use gauze to turn inner cannula counterclockwise until catch is released (unlocked).	Separates inner and outer cannula
7. Gently slide cannula out using an outward and downward arch (Fig. 4.14.2).	Follows curve of tracheostomy tube
8. Place cannula in bowl of half-strength peroxide.	Softens secretions

Action	Rationale

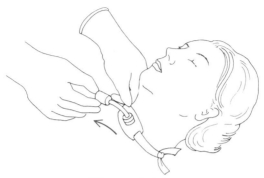

Figure 4.14.2

Action	Rationale
9. Discard gauze.	Avoids contaminating sterile items
10. Unwrap catheter and suction outer cannula of tracheostomy.	Removes remaining secretions
11. Have client take deep breaths or use Ambu bag to deliver 100% oxygen.	Provides oxygenation after suctioning
12. Disconnect suction catheter from suction tubing and discard sterile glove and catheter.	Prevents spread of micro-organisms
13. Remove tracheostomy dressing.	Exposes skin for cleaning
14. Using gauze pads, wipe secretions and crustation from around tracheostomy tube.	Removes possible airway obstruction and medium for infection
15. Use moist swabs to clean area under neck plate at insertion site.	Decreases possible infection
16. Discard gloves.	Prevents spread of micro-organisms
17. Don sterile gloves.	
18. Pick up inner cannula and scrub gently with cleaning brush.	Removes crustation and secretions from outside and inside of cannula

Action	Rationale
19. Use pipe cleaners to clean lumen of inner cannula thoroughly.	Decreases accumulation of mucus in lumen
20. Run inner cannula through peroxide mixture.	Removes remaining debris
21. Rinse cannula in bowl containing sterile saline.	Rinses away peroxide mixture and residual debris
22. Place cannula in sterile gauze and dry thoroughly; use dry pipe cleaner to remove residual moisture from lumen.	Prevents introducing fluid into trachea
23. Slide inner cannula into outer cannula (keeping inner cannula sterile), using smooth inward and downward arch, and rolling inner cannula side to side with fingers.	Facilitates insertion and reduces resistance
24. Hold neck plate stable with other hand and turn inner cannula clockwise until catch (lock) is felt and dots are in alignment.	Assures inner cannula is securely attached to outer cannula
25. If performing tracheostomy dressing or tie change, proceed to Procedure 4.15.	
26. If not performing dressing or tie change, discard materials, wash hands and position client for comfort.	Completes procedure and prevents spread of microorganisms

PROCEDURE 4.15 TRACHEOSTOMY DRESSING AND TIE CHANGE

1. Have assistant hold tracheostomy by neck plate while you clip old tracheostomy ties and remove them.	Prevents accidental dislodgment of tracheostomy during tie replacement
2. Slip end of new tie through tie holder on neck plate and tie a square knot 2 to 3 inches from neck plate (Fig. 4.15.1).	Facilitates removal of tie while holding tracheostomy tube firm

Action   **Rationale**

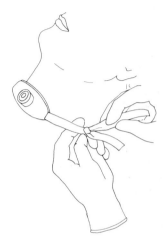

Figure 4.15.1

3. Place tie around back of
   client's neck and repeat
   above step with other end
   of tie, cutting away excess
   tie.

4. Apply tracheostomy   Places dressing in position to
   dressing: catch secretions from tra-
   – Hold ends of tracheos-   cheostomy or surrounding
     tomy dressing (or open   insertion site
     gauze and fold into **V**
     shape).
   – Gently lift neck plate and
     slide end of dressing
     under plate and tie.
   – Pull other end of dress-
     ing under neck plate
     and tie.
   – Slide both ends up to-
     ward neck, using a gen-
     tle rocking motion, until
     middle of dressing (or
     gauze) rests under neck
     plate (Fig. 4.15.2).

Action **Rationale**

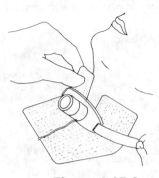

Figure 4.15.2

5. Position client for comfort.
6. Discard materials and   Reduces spread of infection
   wash hands.
7. Raise side rails and leave   Facilitates client safety
   call light within reach.   Permits communication

Evaluation

Goals met, partially met, or unmet?

Desired Outcomes (sample)

Respirations are 14 to 20 breaths/minute, of normal depth,
  smooth, and symmetrical.
Upper lung fields are clear; no cyanosis.
Tracheostomy site remains intact without redness or signs of
  infection.

Documentation

The following should be noted on the client's chart:

- Breath sounds after suctioning
- Character of respirations
- Status of tracheostomy site
- Significant changes in vital signs

- Color, amount, and consistency of secretions
- Tolerance to treatment (*i.e.,* state of incisions, drains)
- Replacement of oxygen equipment after treatment

Sample Documentation

DATE	TIME	
7/3/94	0400	Suctioned moderate amount of thick, cream-colored secretions via trachea. Lungs clear in all fields after suctioning. Tracheostomy care done. Stoma site dry with no redness or swelling. Client slightly short of breath after procedure. Respirations smooth and nonlabored after deep breaths with 100% O_2 taken. O_2 per tracheostomy collar reapplied at 30%. Client tolerated procedure with no pain or excess gagging. Client observed procedure with mirror to learn care procedure.

✋ Tracheostomy/Endotracheal Tube Cuff Management

❎ Equipment

- 10-ml syringe
- Blood pressure manometer
- Three-way stopcock
- Mouth-care swabs, moistener, and mouthwash
- Suctioning equipment
- Nonsterile gloves

Purpose

Maintains minimum amount of air in cuff to ensure adequate ventilation without trauma to trachea

Assessment

Assessment should focus on the following:

Size of cuff
Maximum cuff inflation pressure (check cuff box)
Bronchial breath sounds
Respiratory rate and character
Agency policy or doctor's orders regarding cuff care

Nursing Diagnoses

The nursing diagnoses may include the following:

Ineffective airway clearance related to thick secretions

Planning

Key Goals and Sample Goal Criteria

The client will

Maintain adequate ventilation, evidenced by pink mucous
membranes, smooth nonlabored respirations, and respiratory
rate of 12 to 16 breaths/minute
Experience no undetected tracheal damage

Special Considerations

Some cuffs are low-pressure cuffs and require minimum manipulation; however, client should still be monitored periodically
to ensure proper cuff function.

Pediatric
Tracheal tissue is extremely sensitive in pediatric clients.
Smaller cuffs require lower inflation pressures: be very careful
not to overinflate them.

Implementation

Action	Rationale
Cuff Pressure Check (for long-term cuff inflation)	
1. Wash hands and organize equipment.	Reduces microorganism transfer
	Promotes efficiency
2. Check cuff balloon for inflation by compressing between thumb and finger (should feel resistance).	Indicates cuff is inflated
3. Attach 10-ml syringe to one end of 3-way stopcock. Attach manometer to another stopcock port. Close remaining stopcock port.	Establishes connection between syringe and manometer
4. Attach pilot balloon port to closed port of three-way stopcock (Fig. 4.16).	
5. Instill air from syringe into manometer until 10-mm Hg reading is obtained.	Prevents rapid loss of air from cuff
6. Auscultate tracheal breath sounds, noting presence	Determines if cuff leak is present

Action	Rationale

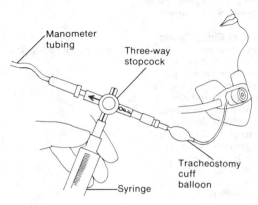

Figure 4.16

of smooth breath sounds or gurgling (cuff leak).

7. If smooth breath sounds are noted:
   – Turn stopcock off to manometer.
   – Withdraw air from cuff until gurgling is noted with respirations.

8. Once gurgling breath sounds are noted, insert air into cuff until gurgling is noted only on inspiration.

Provides minimum leak and minimizes pressure on trachea (airway is larger on inspiration)

9. Turn stopcock off to syringe.

Allows reading of pressure in cuff

10. Note manometer reading as client exhales. Record reading (note if pressure exceeds recommended volume. Do not exceed 20 mm Hg). Notify physician if excessive leak persists or if excess pressure is needed to inflate cuff.

Expiratory cuff pressure indicates minimum occlusive volume (cuff pressure on tracheal wall)

Action	Rationale

11. Turn stopcock off to pilot balloon and disconnect.

Intermittent Cuff Inflation

12. Auscultate tracheal breath sounds noting presence of smooth breath sounds (cuff inflated), or vocalization/hiss (cuff deflated).	Determines if cuff leak is present
13. If smooth breath sounds are noted, withdraw air from cuff until faint gurgling is noted with respirations. If vocalization or hiss is noted, insert air into cuff until faint gurgling is noted with respirations.	
14. Once gurgling breath sounds are noted, insert air into cuff until gurgling is noted only on inspiration.	Provides minimum leak and minimizes pressure on trachea (airway is larger on inspiration)
15. Monitor breath sounds every 2 hours until cuff is deflated.	Determines that minimum leak remains present

Cuff Maintenance Principles

16. Every 2 to 4 hours, check tracheal breath sounds (more frequently if indicated) and note pressure of pilot balloon between fingers.	Determines if minimum or excessive cuff leak is present
17. Every 8 to 12 hours or per agency policy, check cuff pressure and note if minimum occlusive volume increases or decreases.	Indicates if tracheal tissue damage or softening is occurring or if tracheal swelling is present
18. If oral or tube feedings are being received, assess secretions for tube feeding or food particles.	Indicates possible tracheoesophageal fistula
19. To perform cuff deflation: – Obtain and set up suctioning equipment.	Prepares for removal of secretions pooled on top of cuff Facilitates oxygenation

Action	Rationale
– Enlist assistance and perform oral or naso-pharyngeal suctioning.	Removes secretions pooled in pharyngeal area
– Set up Ambu bag (if client is not on ventila-tor and long-term cuff inflation has been used).	Provides for deep ventilations to move secretions
– Have assistant initiate deep sigh with venti-lator or administer deep ventilation with Ambu bag as you remove air from cuff with syringe.	Pushes pooled secretions into oral cavity as cuff is deflated
– Suction pharynx and oral cavity again.	Removes remaining secretions
20. Perform mouth care with swabs and mouthwash.	Freshens mouth and moistens mucous membranes
21. Apply lubricant to lips.	
22. Dispose of supplies appropriately.	
23. Position client for comfort with call light within reach.	Promotes comfort and safety Permits communication

Evaluation

Goals met, partially met, or unmet?

Desired Outcomes (sample)

Respirations are 14 to 20 breaths/minute, of normal depth, smooth, and symmetrical.
Lung fields are clear; no cyanosis.
Minimum occlusive pressure is maintained while cuff is inflated.

Documentation

The following should be noted in the client's chart:

• Cuff pressures noted and tracheal breath sounds
• Suctioning performed and nature of secretions
• Tolerance to procedure (changes in respiratory status and vital signs)

Sample Documentation

DATE	TIME	
1/2/94	1800	Tracheal tube cuff checked with 15-mm Hg minimum occlusive pressure noted. Suctioned scant thin secretions via nasopharynx, then cuff deflated fully. Client remains in bed with head of bed elevated. Respirations even and nonlabored.

☝ Suctioned Sputum Specimen Collection

☒ Equipment

- Gown and mask
- Goggles
- Sterile sputum trap
- Suctioning equipment (see procedure for specific type of suctioning)
- Sterile saline in sterile container and prefilled tubes for irrigation
- Specimen bag and labels
- Sterile gloves
- Nonsterile gloves

Purpose

Obtain sputum specimen for analysis while minimizing risk of contamination

Assessment

Assessment should focus on the following:

Doctor's orders for test to be done and method of obtaining specimen

Breath sounds indicating congestion and need for suction

Previous notes of nurses and respiratory therapists to determine if secretions are thick or if catheter insertion (nasotracheal or nasopharyngeal) was difficult

Nursing Diagnoses

The nursing diagnoses may include the following:

Potential for infection related to pooled secretions

Planning

Key Goals and Sample Goal Criteria

The client will

Maintain clear airway
Receive proper treatment based on noncontaminated sputum
  specimen

Special Considerations

Home Health
Time home visits to coincide with scheduled suctioning and specimen collection. Deliver specimen to laboratory immediately.

Implementation

Action	Rationale
1. Explain procedure to client.	Reduces anxiety
2. Wash hands and organize equipment.	Reduces microorganism transfer
	Promotes efficiency
3. Don clean gloves, goggles, gown, and mask.	Protects nurse from contact with secretions
4. Prepare suction equipment for type of suction to be performed (see appropriate procedure in this chapter).	Promotes efficiency
5. Open sputum trap package.	
6. Remove sputum trap from package cover and attach suction tubing to short spout of trap.	Establishes suction for secretion aspiration
7. Don sterile glove on dominant hand.	Maintains sterility of process
8. Wrap suction catheter around sterile hand.	Maintains control of catheter
9. Holding catheter suction port in sterile hand and rubber tube of sputum trap with nonsterile hand, connect suction to sputum trap (Fig. 4.17.1).	Maintains sterility of procedure

Action	**Rationale**

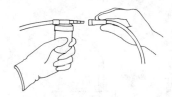

Figure 4.17.1

Action	**Rationale**
10. Suction client until secretions are collected in tubing and sputum trap. (If secretions are thick and need to be removed from catheter, suction small amount of sterile saline until specimen is cleared from tubing.)	Obtains specimen Facilitates collection of thick sputum specimen
11. If insufficient amount of sputum is collected, repeat suction process.	Ensures adequate specimen
12. Using nonsterile hand, disconnect suction from sputum trap.	
13. Disconnect suction catheter and sputum trap, maintaining sterility of suction catheter control port, trap tubing, and sterile glove.	Maintains catheter sterility for further suctioning, if needed
14. Reconnect suction tubing to catheter and continue suction process, if needed.	Clears remaining secretions from airway
15. Discard suction catheter and sterile glove when suctioning is complete.	Prevents spread of microorganisms
16. Connect rubber tubing to sputum trap suction port (Fig. 4.17.2).	Seals specimen closed
17. Place specimen in plastic bag (if agency policy) and label with client's name, date, time, and nurse's initials.	Ensures proper identification of specimen

Action	Rationale

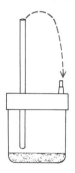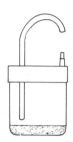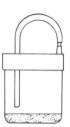

Figure 4.17.2

18. Discard equipment.

Prevents spread of micro-organisms

19. Position client for comfort with side rails up and call light within reach.

Facilitates client comfort and safety

20. Wash hands.

Reduces spread of infection

Evaluation

Goals met, partially met, or unmet?

Desired Outcomes (sample)

Airway is clear of secretions.
Uncontaminated sputum specimen is obtained.

Documentation

The following should be noted on the client's chart:

- Date, time, and type of specimen collection
- Type of suction done
- Amount and character of secretions
- Client tolerance of process

Sample Documentation

DATE	TIME	
1/6/94	1415	Sputum specimen obtained by naso-tracheal suctioning. Large amounts of thick, white mucus obtained; cough reflex stimulated with strong cough noted. Respirations even and nonlabored, breath sounds clear. Specimen sent to lab.

Pulse Oximetry

 Equipment

- Pulse oximeter
- Sensor (permanent or disposable)
- Alcohol wipe/s
- Nail polish remover

Purpose

Noninvasive monitoring of the oxygen saturation of arterial blood

Assessment

Assessment should focus on the following:

Other signs and symptoms of hypoxemia (restlessness; confusion; dusky skin, nailbeds, or mucous membranes)
Quality of pulse and capillary refill proximal to potential sensor application site
Respiratory rate and character
Amount and type of oxygen administration, if applicable

Nursing Diagnoses

The nursing diagnosis may include the following:

Impaired gas exchange related to excessive secretions

Planning

Key Goals and Sample Goal Criteria
The client will

Maintain an SaO₂ (arterial oxygen saturation) between 90% and 100%

Demonstrate knowledge of exogenous factors affecting pulse oximeter readings (*i.e.*, movement-restrictive probe placement, outside light, and anemia)

Special Considerations

Geriatric

Be sensitive to probe placement. This includes tension on probe site as well as tape applied to dry, thin skin.

Pediatric

Choose appropriate sensor.

Stabilization of sensor may only be accomplished by safely immobilizing the monitoring site. An acceptable alternative monitoring site may be the shaft of the penis.

 Transcultural

When choosing the earlobe as a site for pulse oximetry in clients of African descent, be sensitive to the presence of keloids. These ropelike scars, which are the result of an exaggerated wound healing process, may occur as a result of ear piercing. These scars may not allow accurate SaO₂ readings.

Implementation

Action	Rationale
1. Wash hands. Organize equipment.	Reduces microorganism transfer Promotes efficiency
2. Explain procedure to conscious client.	Decreases anxiety and facilitates cooperation
3. Choose sensor.	Sensor types may vary according to weight of client and site considerations
4. Prepare site (see Pediatric Considerations for alternative site). Use alcohol wipe to cleanse site gently. Remove nail polish or acrylic nails if needed when using finger as monitoring site.	Alcohol wipes aid in ensuring that site is clean and dry. Frosted or colored nail polish and acrylic nails may interfere with pulse oximetry reading

Action	Rationale
5. Check capillary refill and pulse proximal to the chosen site.	Compromised peripheral circulation, caused by restriction (probe applied too tightly) or poor circulation due to medications or other conditions, may yield false readings
6. Ascertain the alignment of the light-emitting diodes (LEDs) and the photo detector (light-receiving sensor). These sensors should be directly opposite each other (Fig. 4.18).	Sensors that are not properly aligned will not yield an accurate SaO_2 reading via the pulse oximeter
7. Turn the pulse oximeter to the ON position. REMEMBER: DISPOSABLE SENSORS NEED TO BE ATTACHED TO THE PATIENT CABLE BEFORE TURNING THE PULSE OXIMETER ON.	The emitting sensors (LEDs) will transmit red and infrared light through the tissue
	The receiving sensor (photodetector) will measure the amount of oxygenated hemoglobin (which absorbs more infrared light) and deoxygenated hemoglobin (which absorbs more red light)
	SaO_2 will be computed by the pulse oximeter using these data

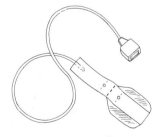
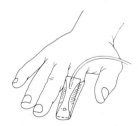

Figure 4.18

Action	Rationale
8. Listen for a beep and note waveform or bar of light on front of pulse oximeter.	Each beep indicates a pulse detected by the pulse oximeter. The light or waveform changes and indicates the strength of the pulse. A weak pulse may not yield accurate SaO_2
9. Check alarm limits. Reset if necessary. Always make certain that both high and low alarms are on before leaving the patient's room.	Alarm limits for both high and low SaO_2 and high and low pulse rate are preset by the manufacturer, but can be easily reset in response to doctor's orders
10. Teach patient common position changes that may trigger the alarm, such as bending the elbow and gripping the side rails or other objects.	Patient participates in care, thus decreasing anxiety
11. Relocate finger sensor at least every 4 hours. Relocate spring tension sensor at least every 2 hours.	Prevents tissue necrosis
Check adhesive sensors at least every shift.	Irritation may occur because of the adhesive

Evaluation

Goals met, partially met, or unmet?

Desired Outcomes (sample)

Client's SaO_2 remains between 90% and 100%.
Client does not exhibit signs or symptoms of hypoxemia.

Documentation

The following should be noted on the client's chart:

- Type and location of sensor
- Presence of pulse proximal to sensor and status of capillary refill

- Percentage of oxygen saturated in arterial blood (SaO_2)
- Rotation of sensor according to guidelines
- Percentage of oxygen client receiving or room air
- Interventions as a result of deviations from the norm

Sample Documentation

DATE	TIME	
7/26/94	1800	Finger sensor (probe) applied to left index finger, capillary refill brisk, radial pulse present. Pulse oximeter yielding SaO_2 of 96% on room air.
	2200	Finger probe applied to right index finger, capillary refill brisk, radial pulse present. Pulse oximeter yielding SaO_2 of 97% of room air.

Nutrition: Fluid and Nutrient Balance

OVERVIEW

- Initiation of intake and output measurement is an appropriate nursing decision any time potential fluid imbalance is present.
- Malnourished clients have a high susceptibility to infection, and nutrition support substances provide a medium

Jean Smith-Temple and Joyce Young Johnson:
Nurses' Guide to Clinical Procedures, Second Edition.© 1994
J. B. Lippincott Company

for possible microorganism growth; thus, good asepsis is a crucial concern.

- Careful monitoring and regulation of fluid administration are essential to prevent a potentially lethal fluid overload.
- Intake and output and daily weights are crucial in assessing nutritional support and fluid balance.
- Infusion of hyperosmotic solutions into the thoracic cavity or aspiration into the pulmonary tree could result in major respiratory compromise; thus, verification of feeding tube or central line placement is a primary concern in nutritional support.
- To prevent possible exposure to infectious organisms, nurses should wear gloves when contact with body fluids is probable.

👆 Intake and Output Measurement

❌ Equipment

- Graduated 1000-ml measuring container
- Graduated water pitcher
- Graduated cups
- Scale
- Nonsterile gloves
- Felt pen or fine-tip marker

Purpose

Facilitates control of fluid balance
Provides data to indicate effects of diuretic or rehydration
  therapy

Assessment

Assessment should focus on the following:

Doctor's orders for frequency of intake and output (I & O;
  hourly, every shift, 24-hourly)
Client status indicating need for I & O: edema, poor skin turgor,
  severely low or high blood pressure, congestive heart failure,
  dyspnea, reduced urinary output, intravenous infusion
Medications being taken that alter fluid status

Nursing Diagnoses

The nursing diagnoses may include the following:

Fluid volume excess related to excess IV fluid intake
Fluid volume deficit related to anorexia

Planning

Key Goals and Sample Goal Criteria

The client will

Demonstrate an output equal to intake (plus or minus insensible loss)

Demonstrate a reduction in ankle edema, evidenced by a decrease in ankle measurement from 6.0 to 5.5 inches within 48 hours

Special Considerations

Strict I & O involves accounting for incontinent urine, emesis and diaphoresis, if possible. Weigh soiled linens to determine fluid loss, or estimate it.

Family members could be important allies in obtaining accurate I & O measurement. Explain procedure and enlist their assistance.

When measuring output, gloves should be worn to protect the caregiver from exposure to contaminated body fluids.

Pediatric

For pediatric clients without bladder control, weigh diapers as a rough estimate of output (1 g will be equal to 1 ml).

Home Health

If the homebound client has difficulty understanding units of measure or seeing calibration lines, make an I & O sheet including columns of drinking glasses, cups of ice, bowls of jello and soup, and so forth, to represent intake and for client to cross off. Have client measure output by number of voidings.

Implementation

Action	Rationale
1. Wash hands and organize equipment.	Reduces microorganism transfer Promotes efficiency
2. Post pad on door or in room, and instruct team members to record intake or output; instruct client and family on use of intake	Ensures complete, accurate record of intake and output

Action	Rationale
and output record, with return demonstration. (If calorie count is in progress, list type of food and fluid consumed as well.)	Allows dietary department to calculate caloric intake correctly based on standard institutional serving sizes

Intake

Action	Rationale
3. Place graduated cups in room and request that all fluids be measured in the cups prior to consumption.	Ensures common units of measurement Minimizes error of measurement
4. Semisolid substance intake should be recorded in percentage or fraction amount. Most institutions use standard portions.	Facilitates accurate calculation of intake
5. Measure all oral intake: – Water: note volume in pitcher at shift's beginning, plus any fluid. added, and subtract fluid remaining in pitcher at shift's end.	Takes into account the wide variety of fluids consumed orally
– Ice chips: multiply volume by 0.5	When melted, the volume of ice is approximately half its previous volume
– All liquids (juice, beverage, broth) should be measured in graduated container.	
– Soup: indicate kind; measure volume or obtain standard volume measurement from food services.	
– Jello, ice cream, sherbet: use institution's standard volume or volume on container.	
6. Measure nasogastric (NG) or gastric tube feedings:	Maintains accurate record by including gastrointestinal (GI) intake besides oral
– Note volume in bottle hanging at beginning of shift (amount left from previous shift) plus any	Indicates volume infusing during current shift

Action	Rationale
feeding added during shift. (Allow prior feeding to infuse almost totally before adding new solution.)	
– Subtract fluid remaining in bag at end of shift (or read infusion total from pump if previous shift has cleared pump total).	Prevents feeding from hanging more than 8 hours
– Liquid—oral or NG— medications should be mixed with a measured volume of water.	Maintains complete I & O measurement
7. Measure all intravenous intake using same methodology as step 6. Volume of each type of intake is often designated on flowsheet (*e.g.,* colloids, blood products).	Maintains complete I & O measurement
8. If NG irrigation is performed and irrigant is left to drain out with other gastric contents, enter irrigant in intake section of flowsheet (or subtract irrigant amount from total output; see step 13).	

Output

Action	Rationale
9. Place one or more (depending on amount of drainage) large graduated containers in room. For small amounts of drainage (wound drains or scant NG drainage), place graduated cups in room with clearly marked labels: *For Drainage Measurement.* Designate if urine measurement from urinals will be used or if urine should be poured into graduated containers.	Maintains accurate output measurement Standardizes measurement units (some containers vary slightly) Prevents inadvertent use of cup for use of intake

Action	Rationale
10. At end of each shift, or hourly if needed, *don gloves* and empty drainage into graduated container. An alternate method of measuring output draining into a graduated container is to mark the level of drainage on a tape strip on the container. Mark drainage level with date and time of each shift—or calibrate in intervals of desired number of hours (Fig. 5.1). When container is nearly full, empty or dispose of container and replace with new container.	Minimizes exposure to body fluids Allows monitoring on a more frequent basis
11. Record amount and source of drainage, particularly with drains from different sites.	Identifies abnormal drainage and source
12. Measure output from: – NG or gastrostomy tubes – Ostomy drainage – Wound drains – Chest tube drainage	Takes into account output from all sources

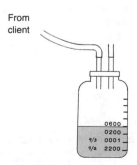

Figure 5.1

Action	Rationale
– Urinary drainage or voidings – Emesis – Liquid stool – Blood or serous drainage and extreme diaphoresis (weigh soiled pads or linens and subtract dry weight to estimate output)	
13. If intermittent or ongoing irrigation is performed, calculate true output (urinary or NG) by measuring total output and subtracting total irrigant infused (record only true output or indicate calculations on forms).	Eliminates errors of double counting output
14. At end of 24-hour period, usually at end of evening or night shift, add total intake and total output. Report extreme input/output discrepancy to doctor (*e.g.*, if input is 1 to 2 liters more than output). Correlate weight gains with fluid intake excesses.	Indicates I & O status over 24-hour period
15. Clean containers and store in client's room. Discard gloves, and wash hands.	Prevents spread of infection

Evaluation

Goals met, partially met, or unmet?

Desired Outcomes (sample)

Blood pressure, pulse, and respirations are within normal limits.
Skin turgor is normal (*i.e.*, pinched skin returns to position immediately).
Edema is reduced from pitting to nonpitting type.

Documentation

The following should be noted on the client's chart:

• Intake from all sources on appropriate graphic sheet
• Output from all sources on appropriate graphic sheet
• Medication or fluid given to improve fluid balance and immediate response noted (*e.g.*, diuresis, blood pressure increase)
• Vital signs and skin status indicating fluid balance or imbalance

---

Sample Documentation

DATE	TIME	
6/9/94	0600	Client excreted 1200 ml urine after Lasix administration. Ankle measurement remains 6 inches with 2+ pitting edema. D$_5$W infusing into right wrist angiocath at 10 ml/hour by infusion pump.

✋ Intravenous Therapy: Vein Selection (5.2)

Intravenous Therapy: Solution Preparation (5.3)

✋ Intravenous Therapy: Catheter/Heparin Lock Insertion (5.4)

❌ Equipment

- Angiocath or butterfly catheter/needle
- IV fluid (if continuous infusion) *or* infusion plug (if heparin lock)
- Armboard (optional)
- Infusion tubing (vented for IV-fluid bag, unvented for IV bottles)
- IV pole (bed or rolling) *or* IV pump/controller
- IV insertion kit or supplies:
  - tourniquet (or blood pressure cuff)
  - tape—1 inch wide (or 2-inch tape, cut)
  - alcohol pads
  - Betadine pad (optional)
  - ointment (optional)
  - dressing—2 × 2-inch gauze, transparent dressing (Opsite)
  - adhesive bandage
  - adhesive labels
- Razor and soap (optional)
- Towel or linen saver

Purpose

Provides venous route for administration of fluids, medications, blood, or nutrients

Assessment

Assessment should focus on the following:

Reason for initiation of IV therapy for particular client
Orders for type and rate of fluid and/or specified IV site
Status of skin on hand and arms; presence of hair or abrasions; previous IV sites
Client's ability to avoid movement of arms or hands for duration of procedure
Allergy to tape, iodine, antibiotic pads, or ointment
Client knowledge of IV therapy

Nursing Diagnoses

The nursing diagnoses may include the following:

Altered fluid balance: deficit, related to dehydration
Alteration in safety related to infection
Potential alteration in cardiac output related to systemic vaso-constriction

Planning

Key Goals and Sample Goal Criteria

The client will

Obtain and maintain fluid and electrolyte balance, as evidenced by good skin turgor, brisk capillary refill, no edema
Maintain intact skin integrity and absence of infection at insertion site, as evidenced by lack of pain, redness, or swelling at site
Verbalize understanding of movement limitations related to IV infusions and complications to be reported to the nurse
Demonstrate no extreme anxiety during or after IV insertion procedure

Special Considerations

Gloves should be worn since contact with blood is likely.
Maintenance of aseptic technique is a prime concern for the nurse performing IV therapy.

Choose tubing and needle appropriate for solution to provide optimal fluid flow: viscous solutions require larger needles.

Small catheters cause less vein wall irritation than large ones: choose the smallest gauge needle that will meet the need.

When working with children, confused clients, or other clients who are restless, obtain an assistant to help hold extremities still.

Because venous blood runs upward toward the heart, attempt to enter a vein at its lower (distal) end so that the same vein can be used later without leakage.

If it is difficult to insert catheter fully, wait until fluid infusion is initiated and then gently insert catheter.

To facilitate accurate 24-hour management, each shift should report to oncoming shift: the amount of IV fluid remaining, the need for new bottle/bag, tubing or site change, or need for site care.

Geriatric

Veins are often fragile. When veins are elevated and clearly visible, needle insertion may be performed without tourniquet.

Pediatric

Microdrip tubing with volume control chambers should be used for strict volume control. Infusion devices are often used for additional safety.

Clear explanations should be given with a demonstration of the equipment (except needles) using a puppet or game. Explain need for a helper to "assist" client in holding extremity stable during needle insertion. Talk to child during procedure.

Scalp vein needles (butterfly catheters) may be used for infants. Armboards may be used for stabilization.

Home Health

If nursing visits are intermittent and IV therapy is continuous, instruct client and family on rate regulation, signs and symptoms of infiltration, and method for discontinuing IV catheter.

Implementation

Action	Rationale

PROCEDURE 5.2 INTRAVENOUS THERAPY: VEIN SELECTION

Action	Rationale
1. Wash hands and organize equipment.	Reduces microorganisms Promotes efficiency
2. Explain procedure, including client assistance needed	Decreases anxiety and ensures cooperation

Action	Rationale
during and after therapy initiation.	
3. Encourage client to use bedpan or commode before beginning.	Avoids interruption during IV insertion process
4. Help client into loose-fitting gown or IV gown.	Promotes ease of gown changes during IV therapy
5. Ask client which is dominant hand.	Facilitates placement of needle in nondominant hand or arm
6. Tie tourniquet on arm 3 to 5 inches below elbow.	Facilitates assessment of distal arm veins and hand veins
7. Ask client to open and close hand or hang arm at side of bed.	Pumps blood to extremity Dilates vein
8. Look for vein with fewest curves or junctions and largest diameter (puffiness).	Allows more complete insertion of catheter and use of large-gauge catheters
9. Find vein on lower arm, if possible. Check anterior and posterior surfaces.	Lower arm has natural splint of radial and ulnar bones
10. If lower arm veins are unsuitable, look at hand and wrist veins.	
11. Look for site with 2 inches of skin surface below it (Fig. 5.2). If a large vein is needed, tie tourniquet just above antecubital area and search upper arm for suitable vein. A doctor's order is usually required before a vein in the lower extremities can be used.	Permits taping with greater stability Upper arm veins are large and support large needle gauges (18 or 16) often needed for blood or blood products Lower extremities are more prone to thrombophlebitis and other peripheral vascular problems
12. Release tourniquet.	Re-establishes blood flow
13. Obtain supplies.	
14. Select smallest catheter size that meets infusion needs and is appropriate for vein size.	Prevents irritation of vein lining, which causes phlebitis and infiltration
15. Include two appropriately sized catheters and one smaller gauge catheter with other supplies.	Prevents delay if second attempt is needed or smaller vein must be used

Action	Rationale

Note: A doctor's order is usually needed for lower extremity IV.

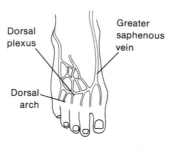

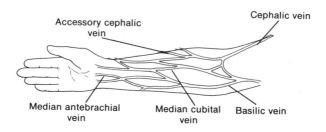

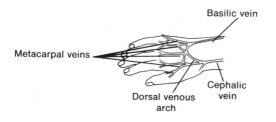

Figure 5.2

PROCEDURE 5.3 INTRAVENOUS THERAPY: SOLUTION PREPARATION

1. Select vein (see Procedure 5.2).
2. Open tubing package and check tubing for cracks or flaws. Check ends for covers and verify that regulator clamp is closed (rolled

Ensures that no defective materials are used and that tubing remains sterile

Allows better fluid control, minimizing air in tubing

Action	**Rationale**

down, clamped off, or
screwed closed).

3. Open IV fluid container:
   – **Bottles:** With one hand,
     hold bottle firmly on
     counter; with other
     hand, lift, then pull metal
     tab down, outward, and
     around until entire ring
     is removed (Fig. 5.3); lift
     metal cap and pull flat
     rubber pad up and off.
     MAINTAIN STERILITY
     OF BOTTLE TOP.

   Prevents injury or bottle
   breakage

   Avoids introducing microorganisms into client's vein

   – **Bags:** Remove outer bag
     covering; hold bag by
     neck in one hand; pull
     down on plastic tab with
     other hand and remove
     (Fig. 5.3).

   Prevents squeezing of fluid or
   air from bag when spike is
   inserted, increasing accuracy of fluid measurement

4. To attach tubing, first remove cap from tubing
   spikes:
   – **Bottles:** Wipe top with
     alcohol; push spike into
     bottle port that is *not*
     attached to white tube.

   Prevents blockage of tube that
   provides air vent

Opening seal on
bottle.

Removing tab
from bag.

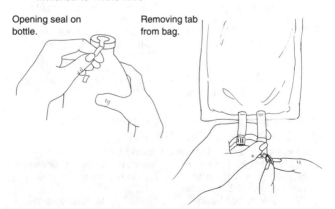

Figure 5.3

Action	Rationale
– **Bags:** Push spike into port until flat end of tubing and bag meet.	Ensures complete connection of bag and tubing
5. Prime the tubing (remove air):	
– Hang bottle or bag on IV pole or wall hook; squeeze and release drip chamber until fluid level reaches ring mark.	Eliminates introduction of air into tubing
– Remove cap from end of tubing.	
– Open roller clamp and flush tubing until air is removed.	Removes air from tubing
– Hold rubber medication plugs and in-line filter (if present) upside down and tap while fluid is running.	Forces air bubbles from plugs and filter
– Close roller clamp.	
6. Replace cap on end of tubing.	Maintains sterility
7. Put tag on bag or bottle, stating client's name, room number, date and time initiated, rate of infusion, and your initials. Apply time strip (see Procedure 5.6).	Identifies when fluid should be replaced (24-hour maximum); prevents fluid contamination. Facilitates monitoring of infusion rate
8. Tag tubing with date and time hung and own initials.	Indicates when tubing replacement is due (every 24 to 48 hours or per agency policy)
9. Proceed to bedside with equipment. Drape tubing over pole.	Maintains sterility of tubing

PROCEDURE 5.4 INTRAVENOUS THERAPY: CATHETER/HEPARIN LOCK INSERTION

For Primary Infusion Line and Heparin Lock

1. Select vein (see Procedure 5.2) and prepare solution (see Procedure 5.3). Place IV tubing on bed beside client.	Selects most appropriate vein. Provides fluid for infusion. Places tubing at easy access

Action	Rationale
2. Lower side rail and assist client into a supine position. Raise bed to high position.	Provides easier access to veins Promotes comfort during procedure Promotes use of good body mechanics
3. Tear 3-inch tape strips. Cut one piece down center.	Narrow strip will secure catheter without covering insertion site
4. Prepare needle/catheter for insertion: **Angiocath:** Examine catheter for cracks or flaws. Slide catheter off and on needle. **Butterfly:** Check needle tip for straight edge without bends or chips.	Ensures that catheter and needle are intact and plastic sheath will thread smoothly into vein Prevents shearing of vein by jagged needle
5. Open several alcohol pads.	Provides fast access to cleaning supplies
6. Place towel under extremity.	Prevents soiling of linens
7. Place tourniquet on extremity.	Restricts blood flow, distending vein
8. Locate largest, most distal vein.	Permits entrance of vein at higher point on future attempts without leakage
9. Don gloves.	Prevents contact with blood
10. With alcohol pad, clean vein area, beginning at the vein and circling outward in a 2-inch diameter.	Maintains asepsis
11. Encourage client to take slow, deep breaths as you begin.	Facilitates relaxation
12. Hold skin taut with one hand while holding catheter with other (Fig. 5.4.1). **Angiocath:** Hold the catheter by holding fingers on opposite sides of needle housing, *not* over catheter hub. (A needleless angiocath will have ribbed lines on the clear needle housing.)	Stabilizes vein and prevents skin movement during insertion Facilitates viewing of initial blood flashback in catheter and reduces additional line contamination

Action	Rationale

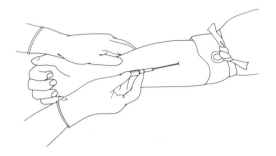

Figure 5.4.1

Butterfly: Pinch "wings" of butterfly together to insert needle.

Decreases pain during needle insertion

13. Maintaining sterility, insert catheter into vein with bevel of needle up. Insert needle parallel to straightest section of vein. Puncture skin at a 30-degree angle, 1 cm below site where the vein will be entered (Fig. 5.4.2).

Allows for full insertion of catheter

Ensures catheter stability

14. When needle has entered skin, lower it until it is al-

Prevents penetration of both walls of the vein

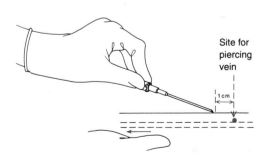

Figure 5.4.2

Action	**Rationale**
most flush with the skin (Fig. 5.4.3).	
15. Following path of vein, insert catheter into side of vein wall. (*If using a needleless angiocath system, insert needle at a 30-degree angle with bevel and push-off tabs in the up position. Place index finger on the push-off tab and thread the catheter to the desired length.*)	
16. Watch for first backflow of blood, then push needle gently into vein.	Indicates needle has pierced vein wall
Angiocath: Push needle into vein about ¼ inch after blood is noted. Slide catheter over needle and into vein before pulling needle out of vein and skin (Fig. 5.4.4).	Prevents piercing both walls of vein with needle
	Permits insertion of catheter without needle to prevent puncture of other vein wall
IF UNABLE TO INSERT CATHETER FULLY, DO NOT FORCE; WAIT UNTIL FLUID FLOW IS INITIATED.	Fluid infusion facilitates dilatation of vein
17. Holding catheter securely, remove cap from IV tubing and insert into hub of catheter; with **HEPARIN LOCK** twist on infusion plug (Fig. 5.4.5*A*).	Prevents dislodging of catheter

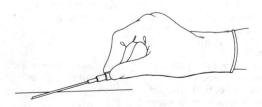

Figure 5.4.3

Action	Rationale

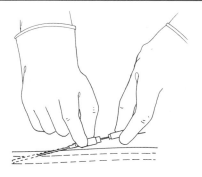

Figure 5.4.4

18. Remove tourniquet.

Prevents vein rupture from infusion of fluid against closed vessel

19. Open roller clamp and allow fluid to flow freely for a few seconds; with **heparin lock,** wipe plug with alcohol and flush with saline (Fig. 5.4.5*B*).

Determines if catheter is in vein or wedged against vessel wall

Fluid infusion prevents clot formation

20. Monitor for swelling or pain.

Indicates infiltration

21. Tape catheter in position that allows free flow of the fluid. Tape catheter in one of the following methods:

Eliminates positional flow of IV fluids

Angiocath: Put small piece of tape under hub of catheter and cross over to secure hub to skin. DO NOT PLACE TAPE OVER INSERTION SITE.

Maintains sterility of insertion site by covering with sterile material only

Butterfly: Put smallest pieces of tape across "wings" of butterfly; put another tape piece across middle to form an **H.** A second method is to put a

Provides catheter stabilization without tape covering insertion site

Action	Rationale

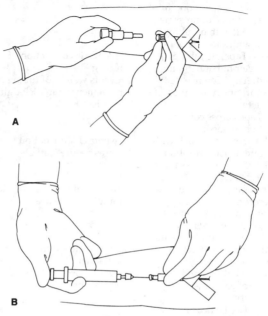

A

B

Figure 5.4.5

small piece of tape under wings and tape over to form a **V**; then place piece of tape across the **V**. (see Fig. 5.8 for an example)

22. Slow IV fluids to a moderate drip.

Prevents accidental fluid bolus while completing site care

23. Place ointment over insertion site, if desired, and cover with adhesive bandage, 2 × 2-inch dressing, or transparent dressing.

Decreases exposure to and growth of microorganism

24. Remove gloves and secure tubing:
Angiocath: Place tape across top of tubing, just

Action	**Rationale**
below catheter. Loop tubing and tape to dressing. Secure length of tubing to arm with short piece of tape. Tape the tubing/catheter hub junction.	Prevents disconnection of tubing
Butterfly: Coil needle tubing around and on top of IV site. – Tape across coil and hub of needle.	Prevents weight of tubing or movement from dislodging needle
Heparin lock: Flush with dilute heparin solution (1:100). Tape across infusion plug.	Prevents clot formation Secures needle/catheter
25. On a piece of tape or label, record: needle size, type, date, and time of insertion and your initials. Place label over top of dressing.	Provides information needed for follow-up care
26. Apply armboard if needed.	Stabilizes sites of frequent movement
27. Discard gloves and dispose of equipment properly.	Prevents spread of micro-organisms.
28. Regulate IV flow manually or set infusion device at appropriate rate (see Procedure 5.6).	
29. Review limitations in range of motion with client. Instruct client to notify nurse of problems or discomfort.	Enlists client's assistance in maintenance of catheter
30. Remove towel and position client for comfort, with call light within reach.	Promotes comfort and safety
31. Check infusion accuracy after 5 minutes and again after 15 minutes. Check volume every 1 to 2 hours.	Determines if rate needs to be adjusted

Evaluation

Goals met, partially met, or unmet?

Desired Outcomes (sample)

Skin is warm with good capillary refill and no edema.
IV intake is consistent with ordered rate.
Electrolytes are within normal limits.
Client performs self-care activities without disruption of IV assembly.
IV insertion site is clean and dry with no pain, redness, or swelling.

Documentation

The following should be noted on the client's chart:

- Client's tolerance of insertion procedure and fluid infusion
- Status of IV site, dressing, fluids, and tubing
- Size and type of catheter/needle
- Type and rate of infusion (if continuous infusion)
- Client teaching accomplished
- Follow-up assessments of the infusion
- Dilute heparin instillation (if heparin lock)

Sample Documentation

DATE	TIME	
12/3/94	1200	Client has 20-gauge Jelco inserted in right lower arm. One liter D_5W infusing at 125 ml/hr. Site intact. Client tolerated insertion procedure and fluid infusion without significant changes in vital signs. Teaching done regarding mobility limitations; client voiced understanding.

Flow Rate Calculation (5.5)

Intravenous Fluid Regulation (5.6)

☒ Equipment

- IV pole (bed or rolling) *or* IV pump/controller
- Calculator (or pencil and pad)
- Watch with second hand

Purpose

Ensures delivery of correct amount of IV fluids

Assessment

Assessment should focus on the following:

Orders for type and rate of fluid
Type of infusion control devices available or ordered
Viscosity of ordered fluids

Nursing Diagnoses

The nursing diagnoses may include the following:

Potential for fluid overload related to incorrect fluid rate

Planning

Key Goal and Sample Goal Criterion
The client will

Receive correct fluid volume

Special Considerations
Viscous solutions may require rate adjustments throughout infusion process based on actual flow due to accumulation in filter or on sides of tubing.

Geriatric and Pediatric
These clients are often volume sensitive and prone to fluid overload, particularly with rapid infusion of large volumes. Infusions must be regulated carefully and checked frequently, and clients must be watched closely for tolerance.

Implementation

Action	Rationale

PROCEDURE 5.5 FLOW RATE CALCULATION

Action	Rationale
1. Check tubing package to determine drop factor of tubing.	Indicates drops per ml for drip rate calculation
2. Determine the infusion *volume in milliliters* (ml) per hour using the following formula:	Simplifies calculations by limiting time to 60 minutes Facilitates monitoring of fluid and time taping container

$$\frac{\text{TOTAL VOLUME}}{\text{TOTAL NUMBER OF HOURS}} = \boxed{\begin{array}{c}\text{Hourly infusion rate} \\ \text{(volume to infuse each hour)}\end{array}}$$

Example: 1000 ml to be infused over 6 hours

$$1000/6 = 167 \text{ ml/hr}$$

3. Determine *flow rate* by using the following formula:

Action	Rationale

$$\frac{\text{TOTAL FLUID VOLUME}}{\text{TOTAL TIME (minutes)}} \times \frac{\text{DROP FACTOR}}{\text{(drops/ml)}} = \boxed{\begin{array}{l}\text{INFUSION}\\\text{RATE}\\\text{(drops/min)}\end{array}}$$

Example: Volume ordered is 1000 ml of D_5W over 6 hours; tubing drop factor is 15 drops/ml

$$\frac{1000 \text{ ml}}{6 (60) \text{ min}} \times 15 \text{ drops/ml} = \frac{15,000 \text{ drops}}{360 \text{ min}} = \begin{array}{l}41.7 \text{ or}\\42 \text{ drops/min}\end{array}$$

Or utilize hourly infusion rate (see above):

$$\frac{167 \text{ ml} \times 15 \text{ drops}}{60 \text{ min/ml}} = \begin{array}{l}41.7 \text{ or}\\42 \text{ drops/min}\end{array}$$

Total fluid volume equals the amount of fluid, expressed in ml, to infuse over the ordered period of time (if order is 1 liter of D_5W over 12 hours, the total volume is 1 liter [1000 ml]).

Total time is the number of minutes (hours × 60) over which the fluid should infuse. IF FLUID IS ORDERED PER HOUR OR YOU CALCULATE VOLUME PER HOUR, THE TOTAL TIME WILL EQUAL 60 MINUTES. Total volume will equal hourly infusion rate.

The drop factor is the number of drops from the chosen tubing that will equal 1 ml. This amount is found on the tubing package and is expressed in drops per ml.

4. *If available, use precalculated infusion chart by:*
   - Looking across chart for drop factor of tubing
   - Coming down chart to line indicating amount of

Indicates drops per minute at point of intersection

TABLE 5.5 Flow Rates for Intravenous Infusions

Drop Factor of Tubing (drops/ml)	1000 ml/6 hr (drops/min)	1000 ml/8 hr (drops/min)
10	28	21
15	42	31
20	56	42
60	167	125

Action	Rationale
fluid infusing per hour (see Table 5.5)	
5. Regulate fluid or set drop rate on fluid regulator (see Procedure 5.6).	

PROCEDURE 5.6 INTRAVENOUS FLUID REGULATION

Action	Rationale
1. Calculate or determine appropriate volume per hour and drip rate (drops per minute; see Procedure 5.5).	
2. Prepare time tape for fluid based on volume of fluid to infuse over 1 hour (Fig. 5.6.1). Use felt pen to mark.	Facilitates close monitoring of fluid infusion Prevents puncture of container
– Tear an 11-inch strip of 1-inch tape.	
– Place tape on IV fluid container beside fluid-level indicators.	
– Mark tape at intervals indicating fluid level after each hour of infusion (for small hourly volumes, mark the volume for a 2- or 3-hour interval instead).	Simplifies marking of fluid amounts (*i.e.*, instead of 75 ml/hr mark 150 ml at 2-hour intervals)
3. Attach appropriate tubing (for infusion pump, with chamber, or Dial-A-Flo) and clear tubing of air. Proceed to appropriate section for step 4.	

1000 ml/10 hr (drops/min)	1000 ml/12 hr (drops/min)	1000 ml/24 hr (drops/min)
17	14	7
25	21	10
34	28	14
100	84	42

Action	Rationale

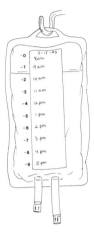

Figure 5.6.1

Manual Rate Regulation

4. Open all clamps except regulator roller/screw.	Limits fluid rate control to regulator
5. Open regulator fully; then slowly close regulator while observing drip chamber—fluid should initially run in a stream (Table 5.6 lists troubleshooting tips).	Determines catheter patency
6. Close regulator screw until fluid is dropping at slow but steady pace.	
7. Count the number of drops falling within 15 seconds and multiply by 4 (see Procedure 5.5).	Determines drops falling per minute
8. Open regulator to increase drop flow if drops-per-minute rate is less than calculated drip rate; close regulator if drops-per-minute rate is more than needed.	

Action	Rationale
9. Count drops again and continue to adjust flow until desired drip rate is obtained.	Produces correct drip rate

TABLE 5.6 Troubleshooting Tips for Intravenous Infusion Management

Problem	Actions
1. Drip chamber is overfilled.	Close regulator clamp, turn fluid container upside down, and squeeze fluid from drip chamber until half full or slightly below.
2. Air is in tubing.	Check adequacy of fluid level in drip chamber and security of tubing connections. Insert needle and syringe into rubber port distal to air and aspirate to remove air.
3. Blood is backing up into tubing.	Be sure fluid is above the level of the IV catheter site and the level of the heart. Check security of tubing connections. Check that infusing fluid has not run out and that catheter is in a vein, not an artery (note pulsation of blood in tubing).
4. Infusion pump alarms indicate flow problem.	Check drip chamber for excess or inadequate fluid level. Check that clamps and regulators are open, air vent is open (if applicable), and tubing is free of kinks. Check IV catheter site for infiltration, blood clot, kinks, and positional obstruction (open fluid regulator fully and change position of arm to see if fluid flows better in various positions). Insert needle and syringe into medication port and gently flush fluid through catheter. If resistance is met, try to aspirate blood/clot into tubing; if unsuccessful, discontinue IV and restart.
5. IV is positional (*i.e.*, runs well only when arm or hand is in a certain position).	Stabilize IV site with armboard or handboard and monitor fluid infusion every 1 to 2 hours.
6. Fluid is dripping but is also leaking into tissue surrounding puncture site.	Discontinue IV and restart in another site. Place warm soak over infiltrated site. Reassess frequently.

Action	Rationale
10. Recheck drip rate after 5 minutes and again after 15 minutes. Proceed to finishing steps 11 to 15.	Detects changes in rate due to expansion/contracting of tubing

Dial-A-Flo Fluid Regulation

See steps 1 to 3 for initial preparation.

Action	Rationale
4. At end of IV tubing attach Dial-A-Flo tubing (Fig. 5.6.2).	
5. Open all clamps and regulator on IV tubing.	
6. Adjust Dial-A-Flo to open position and clear tubing of air (remove cap if needed).	
7. Close fluid regulator roller/screw.	Prevents fluid flow during connection to IV catheter
8. Attach Dial-A-Flo to catheter hub (following initial insertion or during tubing change) and open fluid regulator.	
9. Turn Dial-A-Flo regulator until arrow is aligned with desired volume of fluid to infuse over 1 hour.	Regulates fluid to infuse at desired rate
10. Check drip rate over 15 seconds and multiply by 4 (should coincide with calculated drip rate).	Verifies fluid infusion rate
– Adjust height of pole if necessary.	Gravity facilitates flow
– Recheck drip rate after 5 minutes and again after 15 minutes.	Detects changes in rate due to expansion/contracting of tubing
– Proceed to finishing steps 11 to 15.	

Infusion Controller or Pump Regulation

See steps 1 to 3 for initial preparation.

Action	**Rationale**

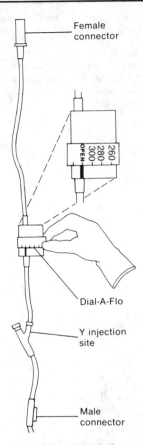

Female connector

OPEN 300 280 260

Dial-A-Flo

Y injection site

Male connector

Figure 5.6.2

Action	**Rationale**
4. Insert tubing into infusion pump/regulator according to pump manual.	Ensures proper functioning of infusion regulator
5. Close door to pump/controller and open all tubing clamps and regulator roller/screw.	Allows pump/controller to regulate fluids

Action	Rationale
6. Set volume dials for appropriate volume per hour *or* drops per minute (check type of pump *carefully*).	Determines amount of fluid pump/controller will deliver
7. Place electronic eye clamp over drip chamber (optional in some infusion regulators; consult manual; Fig. 5.6.3).	Allows pump/controller to monitor fluid flow

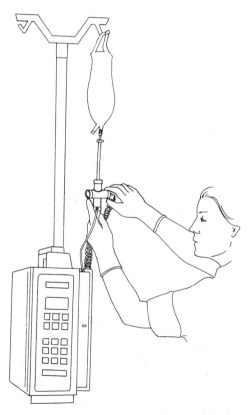

Figure 5.6.3

Action	Rationale
8. Push ON or START button.	Initiates fluid flow and regulation
9. Check drip rate over 15 seconds and multiply by 4 (should coincide with calculated drip rate).	Verifies fluid infusion rate
10. Set volume infusion alarm, if desired (often omitted). If tubing does not contain a regulator cassette, periodically change the sections of tubing placed inside infusion clamp. Proceed to finishing steps 11 to 15.	Notifies nurse when set volume has been infused
	Prevents tubing collapse due to constant squeezing by pump

Volume Control Chamber (Buretrol) Regulation

See steps 1 and 2 for initial preparation.

Action	Rationale
3. Close off regulator 1 (above chamber) and regulator 2 (below chamber).	Controls fluids more precisely
4. Open regulator 1. Fill chamber with 10 ml fluid, prime drip chamber, and clear tubing of air (Fig. 5.6.4A).	Facilitates clearing of air from tubing
5. Fill chamber with volume of fluid to infuse in one hour (or 2 or 3 hours' worth, if volume is small).	Allows for close monitoring of fluid volume (needed for volume-sensitive or pediatric clients)
6. Close regulator 1. Make sure air vent is open (Fig. 5.6.4B).	Fluid will not flow if regulator #1 and air vent are closed
7. Open regulator 2 and regulate drops to calculated rate (drip rate should equal volume per hour if minidrip tubing system is used [check drop factor]), or: – Attach Dial-A-Flo to tubing and leave regulator 2 open, or	Sets volume to infuse over an hour

Action	Rationale

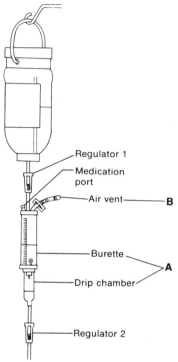

Figure 5.6.4

Action	Rationale
– Place tubing into infusion pump or controller and leave regulator 2 open.	Allows infusion pump/controller to regulate fluid
8. Check drip rate over 15 seconds and multiply by 4 (should coincide with calculated drip rate).	Verifies fluid infusion rate
9. Put a time tape on the chamber (if pump/controller is not used).	Allows for quick, easy check of fluid infusion progress and the need to add fluid to chamber.

Action	**Rationale**
10. Check chamber each hour or two, and add 1 to 2 hours' more fluid volume as needed. IF CLOSE FLUID MONITORING IS NOT NEEDED, CLAMP AIR VENT AND OPEN REGULATOR 1. Proceed to finishing steps 11 to 15.	Maintains fluid infusion and catheter patency Prevents air entrance into tubing Allows fluid to flow directly from bottle/bag into chamber and to client

Finishing Steps

11. Mark beginning hour of fluid infusion on time tape.	Sets times for subsequent checks
12. Check volume every 1 to 2 hours and compare with time tape.	Determines actual volume infusion
13. If volume depleted does not coincide with time mark: – Check time tape for accuracy. – Check settings on pump/controller or Dial-A-Flo and readjust if indicated. – Elevate fluid container on pole. – Check catheter site and position for obstruction (see Table 5.6).	Facilitates flow by gravity
14. Review limitations in range of motion with client. Instruct client to notify nurse of problems or discomfort.	Facilitates early detection of problems with catheter or fluid flow
15. Position client for comfort with call light within reach.	Promotes client comfort and safety

Evaluation

Goals met, partially met, or unmet?

Desired Outcome (sample)

Correct volume of fluid is infused within designated time frame.

Documentation

The following should be noted on the client's chart:

- Time of initiation of fluid infusion
- Type and volume of fluid infusing
- Infusion device used, if applicable
- Status of catheter insertion site
- Problems with infusion procedure and solutions applied (*e.g.*, armboard used, catheter repositioned)
- Client tolerance to fluid infusion
- Client teaching and response

Sample Documentation

DATE	TIME	
2/9/94	1400	Client receiving D_5W; 1000-ml bag infusing at 125 ml/hour per Dial-A-Flow. Tolerating fluid infusion well. Catheter site clean and dry without signs of infiltration or infection. Return demonstration noted arm positions to be avoided during IV fluid infusion.

🖐 Intravenous Tubing Change/Conversion to Heparin Lock (5.7)

🖐 Intravenous Dressing Change (5.8)

❌ Equipment

- Alcohol pads and Betadine pad (optional)
- Infusion tubing (vented for IV fluid bag, unvented for IV bottles)
- Towel
- Tape 1 inch wide (may cut 2-inch tape)
- Dressing: 2 × 2-inch gauze, adhesive bandage or transparent dressing (Opsite)
- IV pole (bed or rolling) *or* IV pump/controller
- Ointment (optional)
- Razor and soap (optional)
- Armboard (optional)
- Adhesive labels
- Nonsterile gloves

Purpose

Decreases opportunity for growth of microorganisms by removing possible medium for infection

Assessment

Assessment should focus on the following:

Doctor's orders for type and rate of fluid
Status of skin on hand and arms, presence of hair or abrasions

Ability to hold arm and hand without movement or resistance
for duration of procedure
Allergy to tape, iodine, antibiotic pads, or ointment

Nursing Diagnoses

The nursing diagnoses may include the following:

Potential for infection related to interruption of skin integrity

Planning

Key Goals and Sample Goal Criteria

The client will

Maintain skin integrity and absence of infection around insertion
site, as evidenced by lack of pain, redness, or swelling at site
Verbalize understanding of movement limitations related to intravenous infusions and complications to be reported to the nurse

Special Considerations

If possible, replace IV fluid and tubing and change dressing at
the same time. This reduces risk of introducing microorganisms. *Many institutions have specified procedures and times for
dressing and tubing change. If unsure, consult policy manual.*

Geriatric and Pediatric

If the client is resistant, confused, or frightened, obtain an assistant to immobilize arm to ensure that IV line is not accidentally dislodged during dressing change.

Home Health

In the homebound client, be constantly alert for subtle signs and
symptoms of infection associated with long-term IV therapy.

Implementation

Action	Rationale

PROCEDURE 5.7 INTRAVENOUS TUBING CHANGE/CONVERSION TO HEPARIN LOCK

Action	Rationale
1. Wash hands and organize equipment.	Reduces microorganism transfer Promotes efficiency

Action	Rationale
2. Open package and check tubing for cracks or flaws. Be sure caps are on all ports and that the regulator clamp is closed (rolled down, clamped off or screwed closed).	Ensures that no defective materials are used and that tubing remains sterile Allows better fluid control minimizing air in tubing
3. Check infusing fluid against doctor's orders.	Validates correct fluid infusion
4. Tape old tubing to IV pole or pump pole with strip of tape and fill drip chamber full (Fig. 5.7.1).	Allows fluid in tubing to infuse into vein while new tubing is being prepared
5. Remove infusing fluid bag/bottle from IV pole or pump (put pump on hold) and disconnect from old tubing.	Provides fluid for new tubing

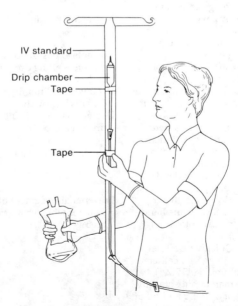

IV standard

Drip chamber

Tape

Tape

Figure 5.7.1

Action	Rationale
6. Attach new tubing to bag/bottle and prime tubing (remove air):	
– Hang bottle or bag on IV pole (or pole or infusion pump hook).	Forces air to bottle/bag top and places fluid at entrance to tubing
– Squeeze and release drip chamber until fluid level reaches ring mark on chamber.	Fills drip chamber and prevents introduction of air into tubing
– Remove cap from end of tubing.	
– Open roller clamp and flush tubing until air is removed.	Allows total removal of air from tubing
– Hold rubber medication plugs and in-line filter (if present) upside down and tap while fluid is running; close clamp.	Forces air bubbles from plugs and filters
7. Loosely cover end of tubing with cap and lay on bed near IV dressing.	Maintains sterility
8. Don gloves.	Prevents exposure to blood
9. Close off flow from old tubing.	Prevents wetting dressing and bed
10. a. Exchange old tubing for new at IV catheter hub:	Removes medium for microorganism growth
– Place alcohol swab under the catheter hub–tubing junction.	Decreases blood soiling of dressing or bed
– Loosen connection at junction of IV catheter and old tubing.	
– Holding catheter firm with one hand, remove old tubing; *and*	Prevents dislodgment of catheter when changing tubing
– Quickly insert new tubing into catheter hub (Fig. 5.7.2*A*), maintaining sterility of catheter and tip of new tubing.	

Action	Rationale
b. Begin flow from new tubing.	Prevents clot formation in catheter
c. Regulate fluid flow or place tubing into pump.	Promotes accurate infusion rate
d. Tape tubing to dressing and arm unless dressing is to be changed.	Decreases accidental pull on catheter
e. Tag tubing with date, time hung, and own initials.	Indicates when tubing replacement is due (every 24 to 48 hours or per agency policy)

11. **Conversion to heparin lock**
    a. Perform steps 1 to 9. Remove old tubing and

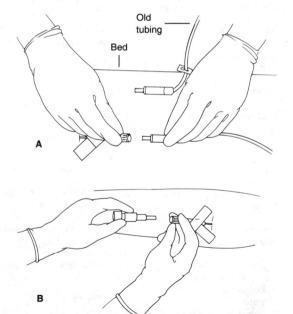

Figure 5.7.2

Action	Rationale
apply infusion plug/heparin lock (Fig. 5.7.2*B*).	
b. Flush catheter with saline or heparin flush.	
c. Tape infusion plug and catheter securely in place or perform dressing change if indicated.	
d. Tag site with date, time, and initials.	
12. Discard old tubing and other trash.	Promotes clean environment
13. If performing dressing change, see Procedure 5.8, Intravenous Dressing Change. If not, place tape across junction of tubing and catheter.	Prevents dislodging of tubing from catheter
14. Raise side rails and position client for safety and comfort.	Promotes client comfort and safety
15. Discard gloves and wash hands.	Reduces microorganism transfer

PROCEDURE 5.8 INTRAVENOUS DRESSING CHANGE

Action	Rationale
1. Wash hands and organize equipment.	Reduces microorganism transfer Promotes efficiency
2. Explain procedure to client.	Decreases anxiety
3. Tear tape strips 3 inches in length, 1 inch wide. Cut one strip down the center. Hang tape pieces from edge of table.	Secures catheter without covering insertion site Places tape in available position without disrupting adhesive
4. Open alcohol/Betadine pads, dressing and adhesive bandage, and ointment.	Provides fast access to supplies
5. Lower side rail and assist client into a supine position.	Provides easy access to IV site Promotes comfort during procedure

Action	Rationale
6. Raise bed to high position.	Decreases strain on nurse's back
7. Place towel under extremity.	Prevents soiling of linens
8. Don gloves.	Protects from potential contamination
9. Remove dressing and all tape except tape holding catheter.	Prevents dislodging of catheter while cleaning site
10. Using alcohol first and then Betadine swabs, clean catheter-insertion site beginning at catheter and cleaning outward in a 2-inch diameter circle.	Removes blood and drainage from site and surrounding area
11. Holding catheter secure with one hand, remove remaining tape and clean under catheter.	Prevents catheter dislodgment
12. Allow area to dry and secure catheter in position:	
– **Angiocath:** With tape edges sticking to thumb and fingertip, slide small strip of tape under catheter hub with	Provides greater control of tape Insertion site should be covered with sterile material only

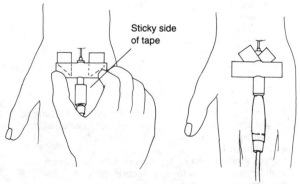

Sticky side of tape

Figure 5.8

Action	Rationale
adhesive side up (Fig. 5.8*A*); cross tape over hub to secure catheter, but DO NOT place tape over insertion site; put other small strip of tape across catheter hub (Fig. 5.8*B*).	Adds stability to catheter
– **Butterfly:** Put smallest pieces of tape across wings of butterfly and another tape piece across middle to form an **H;** or put small piece of tape under wings, tape over to form a **V,** and then place piece of tape across the **V.**	Eliminates positional flow of IV fluids Allows for catheter stabilization without tape covering insertion site
13. Place ointment over insertion site, if desired, and cover site with adhesive bandage, 2 × 2-inch dressing, or Opsite (if client is allergic to iodine, use Neosporin ointment).	
14. Remove gloves and secure tubing:	
– **Angiocath:** Place tape across top of tubing just below catheter, loop tubing and tape to dressing, and secure tubing to arm with short piece of tape (taping the tubing/ catheter hub junction is optional).	Prevents disconnection of tubing
– **Butterfly:** Coil catheter tubing around on top of IV site; tape across coil and catheter hub.	Prevents weight of tubing or movement from dislodging catheter
– **Heparin lock:** Flush with heparin flush solution and tape across infusion plug.	Prevents clot formation and secures catheter

Action	Rationale
15. Apply armboard if needed.	Stabilizes sites of frequent movement
16. On a piece of tape or label, record needle size, type, date and time of site care and your initials; place label over top of dressing.	Provides information needed for follow-up care
17. Raise side rails and position client for comfort.	Promotes client comfort and safety
18. Explain limitations of movement to client with return demonstrations, as well as need to report pain or swelling at site.	Decreases client anxiety regarding proper maintenance of IV needle Promotes early detection of infiltration or other complications
19. Discard or restore supplies; wash hands.	Decreases the spread of organisms

Evaluation

Goals met, partially met, or unmet?

Desired Outcomes (sample)

No evidence of infection exists around insertion site, and skin integrity is intact. Client verbalizes understanding of movement limitations related to intravenous infusions and of complications to be reported to the nurse.

Documentation

The following should be noted on the client's chart:

- Location and status of IV site, dressing, fluids, and tubing
- Size and type of catheter/needle
- Reports of pain at site
- IV site care rendered and client tolerance to care
- Client teaching

Sample Documentation

DATE	TIME	
4/9/94	1200	Tubing changed to IV of D$_5$W infusing at 125 ml/hr in right lower arm. Site care done, #20 Jelco present, site clean without swelling or pain. Client tolerated procedure well. Reinforced teaching regarding mobility limitations; client demonstrated understanding.

☝ Central Line Maintenance

✖ Equipment

- Sterile gloves
- Sterile gauze pads (4 × 4 inches) or transparent dressing
- Face mask (optional)
- 2-inch tape
- Alcohol pads
- Betadine swabs (optional)
- IV fluids and tubing or heparin flush or saline flush
- Prep razor
- Suture with needle holder
- CVP insertion kit containing:
  - sterile gloves (multiple sizes)
  - Betadine swabs or solution and gauze
  - sterile towels/drapes
  - 10-ml syringe (slip-tip)
  - ⅝-, 1-, and 1½-inch needles
- Lidocaine/Xylocaine (without epinephrine) 1% or 2%
- Central line with introducer (*e.g.*, single-lumen or multilumen catheter, Hickmann catheter, angiocath)

Purpose

Permits administration of medications and nutritional support that should not be given via a peripheral route or when peripheral routes cannot be obtained

Assessment

Assessment should focus on the following:

Type of catheter
Location of catheter
Type of infusion(s)
Agency policy regarding central line care

Nursing Diagnoses

The nursing diagnoses may include the following:

Fluid volume deficit related to nausea and vomiting
Nutrition, altered: Less than body requirements related to anorexia

Planning

Key Goals and Sample Goal Criteria

The client will

Maintain skin turgor during total parenteral nutrition (TPN) administration
Gain 2 to 3 kg per week

Special Considerations

If central line was inserted for infusion of TPN, infuse only $D_{10}W$ or D_5W until TPN is available.
If multilumen catheter is used, select and mark a catheter port for TPN only.
Policy varies greatly regarding use of saline or Heparin solution for flushing catheter; consult agency policy manual.

Home Health
In the homebound client, a central line is likely to be in place for a long time. Therefore, be constantly alert for early signs and symptoms of infection.

Implementation

Action	Rationale
Assisting with Insertion	
1. Wash hands and organize equipment.	Reduces microorganism transfer Promotes efficiency
2. Arrange supplies on tray, using appropriate-size gloves for physician.	
3. Reinforce explanation of procedure to client. Clarify that his/her face will be	Reduces client anxiety

Action	Rationale
covered with towels or drapes but that you will be nearby.	
4. Put bed and client in Trendelenburg position. If client has respiratory distress, place in supine position with feet elevated 45 to 60 degrees (modified Trendelenburg).	Dilates vessels in upper trunk and neck Puts less pressure on diaphragm and facilitates breathing
5. Hold client's hand (obtain assistant and restrain both hands if client is resistant or confused).	Provides comfort Prevents procedure disruption or contamination of field
6. Don face mask and apply mask to client (optional).	Decreases contamination of insertion site
7. Inform client of progression of the procedure, particularly when needle stick is to occur.	Prepares client for discomfort Decreases startle reaction
8. Monitor client for respiratory distress, complaints of chest pain, dysrhythmias, or other complications.	Facilitates early detection of pneumothorax, air or catheter embolism, or other complication
9. After the vein has been punctured, the doctor will exchange the catheter for the syringe; at this time, instruct the client to take a deep breath and bear down (Valsalva's maneuver).	Prevents air from being sucked into vein by increasing the intrathoracic pressure
10. Once the catheter is in place and sutured, attach IV fluid tubing (many catheters have 3 to 4 inches of tubing attached), apply sterile gauze pads, loop tubing loosely on top of pads, and tape dressing down.	Maintains sterility of insertion site Secures tubing to prevent direct pull on catheter
11. Infuse fluid slowly (5 to 10 ml/hour); begin regular infusion rate after catheter position has been con-	Verifies catheter is in vena cava (or right atrium) prior to infusion of fluid

Action	Rationale

firmed by chest radiograph. (Use of intermittent infusion plugs/heparin locks may be noted, with saline or heparin flushes.)

12. Position client for comfort with call light within reach; instruct client to call nurse if any respiratory distress or pain is experienced.

Promotes client safety and early detection of complications

Monitoring and Maintenance

1. Mark each lumen of multilumen catheter with name of fluid/medication infusing.

Prevents mixing of medications

2. Lumens without continuing infusion of fluids are capped with infusion plug and flushed every 8 hours with heparin solution (usually 1:100 dilution); depending on length of tubing and size of catheter, 1 to 3 ml are used (use 6 ml or ordered amount of flush for Hickman catheter and short small needle—⅝ inch, 25 gauge).

Prevents obstruction of catheter lumen with blood clot

Minimizes leakage of plug or damage to catheter

3. Flush tubings, between infusion of medications and drawing of blood, first using saline, and then heparin.

Prevents medication interaction or lumen obstruction with blood

4. ALWAYS ASPIRATE BEFORE INFUSING MEDICATIONS OR FLUSHING TUBINGS.

Assures patency of line and validates presence in vessel

5. Monitor for clot formation in lumen:
   If resistance is met when flushing tubing, DO NOT FORCE; aspirate and remove clot if possible; if not, notify doctor.

Prevents clot from reaching client and causing emboli

Action	Rationale
6. Monitor respirations and breath sounds every 4 hours.	Promotes early detection of fluid entering chest cavity or of pulmonary embolism
7. Maintain IV fluids above the level of the heart. Do not allow fluid to run out and air to enter tubing (see Table 5.6 and Procedure 5.6).	Prevents blood reflux into tubing Prevents infusion of air

Tubing Change

1. Review Procedure 5.7. Prepare fluid and tubing (see Procedure 5.3).	Minimizes exposure to micro-organisms
2. Don gloves.	Protects from potential contamination
3. Expose catheter hub or rubber port of multilumen catheter.	Precedes connection of tubing
4. Ask client to take a deep breath and bear down (Valsalva's maneuver).	Increases intrathoracic pressure Prevents air from entering vein
5. Disconnect old tubing and quickly connect new tubing.	
6. Open fluid and adjust to appropriate infusion rate.	
7. Proceed to dressing change, if needed.	

Dressing Change

1. Explain procedure to client.	Reduces anxiety
2. Wash hands and gather equipment.	Reduces microorganism transfer Promotes efficiency
3. Open packages, keeping supplies sterile.	Prevents contamination of catheter site
4. Don clean gloves and mask.	
5. Remove tape.	
6. Don sterile gloves.	
7. Beginning at catheter and wiping outward to the surrounding skin, clean insertion site with alcohol and Betadine.	Decreases contamination Removes microorganisms from site

Action	Rationale
8. Place ointment over insertion site (optional) and cover with sterile gauze.	
9. Cover gauze with tape, wrap tubing on top of tape, and cover tubing with tape.	Secures dressing Prevents pull on catheter
10. Remove gloves and mask.	
11. On a piece of tape or label, record date and time of site care and your initials. Place label over top of dressing.	Determines next site care (required every 48 to 72 hours)
12. Raise side rails and position client for comfort.	Promotes client safety and comfort

Evaluation

Goals met, partially met, or unmet?

Desired Outcomes (sample)

Client remains free of embolism, pleural effusion, and infection, both systemic and at catheter site.
Central line remains patent.

Documentation

The following should be noted on the client's chart:

- Date and time of catheter insertion
- Type and location of catheter
- Care and maintenance procedures performed
- Equipment used with catheter
- Client tolerance to procedures

Sample Documentation

DATE	TIME	
1/9/94	0400	Dressing changed at right subclavian triple-lumen catheter site. No redness, edema, or drainage at site. Povidone ointment applied. IV fluid bag and tubing changed. D_5W infusing via IVAC pump at 50 ml/hr.

✋ Total Parenteral Nutrition Management

☒ Equipment

- IV tubing with filter (for total parenteral nutrition; TPN)
- IV tubing without filter for lipids, if ordered
- Infusion pumps, if available
- Appropriate labels
- Sterile gloves

Purpose

Permits administration of nutritional support when gastrointestinal tract is traumatized or nonfunctional

Assessment

Assessment should focus on the following:

Doctor's orders for TPN type (central or peripheral), contents, and rate

Doctor's orders for lipid infusion frequency and rate

Current nutritional status (weight, height, skin turgor, edema)

Laboratory values, particularly albumin level, glucose, and potassium

Nursing Diagnoses

The nursing diagnoses may include the following:

Nutrition, altered: Less than body requirements related to anorexia

Planning

Key Goals and Sample Goal Criteria

The client will

Maintain skin turgor during TPN administration
Gain 2 to 3 kg per week

Special Considerations

High glucose levels in TPN provide a good medium for bacterial growth; thus, strict asepsis is needed to prevent septicemia.

Geriatric and Pediatric
Children and the elderly tend to be very sensitive to volume changes; thus, volume should be infused cautiously.
They are also susceptible to infection; therefore, check temperatures frequently.

Home Health
If total parenteral nutrition is to infuse very slowly and client's residence is unusually warm (*e.g.,* summer months without air conditioning), request that the supplier divide solution into two containers to decrease opportunity for growth of microorganisms.

Implementation

Action	Rationale
Central Parenteral Nutrition	
1. Wash hands and organize equipment.	Reduces microorganism transfer
	Promotes efficiency
2. Assist in starting central line (see Procedure 5.9) and monitor client appropriately.	Provides venous access for TPN
3. Don gloves.	Reduces contamination
4. Mark port intended for TPN and close it with infusion plug; or prepare infusion of $D_{10}W$ or D_5W to be used until TPN solution	Preserves sterility of port for TPN
	Maintains tubing for TPN

Action	Rationale
is available. DO NOT INFUSE MEDICATIONS OR OTHER SOLUTIONS THROUGH PORT.	Minimizes contamination of tubing
5. Compare TPN label with doctor's orders.	Verifies correct dosage of nutrients
6. Check client's name band against TPN label.	Verifies correct client
7. Prepare TPN:	
– If refrigerated, allow bag/bottle to stand at room temperature 15 to 30 minutes.	Prevents infusion of cold fluid with resulting discomfort and chilling
– Put time tape bag/bottle.	
– Close drip regulator on filtered tubing.	
– Remove cap from filtered IV tubing to expose spike.	
– Remove tab/cover from TPN bag/bottle.	
– Insert tubing spike.	
– Prime drip chamber.	
– Open drip regulator.	
– Clear air from tubing.	
– Close drip regulator.	
– Place tubing at bedside.	
8. Prepare lipids (if lipids and TPN are to infuse simultaneously):	
– Put time tape bottle (every 2 hours if small hourly infusion).	Facilitates correct infusion rate
– Insert vented, nonfiltered tubing spike into lipid container.	
– Prime drip chamber and clear air from tubing.	Prevents infusion of air into chest
– Place needle (21 gauge) on end of tubing and plug into medication plug at distal end of TPN tubing (Fig. 5.10).	
9. Attach TPN tubing to central line port (see Fig. 5.10).	

Action   **Rationale**

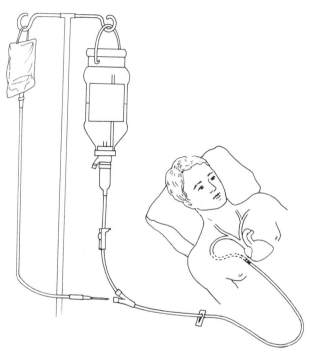

Figure 5.10

Action	Rationale
10. Discard gloves and disposable materials; position client for comfort with call bell within reach.	Promotes clean environment Facilitates communication and client safety
11. Set pumps to deliver appropriate volumes per hour.	
12. Calculate and check drip rate and monitor infusion every 1 to 2 hours. (If infusion is behind sched-	Verifies correct infusion rate

Action	Rationale
ule, DO NOT SPEED UP INFUSION RATE. Correct infusion rate and resume proper administration.)	Prevents volume overload or glucose bolus
13. Perform client teaching regarding:	
– Need to keep solution higher than chest, avoid manipulating catheter	Facilitates proper flow of solution
– Need to report any pain, respiratory distress, warmth, or flushing	Indicates possible catheter dislodgment or infection
14. Monitor:	
– Vital signs with temperature check every 4 to 8 hours (depending on orders)	Facilitates early detection of infection or complications
– Blood glucose level every 12 to 24 hours (more frequently if client is diabetic)	Detects glucose intolerance
– Urine glucose and electrolytes in pediatric clients (and watch for signs of hyperglycemia)	
– Central line site every shift; provide care every 48 to 72 hours (see Procedure 5.9)	
– For dyspnea (i.e., rales in lung bases)	Indicates possible fluid overload
15. Weigh client daily and monitor total protein and albumin levels.	Indicates benefits of nutritional intake
16. Place TPN and lipids on rolling infusion pumps and encourage client ambulation, if allowed.	Facilitates pulmonary toilet Facilitates muscle development Promotes sense of well-being

Evaluation

Goals met, partially met, or unmet?

Desired Outcomes (sample)

Skin turgor is good; no edema is present.
Albumin and potassium levels are within normal range; glucose
    level is within acceptable range.

Documentation

The following should be noted on the client's chart:

- Time TPN bottle/bag is hung, number of bottles/bags, and
  rate of infusion
- Time lipid bottle is hung and rate of infusion
- Site of IV catheter and verification of patency
- Status of dressing and site, if visible
- Laboratory results of electrolytes
- Client tolerance to TPN

Sample Documentation

DATE	TIME	
3/9/94	2400	Bag #3 of TPN infusing at 80 ml/hour into middle port of right subclavian triple-lumen catheter. Lipids piggy-backed into TPN tubing and infusing at 21 ml/hour. Catheter insertion site intact with good blood return. Fingerstick blood sugar 110.

🖐 Blood Transfusion Management

🗙 Equipment

- Blood transfusion tubing (Blood Y set with in-line filter)
- 250- to 500-ml bag/bottle normal saline
- Packed cells or whole blood, as ordered
- Blood warmer or coiled tubing and pan of warm water (optional)
- Order slips for blood
- Flow sheet for vital signs (for frequent checks)
- Nonsterile gloves
- Materials for IV start (see Procedures 5.3 and 5.4).

Purpose

Increases client's hemoglobin and hematocrit for improved circulation and oxygen distribution

Assessment

Assessment should focus on the following:

Baseline vital signs; circulatory and respiratory status
Skin status (*e.g.*, rash)
Doctor's orders for type, amount, and rate of blood administration
Size of IV catheter or need for catheter insertion
History of blood transfusions and reactions, if any
Religious or other personal objections to client's receipt of blood
Compatibility of client to blood (matching blood sheet numbers to name band; see p. 221)

Nursing Diagnoses

The nursing diagnoses may include:

Decreased activity tolerance related to weakness (associated with low hemoglobin and hematocrit levels)

Altered circulation related to gastrointestinal hemorrhage

Planning

Key Goals and Sample Goal Criteria

The client will

Demonstrate adequate circulation evidenced by capillary refill time of 2 to 3 seconds, pink mucous membranes, and warm, dry skin

Increase activity tolerance from ambulation in room to ambulation to nurses' station, without tachycardia or tachypnea, within 72 hours

Special Considerations

Some agencies require that two registered nurses perform blood–client identification checks. Refer to agency policy.

Clients with a history of previous transfusions must be watched carefully for a transfusion reaction.

The maximum transfusion time for packed cells or whole blood is 4 hours.

The transfusion must be started within half an hour after getting the blood from the blood bank; otherwise, the blood cannot be reissued.

Geriatric

Fluid-sensitive clients may not tolerate a rapid change in blood volume; they must receive the transfusion as slowly as possible.

Pediatric

Small children and confused or comatose clients must be watched closely for a transfusion reaction because they often cannot communicate discomfort.

Home Health

Remain with the client during the entire transfusion and for 1 hour afterward.

Because you may be the only licensed caregiver in the home at the time, double-check the date, time, and transfusion information on the blood bag and blood bank slip at two separate points in time or ask the client or relative to verify that the transfusion data are identical.

Have adrenalin on hand in case an anaphylactic reaction occurs.

Implementation

Action	Rationale
1. Wash hands and organize equipment.	Reduces microorganism transfer Promotes efficiency
2. Explain procedure to client, particularly the need for frequent vital sign checks.	Decreases client anxiety
3. **Prepare tubing:**	
– Open tubing package and close drip regulator (which may be a clamp, roller, or screw). Note red and white caps over tubing spikes.	Prepares for infusion of saline before and after transfusion
– Remove white cap to reveal spike on one side of blood tubing (Fig. 5.11A).	
– Remove tab from normal saline bag/bottle and insert tubing spike.	
– Remove cap from end of tubing, open saline regulator 1, prime drip chamber with saline, and flush tubing to end.	Prevents air entering tubing Clears air from tubing
– Close fluid regulator.	
– Replace cap on tubing end and place on bed near IV catheter.	Retains sterility
(If infusing blood rapidly, connect to warming-coil tubing and flush tubing to end. Place coil in warm water bath.)	Prepares medium for warming blood before infusing Prevents infusion of cold blood and lowering of body temperature

Action   **Rationale**

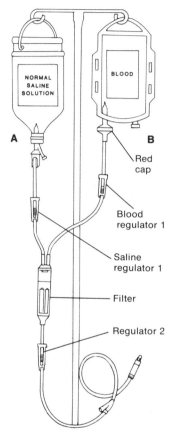

Figure 5.11

4. Don gloves and insert IV   Permits access for connection
   catheter, if needed (see Pro-   of blood tubing
   cedure 5.4); or if IV catheter   Decreases hemolysis
   is present and is of ade-   Allows free flow of blood
   quate size (catheter should
   be 20 gauge or larger).

Action	Rationale
remove dressing enough to expose catheter hub.	
5. Connect blood tubing to catheter hub (discard infusion plug or place needle cap over previous infusion-tubing tip).	Connects blood directly to catheter Preserves previous infusion for future use
6. Open fluid regulator fully and regulate to a rate that will keep vein open (15 to 30 ml/hour) until blood is available.	Verifies and maintains patency of catheter
7. **Check for correct identification information.** When blood arrives, check blood and client information with a second nurse; compare blood package with:	Prevents transfusion of unmatched blood. Failure to identify the blood product or client properly is often linked to severe transfusion reactions
– *Order slip*, checking client name, hospital number, blood type, expiration date	Verifies that the patient name, ABO group, Rh type, and unit number match
– *Client's name band:* name and hospital number (or emergency department) name band if typing and crossmatching were done in emergency department) *If discrepancies are noted, notify the blood bank immediately and postpone transfusion until problems are resolved.*	Ensures transfusion to correct client
8. Complete blood bank slip with date and time of transfusion initiation and nurses' checking information.	Provides legal record of blood verification
9. Check and record pulse, respirations, blood pressure, and temperature.	Provides baseline vital signs prior to blood transfusion
10. Remove red cap to reveal spike on other side of blood tubing and push	

Action	Rationale
spike into port on blood bag (Fig. 5.11*B*).	
11. Close regulator 1 on normal saline side of tubing and open regulator 1 on blood side of tubing.	Prevents saline infusing into blood bag Allows blood tubing to fill with blood Most reactions occur within the first 15 minutes
12. Regulate drip rate to deliver:	
a. A maximum of 30 ml of blood within the first 15 minutes	Delivers blood volume in 2 to 4 hours
b. ½ to ¼ of the volume of blood each hour (62 to 125 ml per hour—depending on client tolerance to volume change and volume of blood to be infused; if client has poor tolerance to volume change, some blood banks will divide units in half so that 8 hours may be used to infuse one unit of packed cells.	Allows slower infusion of total unit without violating 4-hour transfusion time limit
13. Check vital signs and temperature again 15 minutes after beginning the transfusion, then half an hour or hourly until transfusion is completed (refer to agency policy); check at the completion of delivery of each unit of blood.	Detects transfusion reaction (Most reactions occur within the first 15 minutes.)
14. When blood transfusion is complete:	
– Clamp off blood regulator 1.	Clears bloodline for infusion of other fluids
– Turn on normal saline.	
– Remove empty blood bag/bottle. Recap spike.	Maintains sterility for future transfusions
– Fill in time of completion on blood bank slip and place copy of slip	Complies with agency regulations for confirmation of blood administration

Action	Rationale
with empty bag or bottle.	
– Place other copy of slip on chart. (If no further blood is to be given, replace blood transfusion tubing with IV tubing or infusion plug.)	
15. During and after transfusion, monitor client closely for signs of a transfusion reaction, which include the following:	Prevents severe complications from undetected reaction
– **Allergic reaction,** evidenced by rash, chills, fever, nausea, or severe hypotension (shock)	Indicates incompatibility between transfused red cells and the host cells
– **Pyrogenic reaction** (usually noted toward end or after transfusion), evidenced by nausea, chilling, fever, and headache	Indicates sepsis and subsequent renal shutdown
– **Circulatory overload,** evidenced by cough, dyspnea, distended neck veins, and rales in lung bases	Indicates acute pulmonary edema or congestive failure
16. *If allergic or pyrogenic reaction is noted:*	
– Turn off blood transfusion.	Decreases further infusion of incompatible or contaminated blood
– Remove blood tubing and replace with tubing primed with normal saline.	Maintains catheter patency
– Turn on normal saline at slow rate.	
– Contact doctor immediately.	
17. *If fluid overload is noted:*	
– Slow blood transfusion rate and contact doctor.	Decreases workload of the heart and avoids further overload

Action	Rationale
– Take vital signs frequently (every 10 to 15 minutes until stable), and perform emergency treatment as needed or ordered.	Detects and treats resulting shock or cardiac insufficiency
– Remove and send remaining blood and blood tubing to blood bank with completed blood transfusion forms.	
– Send first voided urine specimen to laboratory.	Confirms hemolytic reaction, if red blood cells present
– Monitor input and output (particularly urinary output).	Detects renal shutdown secondary to reaction
– Check vital signs every 4 hours for 24 hours (or per institutional policy).	Facilitates early detection of complications
18. Position client for comfort.	
19. Discard supplies, remove gloves and wash hands.	Prevents spread of microorganisms

Evaluation

Goals met, partially met, or unmet?

Desired Outcomes (sample)

Blood pressure, pulse, respirations, and temperature are within normal range for client.
Client's activity tolerance has increased to ambulation in hallway without dyspnea.

Documentation

The following should be noted on the client's chart:

- Date and initiation and completion time for each unit of blood transfused
- Type of blood infused (packed cells or whole blood)
- Initial and subsequent vital signs
- Presence or absence of transfusion reaction and actions taken
- State of client after transfusion and current IV fluids infusing, if any

Sample Documentation

DATE	TIME	
1/9/94	0400	One unit of packed red blood cells (Unit # R46862, O positive) hung at 0345; blood pressure, 120/70; pulse, 80 and regular; respirations, 20 and nonlabored; temperature, 98.4° F after first 15 minutes of transfusion. Blood regulated at 100 ml/hour to infuse over 3 hours. No signs of transfusion reaction or fluid overload noted.

Nasogastric/Nasointestinal Tube Insertion

Equipment

- Nasogastric (NG) tube (14 to 18 French sump tube) or nasointestinal (8 to 12 French, small-bore feeding tube)
- Lubricant
- Ice chips or glass of water
- Appropriate-sized syringe:
  - *NG*: 30 or 60 cc syringe with catheter tip
  - *Small bore*: 20- to 30-cc luer-lock syringe
- Nonsterile gloves
- Stethoscope
- 1-inch tape (two 3-inch strips and one 1-inch strip)
- Washcloth, gauze, cotton balls, cotton-tip swab
- Petroleum jelly
- Emesis basin
- Tissues

Purpose

Permits nutritional support through gastrointestinal tract
Allows evacuation of gastric contents
Relieves nausea

Assessment

Assessment should focus on the following:

Doctor's order for type of tube and use of tube
Size of previous tube used, if any
History of nasal or sinus problems

Nursing Diagnoses

The nursing diagnoses may include the following:

Nutrition, altered: less than body requirements, related to dysphagia

Nausea and vomiting related to absence of bowel sounds and peristalsis

Planning

Key Goals and Sample Goal Criteria

The client will

Gain 2 to 3 kg per week after initiation of tube feeding

Experience no episodes of nausea and vomiting within 1 hour of NG suction initiation

Special Considerations

Pediatric

Be prepared to restrain client to prevent pulling on NG tube.

If NG tube is plastic, change every 3 days.

The tube should be taped to side of client's face rather than nostril to prevent nasal ulceration.

Implementation

Action	Rationale
1. Wash hands and organize equipment.	Reduces microorganism transfer Promotes efficiency
2. Explain procedure to client.	Reduces anxiety Promotes cooperation and participation
3. Place client in semi-Fowler's position.	Facilitates passage of tube into esophagus instead of trachea
4. Check and improve nasal patency: – Ask client to breathe through one naris while the other is occluded.	Determines patency of nasal passage

Action	Rationale
– Repeat with other naris	Determines patency of nasal passage
– Have client blow nose with both nares open	Clears nasal passage without pushing microorganisms into inner ear
– Clean mucus and secretions from nares with moist tissues or cotton-tip swabs	Clears nasal passage

5. Measure length of tubing needed by using tube itself as a tape measure:

Action	Rationale
– Measure distance from tip of nose to earlobe, placing the rounded end of the tubing at earlobe (Fig. 5.12.1*A*).	Indicates distance from nasal entrance to pharyngeal area
– Continue measurement from earlobe to sternal notch (Fig. 5.12.1*B*).	Indicates distance from pharyngeal area to stomach
– Mark location of sternal notch along the tubing with small strip of tape.	Indicates depth to which tube should be inserted
– Place tube in ice-water bath (optional).	Makes tube less pliable
(If a feeding tube with	Facilitates insertion of tube

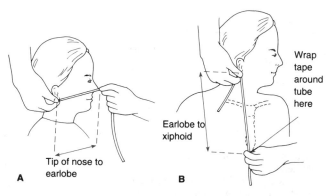

Wrap tape around tube here

Earlobe to xiphoid

Tip of nose to earlobe

A

B

Figure 5.12.1

Action	Rationale
weighted tip is used [small-bore feeding tube], insert guide wire and prepare the tube as instructed on package insert [usually by flushing with 10 to 20 cc of irrigation saline]).	
6. Don gloves and dip feeding tube in water to lubricate tip.	Reduces contamination Promotes smooth insertion of tube
7. Ask client to tilt head backward; insert tube into clearest naris.	Facilitates smooth entrance of tube into naris
8. As you insert tube deeper into naris have client hold head and neck straight and open mouth.	Decreases possibility of insertion into trachea Allows nurse to see when tube is in pharynx
9. When tube is seen and client can feel tube in pharynx, instruct client to swallow (offer ice chips or sips of water).	Facilitates passage of tube into esophagus
10. Insert tube further into esophagus as client swallows (if client coughs or tube curls in throat, withdraw tube to pharynx and repeat attempts); between attempts, encourage client to take deep breaths.	Prevents trauma from forcing tube and prevents tube from entering trachea Maintains good oxygenation

11. When tape mark on tube reaches entrance to naris, stop tube insertion and check placement:
  – Have client open mouth for tube visualization.
  – Aspirate with syringe and monitor for gastric drainage (or old tube feeding if reinsertion).
  – Connect syringe with 10 to 20 cc (10 cc for pediatric clients) air to tube and push air in while
	Indicates tube is in stomach and not curled in mouth or in tracheobronchial tree
	
	Preserves guide wire for reinsertion of tube, if needed

Action	Rationale
listening to stomach with stethoscope (see Fig. 5.13); if gurgling is heard, secure tube. (If tube is a feeding tube, remove the guide wire and store it.)	

12. To secure tube:
  – Split 2 inches of long tape strip, leaving 1 inch of strip intact.
  – Apply 1-inch base of tape on bridge of nose.
  – Wrap first one, then the other, side of split tape around tube (Fig. 5.12.2).
	Maintains tube placement with client activity

13. Tape loop of tube to side of client's face (if feeding tube) or pin to client's gown (if sump tube).	Decreases pull on client's nose and possible dislodgment
14. Obtain order for chest radiograph; delay tube feeding or flushing with	Confirms placement of tube in stomach or duodenum for type of tube

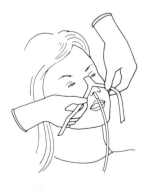 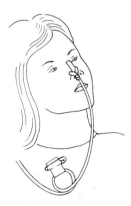

Figure 5.12.2

Action	Rationale
fluid until doctor has read radiograph.	Prevents infusion of fluid into lungs
15. Remove stylet from small-bore feeding tube after correct placement is confirmed by X-ray film.	
16. Begin suction or tube feeding as ordered.	

Evaluation

Goals met, partially met, or unmet?

Desired Outcomes (sample)

Client gains 2 to 3 kg per week.
Client has no complaints of nausea or vomiting.

Documentation

The following should be noted on the client's chart:

- Date and time of tube insertion
- Color and amount of drainage return
- Size and type of tube
- Client tolerance to procedure
- Confirmation of tube placement by radiograph
- Suction applied or tube feeding started and rate

Sample Documentation

DATE	TIME	
3/9/94	1230	Sump tube (#18) inserted via left naris with no obstruction or difficulty, tolerated with no visible clinical problems. Gurgling audible with insertion of air; radiograph obtained with placement confirmed by Dr. Wey. Connected to suction at 80 mm Hg with scant green drainage noted.

📳 Nasogastric Tube Maintenance (5.13)

📳 Nasogastric Tube Discontinuation (5.14)

❎ Equipment

- Syringe and container with saline
- Tape or tube holder
- Washcloth, gauze, cotton balls, cotton-tip swabs
- Petroleum jelly or ointment
- Towel or linen saver
- 500- or 1000-ml bottle saline or ordered irrigant
- Stethoscope
- Mouth moistener
- Nonsterile gloves

Purpose

Minimizes damage to naris from tube
Maintains proper tube placement
Promotes proper gastric suctioning or tube feeding
Terminates nasogastric (NG) therapy properly

Assessment

Assessment should focus on the following:

Size and type of tube
Purpose of tube

Doctor's orders regarding type and frequency of tube irrigation
Type and rate of tube feeding

Nursing Diagnoses

The nursing diagnoses may include the following:

Decreased oral intake related to dysphagia

Planning

Key Goal and Sample Goal Criterion
The client will

Have no episodes of nausea or vomiting

Special Considerations
General
Aspiration is a primary problem with nasogastric tubes. Clients
at risk for aspiration are those with decreased levels of consciousness, absent or diminished cough reflex, and those who
are noncommunicative and recumbent most of the time
(Young and White, 1992)

Home Health
When NG therapy is long term, include in plan of care replacement of tube at specified intervals to avoid complications.
Home caregivers should be taught signs of and ways to avoid
aspiration.

Implementation

Action	Rationale

PROCEDURE 5.13 NASOGASTRIC TUBE MAINTENANCE

Action	Rationale
1. Question client regarding discomfort from tube and determine need for adjustments.	Facilitates client comfort
2. Observe tube insertion site for signs of irritation or pressure.	Indicates need to adjust or remove tube from current site Reduces contamination

Action	Rationale
3. Don gloves.	
4. Check tube placement before irrigation or medication administration and every 4 to 8 hours of tube feeding:	
– Have client open mouth for tube visualization.	Indicates tube is in stomach and not curled in mouth or in tracheobronchial tree
– Aspirate and monitor for gastric contents (or old tube feeding if reinsertion).	
– Connect syringe with 15 to 20 cc air to NG tube and push air in while listening to stomach with stethoscope; if gurgling is heard, secure tube (Fig. 5.13).	

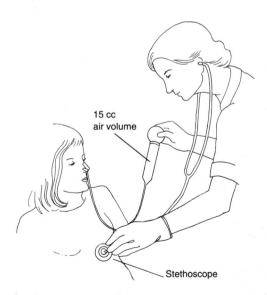

15 cc
air volume

Stethoscope

Figure 5.13

Action	Rationale
5. Cleanse nares with moist gauze or cloth and apply ointment or oil to site.	Maintains skin integrity and patency of nares
6. Every 4 hours, perform mouth care: apply moistener to oral cavity and ointment to lips.	Maintains integrity of oral mucous membranes
7. Irrigate tube (if permitted by doctor) with 20 to 30 ml of saline every 3 hours:	Maintains patency of tube
– Connect saline-filled syringe to tube.	
– Slowly and gently push fluid into tube.	Prevents rupture of tube
– Aspirate fluid gently; note appearance and discard.	Removes irrigant and detects possible gastric bleeding
– Repeat irrigation and aspiration.	
– Reconnect tube to suction or tube feeding.	
8. Remove and reapply tape if loose or extremely soiled.	Prevents dislodgment of tube Promotes cleanliness
9. If entrance to naris is irritated, place tube in other naris, if clear.	Prevents additional skin breakdown
10. Reconnect to tube feeding (see Procedure 5.15) or suction.	

Gastric Suction

Action	Rationale
11. Every 2 hours, check suction for appropriate suction pressure (usually 80 to 100 mm Hg = low suction) and frequency (*i.e.*, constant or intermittent).	
12. Monitor drainage in tubing and bag for color, consistency, and odor.	Indicates presence of bleeding or infection or need for irrigation
13. Each shift, mark drainage level (if bottle or cannister is used) or empty and	Monitors amounts of drainage

Action	**Rationale**

measure amount of
drainage.

14. To empty drainage bag (if
75% to 100% full), first
turn off suction and wait
until suction meter re-
turns to 0. Measure and
record drainage.

Removes suction pressure, so
canister can be emptied

If Using Canister Suction
(wall or floor suction)
  – Loosen seal and remove
    cap (disconnect tubing
    leading to NG tube if
    disposable lining is
    used).
  – Empty contents into
    graduated container
    and rinse canister (or
    discard plastic liner
    and obtain fresh one).
  – Reseal cap and recon-
    nect NG tubing.

If Using Vacuum Suction
  – Open door to suction
    machine (Omnibus).
  – Remove bag.
  – Remove cap from bag
    port.
  – Pour contents into grad-
    uated container.
  – Replace cap and place
    bag into suction
    machine.
  – Reseal door to suction
    machine.
  – Reset and initiate
    appropriate suction
    pressure.

15. Every 24 hours (or per
institutional policy) re-
place drainage bag (if
used) and clean canister.

Reduces accumulation of
microorganisms

Action	Rationale
16. Discard supplies and wash hands.	Reduces contamination

PROCEDURE 5.14 NASOGASTRIC TUBE DISCONTINUATION

1. Explain procedure to client.	Decreases anxiety
2. Place client in semi-Fowler's position.	Opens glottis for easy removal
3. Don gloves.	Reduces contamination
4. Remove tape securing tube to cheek or attaching tube to gown and remove or loosen tape across bridge of nose.	Facilitates smooth removal of tube
5. Remove tube:	
– Place towel under nose and drape over tube.	Shields appearance of tube from client during removal
– Clamp tube by pinching off or folding over.	Prevents aspiration while withdrawing tube (accidental leaking of gastric contents from tube into lungs)
– Slowly withdraw tube until completely removed.	
– Wrap tube in towel and place in trash bag.	
6. Clean nares and apply ointment.	Promotes skin integrity
7. Perform mouth care.	
8. Position client with head of bed elevated 45 degrees and call light within reach.	Facilitates comfort and gastric drainage
9. Encourage client to call if nausea or discomfort is experienced.	Facilitates early detection of gastric distension or distress
10. Monitor bowel sounds and note flatulence.	Indicates adequate bowel activity

Evaluation

Goals met, partially met, or unmet?

Desired Outcomes (sample)

Tubing patency is maintained.
Client experiences no nausea or vomiting.

Documentation

The following should be noted on the client's chart:

- Type of NG tube and therapy (suction or tube feeding)
- Status of tubing patency and security
- Type and amount of drainage (or of residual if tube feeding)
- Time of NG tube removal
- Client tolerance of continued therapy or tube removal

Sample Documentation		
DATE	**TIME**	
2/5/94	1400	Nasogastric suction intact per Omnibus suction at 80 mm continuous suction pressure. Thick green drainage noted, with scant amounts this shift. Sump tube intact in right naris with surrounding skin intact. Bilateral nares cleaned with petroleum jelly.
2/5/94	1800	NG tube removed per orders. Mouth care performed with mouthwash. Active bowel sounds noted. Sips of water provided and tolerated without nausea.

Tube Feeding Management/Medication by Nasogastric Tube

X Equipment

- Ordered tube feeding
- Syringe
- Tube feeding pump or infusion pump
- Appropriate feeding bag and tubing for pump
- Glass or cup
- Nonsterile gloves

Purpose

Provides nutritional support using the gastrointestinal tract

Assessment

Assessment should focus on the following:

Nutritional status (skin turgor, urine output, weight, caloric intake)
Elimination pattern (diarrhea, constipation, date of last stool)
Response to previous nutritional support

Nursing Diagnoses

The nursing diagnoses may include the following:

Nutrition, altered: Less than body requirements related to anorexia
Decreased nutritional intake related to esophageal obstruction

Planning

Key Goals and Sample Goal Criteria

The client will

Maintain current weight or gain 2 to 3 kg per week
Have decreased edema
Show albumin level within normal limits

Special Considerations

If client has endotracheal or tracheostomy tube and is receiving
NG tube feedings, check tracheostomy cuff inflation. If cuff is
deflated, inflate and maintain for 30 minutes after feeding to
prevent aspiration.

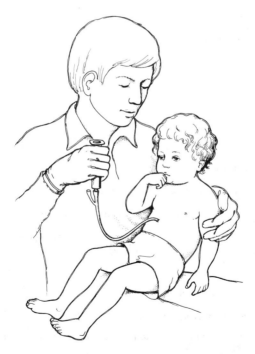

Figure 5.15.1

Many tube feeding formulas cause diarrhea, thus volume and concentration are increased slowly. If diarrhea persists, report to doctor and administer antidiarrhea medication, if ordered.

Be careful with gastrostomy tube irrigations. Depending on the surgery, irrigation may be contraindicated. Verify this with the doctor.

Pediatric

Feeding time is normally a time for interaction with an infant or child; thus, it is crucial that the nurse or family member administering the tube feeding hold, cuddle, and establish eye contact with the child during feeding (Fig. 5.15.1). The feeding formula should be at room temperature. The rate for intermittent feeding should be approximately 10 ml/minute.

Implementation

Action	Rationale
1. Wash hands and organize supplies.	Reduces contamination Promotes efficiency
2. Explain procedure to client and insert feeding tube, if needed (see Procedure 5.12).	
3. Verify tube placement by radiograph.	Indicates tube is in stomach Prevents infusion of tube feeding into pharynx or pulmonary tree
– Aspirate and monitor for gastric contents (or old tube feeding if reinsertion), *or*	
– Pinch tube off at the end and connect syringe with 15 to 20 cc air to tube and push air in while listening with stethoscope over epigastric area for gurgling.	
Proceed to step 4 for continuous feedings, or to step 13 for intermittent feedings.	

Continuous Tube Feeding (steps 4 to 12 only)

4. Prepare tube feeding:	Prevents muscle cramps from infusion of cold solution
– Remove feeding from refrigerator 30 minutes	

Action	Rationale
before hanging (if applicable).	
– Rinse bag and bag tubing with water.	Checks for bag or tubing leaks
– Clamp bag tubing closed.	
– Pour 4 hours' worth of feeding in bag (1 hours' worth if medication is added).	Prevents spoilage of feeding hanging without refrigeration
– Open bag tubing and allow feeding to flow to end.	Clears air from tubing
– Clamp tubing and insert into pump mechanism, if used (Fig. 5.15.2).	
– Time tape bag (see Procedure 5.6).	

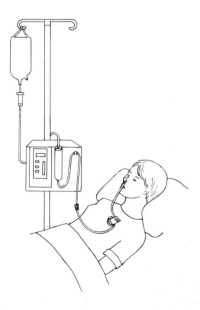

Figure 5.15.2

Action	Rationale
5. Attach feeding bag tubing to feeding tube.	
6. Set pump to deliver appropriate volume; unclamp bag tubing and start pump or regulate manually after calculating drip rate (see Procedures 5.5 and 5.6).	
7. Check infusion hourly or every 2 hours: check time tape and drip rate.	Ensures infusion of proper volume per hour
8. Every 4 hours:	
– Check for residual: stop infusion, slowly aspirate gastric contents, and note amount of residual—may be difficult with small feeding tubes.	Determines degree of absorption of feeding
(If residual is greater than specified amount per doctor's orders [commonly 100 ml], discard aspirated volume to stomach, cease feedings, and notify doctor).	Prevents distension of abdomen and possible aspiration
– Monitor bowel sounds in all abdominal quadrants.	Determines presence of bowel activity (peristalsis)
– Perform mouth care.	Freshens mouth Prevents accumulation of microorganisms
9. Irrigate tube every 3 hours (or after any medication) with 20 to 30 ml saline, or as indicated by doctor's orders or hospital policy.	Maintains patency of tube
10. Once each shift, while irrigating NG tube after completing a supply of tube feeding, rinse bag and tubing with water.	Clears accumulated feeding from bag and tubing
11. Every 24 hours (or 48, if institutional policy), re-	Removes medium for microorganism growth

Action	**Rationale**
place old bag and tubing with new.	
12. Elevate head of bed 30 to 45 degrees and maintain throughout feedings.	Decreases aspiration of feeding into lungs

Intermittent Tube Feeding

Action	**Rationale**
13. Follow steps 1 to 3.	
14. Determine amount of water, if any, to be infused and pour into glass or cup.	
15. Don gloves.	
16. If client previously received feeding, check for and note amount of residual; this may be difficult with small feeding tubes. (If residual is greater than specified amount per doctor's orders [commonly 100 ml], discard aspirated volume—unless prohibited by doctor's orders or agency policy—delay feeding, and notify doctor.)	Prevents distension of abdomen and possible aspiration of feeding into lungs
16. Attach syringe to NG tube and aspirate small amount of contents to fill tube and lower portion of syringe.	Prevents infusion of air into stomach
17. Infuse feeding or medication (see steps 21–24): – Hold syringe 6 inches above tube insertion site (nose or abdomen; Fig. 5.15.1) – Fill syringe with feeding and allow to flow slowly into NG tube; follow with water (30-ml flush if no water is ordered).	Assists flow of feeding by gravity

Action	Rationale
DO NOT ALLOW SYRINGE TO EMPTY UNTIL FEEDING AND WATER INFUSION ARE COMPLETED.	Prevents entrance of air into tubing and stomach
18. Clamp NG or gastrostomy tube and place client in semi-Fowler's position.	Decreases reflux of feeding and possible aspiration into lungs
19. Monitor bowel sounds, stools, and residual continuously.	Detects loss of or decrease in GI function
20. Check NG tube placement and residual prior to each tube feeding.	Prevents aspiration of secretions into tracheobronchial tree

Medication Administration Through NG Tube

Action	Rationale
21. Check tube placement.	Prevents obstruction of tube with large medication particles or thick solution
22. Crush pill (if crushable) and mix with fluid to make a thin solution with small sediment. (*Note*: Be sure guidelines for drug administration are being followed.)	
23. Mix viscous solutions with water or saline (30 to 60 ml).	Prevents clogging of tube
24. Follow medication infusion with 30 ml saline or water.	Prevents obstruction of tubing

Evaluation

Goals met, partially met, or unmet?

Desired Outcomes (sample)

Tube feeding is infused at appropriate volume and rate.
Client has no complaints of nausea or signs of aspiration.
Client gains 2 to 3 kg per week.

Documentation

The following should be noted on the client's chart:

- Type of NG tube and tube feeding
- Status of tubing patency and security
- Type and amount of residual
- Client tolerance of continued therapy or tube removal

Sample Documentation

DATE	TIME	
7/8/94	1400	Tube feeding initiated at 0800 with Ensure, 50 ml per hour. Infusing per Dobhoff feeding tube, regulated by infusion pump. Active bowel sounds noted; no complaints of nausea. Residual of 30 ml noted after 4 hours of infusion. Tubing flushed with 30 ml water.

Elimination

OVERVIEW

- Adequate elimination of body waste is an essential function to sustain life.
- Inadequate bladder and bowel elimination ultimately affects the body's delicate balance of fluid, electrolyte, and acid–base level.
- Various means are available clinically to help assess and maintain adequate elimination status.
- Factors that affect bowel and bladder elimination status include food and fluid intake; age; psychological barriers; medications; personal hygiene habits; educational level;

Jean Smith-Temple and Joyce Young Johnson:
Nurses' Guide to Clinical Procedures, Second Edition.© 1994
J. B. Lippincott Company

cultural practices; pathology of the renal, urinary, or gastrointestinal system; surgery; hormonal variations; muscle tone of supporting organs and structures; and concurrent medical problems, such as decreased cardiac output or motor disturbances.

- Alterations in bowel and bladder elimination mandate careful assessment and monitoring of the upper and lower abdomen, as well as of amounts and appearance of body excretions.

- Procedures related to adequate bladder elimination usually require the use of sterile technique to prevent contamination to the highly susceptible urinary tract.

- Because clients on peritoneal dialysis or hemodialysis are using final means of adequate renal excretion, it is crucial that the nurse perform these procedures with precision.

- Various concentrations of dialysate affect osmolality, rate of fluid removal, electrolyte balance, solute removal, and cardiovascular stability.

- Elimination is very personal to the client; therefore, privacy and professionalism should be maintained when assisting clients with elimination needs.

- Clients with colostomies frequently experience body-image and self-concept alterations. Psychological support and teaching are crucial in resolving these problems.

- All procedures involving elimination of body waste require use of gloves and occasionally other protective barriers.

- Before planning a procedure, the nurse should determine if same-sex or opposite-sex contact with genitalia is culturally offensive to the client.

Midstream Urine Collection

✖ Equipment

- Basin of warm water
- Soap
- Washcloth
- Towel
- Antiseptic swabs or cotton balls
- Sterile specimen collection container
- Specimen container labels
- Bedpan, urinal, bedside commode, or toilet
- Nonsterile gloves
- Pen

Purpose

Obtains urine specimen by aseptic technique for microbiological analysis

Assessment

Assessment should focus on the following:

Characteristics of the urine
Symptoms associated with urinary tract infections (*e.g.,* pain or discomfort upon voiding, urinary frequency)
Temperature increase
Ability of client to follow instructions for obtaining specimen
Time of day of specimen collection
Fluid intake and output

Nursing Diagnoses

The nursing diagnoses may include the following:

Potential for infection related to poor technique in cleaning perineum

Alteration in urinary elimination: frequency related to urinary tract infection

Planning

Key Goal and Sample Goal Criterion
The client will

Demonstrate no signs of urinary tract infection (such as discomfort upon voiding, elevated temperature, abnormal urine constituents, and abnormal urine characteristics) within 3 days of admission

Special Considerations
Midstream urine collection is frequently performed by the client; however, instructions for the procedure must be clear to obtain reliable laboratory results. Perhaps the most frequent error the client commits is poor cleaning technique. Be certain women understand to cleanse from the front to the back of the perineum, and men from the tip of the penis downward.
If possible, a specimen should be obtained upon first voiding in the morning.

Implementation

Action	Rationale
1. Wash hands.	Reduces microorganism transfer
2. Explain procedure to client.	Decreases anxiety
3. Provide for privacy.	Decreases embarrassment
4. Don clean gloves.	Reduces nurse's exposure to body secretions
5. Wash perineal area with soap and water, rinse, and pat dry.	Reduces microorganisms in perineal area
6. Cleanse meatus with antiseptic solution in same manner as for catheterization in males (see Procedure 6.3, steps 15 to 17) and females (see Procedure 6.4, steps 23 and 24).	Reduces microorganisms at urethral opening

Action	Rationale
7. Ask client to begin voiding.	Flushes organisms from ure- thral opening
8. After stream of urine be- gins, place specimen con- tainer in place to obtain 30 ml of urine.	Collects urine at point in which urine is least contaminated
9. Remove container before client stops voiding.	Prevents end stream organ- isms from dripping into container
10. Allow client to complete voiding using urinal, bedpan, or toilet.	
11. Wash perineal area again if stain-producing antisep- tic was used.	Removes antiseptic solution Promotes general comfort
12. Label specimen container with date and time as well as client identification information.	
13. Discard equipment and gloves.	Reduces spread of infection
14. Wash hands.	Reduces contamination

Evaluation

Goals met, partially met, or unmet?

Desired Outcomes (sample)

Client shows no signs or symptoms of urinary tract infection.
Client verbalizes relief of discomfort within 3 days.

Documentation

The following should be noted on the client's chart:

- Signs or symptoms of urinary infection
- Amount, color, odor, and consistency of urine obtained
- Specimen collection time
- Total amount voided
- Teaching performed regarding technique for cleaning genitalia

Sample Documentation

DATE	TIME	
1/11/94	1100	Clean-catch urine specimen obtained and sent to laboratory—30 ml of cloudy, yellow urine with slight foul odor noted. Client reports slight perineal burning.

✋ Urine Specimen Collection From an Indwelling Catheter

☒ Equipment

- Sterile 3-ml syringe with 23- or 25-gauge needle
- Nonsterile gloves
- Alcohol swab
- Sterile specimen container
- Container labels
- Pen
- Catheter clamp

Purpose

Obtains sterile urine specimens for microbiological analysis

Assessment

Assessment should focus on the following:

Characteristics of the urine
Symptoms associated with urinary tract infections (pain or discomfort)
Temperature increase
Fluid intake and output

Nursing Diagnoses

The nursing diagnoses may include the following:

Potential for infection related to long-term indwelling catheter
Alteration in comfort: perineal pain related to urinary tract infection

Planning

Key Goals and Sample Goal Criteria

The client will

Demonstrate no signs of urinary tract infection (*i.e.,* perineal discomfort, elevated temperature, abnormal urine constituents, and abnormal urine characteristics)

Verbalize lack of perineal discomfort within 3 days

Special Consideration

If a specimen is needed and a new catheter is to be inserted, obtain the specimen during catheter insertion procedure. See Procedure 6.3, Male Catheterization, or Procedure 6.4, Female Catheterization.

Geriatric and Pediatric

If a specimen is needed from a confused or a pediatric client unable to follow directions, obtain assistance to maintain sterility of the specimen and catheter.

Implementation

Action	Rationale
1. Wash hands.	Reduces microorganism transfer
2. Explain procedure to client.	Decreases anxiety
3. Provide for privacy.	Decreases embarrassment
4. Don clean gloves.	Reduces nurse exposure to body secretions

Proceed to step 12 for open-system method

Closed-system Method

5. Fold or clamp drainage tubing about 4 inches below junction of drainage tubing and catheter.	Facilitates trapping of urine in tubing at specimen port
6. Allow urine to pool in drainage tubing; if urine does not pool in tubing immediately, leave it clamped for urine to collect over period of time (usually 10 to 30 minutes).	Allows urine to pool in tubing at specimen port

Action	**Rationale**
7. Cleanse specimen collection port of drainage tubing with alcohol swab or antiseptic solution recommended by agency. (If no collection port is visible, catheter tubing is probably designed with a self-sealing material so that specimen may be obtained from catheter itself by cleansing and piercing catheter tubing close to junction. However, check package label and instructions. If catheter tubing is self-sealing, cleanse catheter tubing close to junction of drainage tubing.)	Reduces microorganisms at insertion port
8. Carefully insert sterile needle of syringe into specimen-collection port or self-sealing catheter tubing at a 45-degree angle; insert needle slowly, taking care not to puncture other side of catheter tubing (Fig. 6.2).	Prevents accidental puncture of drainage tubing or catheter

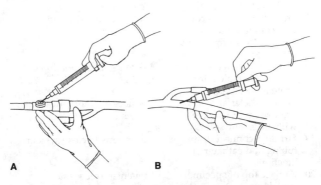

A   B

Figure 6.2

Action	Rationale
9. Pull back on plunger of syringe and obtain 3 to 10 ml of urine.	Draws urine into syringe
10. Slowly squirt urine into collection container; do not touch inside of specimen container.	Places urine in container maintaining sterility of container and specimen
11. Complete steps 20 to 24.	

Open-system Method

Action	Rationale
12. Place linen saver under tubing at junction of catheter and drainage tubing.	Prevents soiling linen
13. Remove cap from specimen bottle and place bottle on linen saver.	
14. Cleanse junction with antiseptic solution such as Betadine (or antiseptic recommended by agency).	Reduces microorganisms
15. Carefully disconnect catheter from drainage tubing at junction. Hold drainage tubing and catheter 1.5 to 2 inches from junction, being careful not to contaminate either end.	Disconnects catheter to allow for specimen collection Avoids system contamination
16. Place specimen container under catheter opening and allow urine to run into container; do not allow catheter tip to touch container.	Allows urine to run into container Avoids contamination
17. Place specimen container on bedside table after urine is obtained.	Prevents contamination of catheter line
18. Wipe catheter and drainage tubing again with antiseptic solution.	Reduces microorganism transfer
19. Firmly reconnect drainage tubing and catheter at junction.	Reconnects to close system
20. Replace top of specimen container.	Prevents urine waste

Action	Rationale
21. Label container with date and time of collection as well as client identification information.	Eliminates errors in client identification
22. Fill out agency requisition form for specimen.	Facilitates proper logging and charging in lab
23. Send to laboratory immediately.	Avoids sending old specimen in which urine constituents may have changed
24. Discard gloves and wash hands.	Prevents spread of microorganisms

Evaluation

Goals met, partially met, or unmet?

Desired Outcomes (sample)

Client shows no signs of urinary tract infection.
Client verbalizes lack of perineal discomfort within 3 days.

Documentation

The following should be noted on the client's chart:

- Amount, color, odor, and consistency of urine obtained
- Specimen collection time
- Total amount of urine collected
- Signs or symptoms of urinary infection
- Disposition of specimen to lab

Sample Documentation

DATE	TIME	
1/3/94	1100	Sterile urine specimen obtained via indwelling catheter and sent to laboratory. Specimen is 30 ml of cloudy, yellow urine with slight foul odor noted. Client reports slight perineal burning.

☝ Male Catheterization

☒ Equipment

- Urethral catheterization set (includes sterile gloves, specimen-collection container, catheter, two drapes, graduated measurement receptacle, antiseptic solution, cotton balls, forceps, lubricating jelly)
  or
- Indwelling catheterization set (all of the items in urethral catheterization kit, except the graduated measurement receptacle, plus a drainage-collection system [tubing and bag that connect to the catheter] and a prefilled saline syringe for inflation)
- Basin of warm soapy water
- Washcloth
- Large towel
- Nonsterile gloves
- Sheet for draping
- Linen saver
- Roll of tape
- Bedpan, urinal, or second collection container
- Specimen container, if specimen is needed
- Goggles (for young boy unable to maintain urinary control during procedure)

Purpose

Facilitates emptying of bladder
Facilitates obtaining sterile urine specimens
Facilitates determining amount of residual urine in bladder
Allows for continuous, accurate monitoring of urinary output
Provides avenue for bladder irrigations

Assessment

Assessment should focus on the following:

Type of catheterization ordered (straight, Foley, residual)

Status of bladder (distension prior to catheter insertion)
Abnormalities of genitalia or prostate gland
History of conditions that may interfere with smooth insertion
(*e.g.*, prostate enlargement, urethral stricture)
Client allergy to iodine-based antiseptics (*e.g.*, Betadine)

Nursing Diagnoses

The nursing diagnoses may include the following:

Alteration in urinary elimination: decreased output related to
reduction in total fluid volume
Alteration in comfort: lower abdominal pain related to bladder
distension

Planning

Key Goals and Sample Goal Criteria

The client will

Attain and maintain a urine output of at least 250 ml per shift
Verbalize relief of lower abdominal pain within 1 hour of
catheter insertion

Special Considerations

Never force a catheter if it does not pass through the urethral
canal smoothly. If the catheter still does not pass smoothly
after using the suggested troubleshooting methods, discontin-
ue the procedure and notify the physician. Forcing the
catheter may result in damage to the urethra and surrounding
structures.

Geriatric
A common pathologic feature in elderly men is enlargement of
the prostate gland. The enlargement frequently makes insert-
ing a catheter difficult.

Pediatric
In the infant, the bladder is higher and more anterior than in the
adult. Common catheter sizes are 8 and 10 French.
Catheterization is a very threatening and anxiety-provoking experience for children. They need explanations, support, and
understanding.

Home Health

Because indwelling catheterization is used on a long-term basis
for the homebound client, potential is high for infection: Be
alert for early signs and symptoms of infection and adhere to a
strict schedule for changing catheters.

Explore the possibility of an external catheter as an alternative
to the indwelling catheter.

If the client uses intermittent self-catheterization, store sterilized
catheters in sterilized jars.

Implementation

Action	Rationale
1. Wash hands.	Reduces microorganism transfer
2. Explain procedure to client.	Decreases anxiety
3. Determine if client is allergic to iodine-based antiseptics.	Avoids allergic reactions
4. Provide for privacy.	Decreases embarrassment
5. Don nonsterile gloves.	Reduces nurse's exposure to body secretions
6. If catheterization is for residual urine, ask client to void in urinal, and measure and record the amount voided; empty urinal.	Determines amount of urine client is able to void without catheterization Determines exact amount
7. Place linen saver under buttocks.	Avoids wetting linens
8. Wash genital area with warm water, rinse, and pat dry with towel.	Decreases microorganisms around urethral opening
9. Discard gloves, bath water, wash cloth, and towel; then wash hands.	Decreases clutter Reduces microorganism transfer
10. Drape client so that only penis is exposed.	Provides privacy Reduces embarrassment
11. Set up work field: – Open catheter set and remove from outer plastic package	Removes kit without opening inner folds

Action	Rationale
– Tape outer package to bedside table with top edge turned inside.	Provides waste bag
– Place catheter kit beside client's knees and carefully open outer edges.	Places items within easy reach
– Ask client to open legs slightly.	Relaxes pelvic muscles
– Remove full drape from kit with fingertips and place across thighs, plastic side down, just below penis; keep other side sterile.	Provides sterile field
– If catheter and bag are separate, use sterile technique to open package containing bag and place bag on work field.	
12. Don sterile gloves.	Avoids contaminating other items in kit
13. Prepare items in kit for use during insertion as follows:	
– Pour iodine solution over cotton balls.	Prepares cotton balls for cleaning
– Separate cotton balls with forceps.	Promotes easy manipulation
– Lubricate 6 to 7 inches of catheter tip and place carefully on tray so that tip is secure in tray.	Prevents local irritation of meatus on catheter insertion Promotes ease of insertion
– If inserting indwelling catheter, attach prefilled syringe of sterile water to balloon port of catheter.	Connects to balloon port the syringe needed to inflate balloon
– Inject 2 to 3 ml of sterile water from prefilled syringe into balloon and observe balloon for leaks as it fills.	Tests balloon for defects
– Discard and obtain another kit if any leaks are noted.	Prevents catheter dislodgment after insertion

Action	Rationale
– Deflate balloon and leave syringe connected.	Leaves syringe within reach
– Attach catheter to drainage container tubing (or if drainage tubing is already attached to the catheter, place tubing and bag securely on sterile field, close to the other equipment.	Facilitates organization while maintaining sterility
– Check clamp on collection bag to be sure it is closed. Place catheter and collection tray close to perineum.	Prevents loss of urine prior to measurement
– Open specimen collection container and place on sterile field.	Places container within easy reach for specimen
14. Remove fenestrated drape from kit and place penis through hole in drape with nondominant hand. KEEP DOMINANT HAND STERILE.	Expands sterile field
15. Pull penis up at a 90-degree angle to client's supine body.	Straightens urethra
16. With nondominant hand, gently grasp glans (tip) of penis; retract foreskin, if necessary.	Provides grasp of penis preventing contamination of sterile field later
17. With forceps in dominant hand, cleanse meatus and glans with cotton balls, beginning at urethral opening and moving toward shaft of penis; make one complete circle around penis with each cotton ball, discarding cotton ball after each wipe (Fig. 6.3).	Cleanses meatus without cross-contaminating or contaminating sterile hand
18. After all cotton balls have been used, discard forceps.	Prevents contamination of sterile field

Action	Rationale

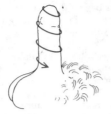

Figure 6.3

19. With thumb and first finger, pick catheter up about 1.5 to 2 inches from tip.

Gives nurse good control of catheter tip (which easily bends)

20. Carefully gather additional tubing in hand.

Gives nurse good control of full catheter length

21. Ask client to bear down as if voiding and take slow, deep breaths; encourage him to continue to breathe deeply until catheter is fully inserted.

Opens sphincter. Relaxes sphincter muscles of bladder and urethra

22. Insert tip of catheter slowly through urethral opening 7 to 9 inches (or until urine returns).

Inserts catheter

23. Lower penis to about a 45-degree angle after catheter is inserted about halfway and hold open end of catheter over collection container (if it is not connected to a drainage bag).

Places penis in position for urine to be released into collection container so that accurate amount is measured

24. If resistance is met:
    – Stop for a few seconds.

Allows sphincters to relax and reduces anxiety

    – Encourage client to continue taking slow, deep breaths.
    – Do not force; remove catheter tip and notify doctor if above sequence is unsuccessful.

Prevents injury to prostate, urethra, and surrounding structures

Action	**Rationale**
25. After catheter has been advanced an appropriate distance, advance another 1 to 1.5 inches.	Ensures catheter advances far enough not to dislodge
26. For straight catheterization: – Obtain urine specimen in specimen container, if ordered.	Obtains sterile specimen
– Allow urine to drain until it stops or UNTIL MAXIMUM NUMBER OF MILLILITERS SPECIFIED BY AGENCY (usually 1000 to 1500 ml) have drained into container; use second container, bedpan, or urinal, if necessary.	Empties bladder Obtains residual urine amount
27. For an indwelling catheter, inflate balloon with attached syringe and gently pull back on catheter until it stops (catches).	Secures catheter placement
28. Secure catheter loosely with tape to lower abdomen on side from which drainage bag will be hanging (preferably away from door); make certain that tubing is not caught on railing locks or obstructed.	Stabilizes catheter Prevents accidental dislodgment
29. Clear bed of all equipment.	Removes waste from bed
30. Reposition client for comfort and replace linens for warmth and privacy.	Promotes general comfort
31. Raise side rails.	Prevents falls
32. Measure amount of urine in collection container or drainage bag and discard.	Provides assessment data
33. Gather all additional equipment and discard with gloves.	Promotes clean environment
34. Wash hands.	Reduces microorganism transfer

Evaluation

Goals met, partially met, or unmet?

Desired Outcomes (sample)

A urine output of at least 250 ml per shift is attained and maintained during hospital stay.

Client verbalizes relief of lower abdominal pain within 1 hour of catheter insertion.

Documentation

The following should be noted on the client's chart:

- Presence of distension prior to catheterization
- Assessment of genitalia, if abnormalities noted
- Type of catheterization
- Size of catheter
- Amount, color, and consistency of urine returned upon catheterization
- Amount of urine returned prior to catheterization (if residual urine catheterization)
- Difficulties encountered, if any, in passing the catheter smoothly
- Reports of unusual discomfort during insertion
- Specimen obtained

Sample Documentation

DATE	TIME	
4/6/94	1100	Catheter (#16 French Foley) inserted without resistance or report of discomfort. Procedure yielded 700 ml straw-colored urine without sediment or foul odor.

✋ Female Catheterization

☒ Equipment

- Urethral catheterization set (includes sterile gloves, specimen collection container, catheter, two drapes, graduated measurement receptacle, antiseptic solution, cotton balls, forceps, lubricating jelly)
  or
- Indwelling catheterization set (all of the items in urethral catheterization kit, except the graduated measurement receptacle, plus a drainage-collection system [tubing and bag that connect to the catheter] and a prefilled saline syringe for balloon inflation)
- Basin of warm soapy water
- Washcloth
- Large towel
- Nonsterile gloves
- One sheet for draping
- Linen saver
- Roll of tape
- Bedpan, urinal, or second collection container
- Specimen container, if specimen is needed
- Extra lighting

Purpose

Facilitates emptying of bladder
Facilitates obtaining sterile urine specimens
Facilitates determining amount of residual urine in bladder
Allows for continuous, accurate monitoring of urinary output
Provides avenue for bladder irrigations

Assessment

Assessment should focus on the following:

Type of catheterization ordered (straight, Foley, residual)

Status of bladder (distension prior to catheter insertion)
Abnormalities of genitalia
Client allergy to iodine-based antiseptics (*e.g.*, Betadine)

Nursing Diagnoses

The nursing diagnoses may include the following:

Alteration in urinary elimination: decreased output related to reduction in total fluid volume
Alteration in comfort: lower abdominal pain related to bladder distension

Planning

Key Goals and Sample Goal Criteria

The client will

Attain and maintain a urine output of at least 250 ml per shift
Verbalize relief of lower abdominal pain within 1 hour of catheter insertion

Special Considerations

Pediatric
Catheterization is a very threatening and anxiety-producing experience. Children need explanations, support, and understanding.
In the baby girl, the urethra hooks around the symphysis in a C shape. Common catheter size is 8 or 10 French.

Home Health
When indwelling catheterization is used on a long-term basis, there is a high potential for infection: Be alert for early signs and symptoms of infection and adhere to a strict schedule for changing catheters.
If the client uses intermittent self-catheterization, store sterilized catheters in sterilized jars.

Implementation

Action	Rationale
1. Wash hands.	Reduces microorganism transfer

Action	Rationale
2. Explain procedure to client, emphasizing need to maintain sterile field.	Decreases anxiety
3. Determine if client is allergic to iodine-based antiseptics.	Avoids allergic reactions
4. Provide for privacy.	Decreases embarrassment
5. Don nonsterile gloves.	Reduces nurse's exposure to body secretions
6. If catheterization is for residual urine, ask client to void in urinal, and measure and record the amount voided; empty urinal.	Determines amount of urine client is able to void without catheterization Determines exact amount Promotes tidiness
7. Place linen saver under buttocks.	Avoids wetting linens
8. Place light to enhance visualization.	Promotes clear identification of anatomical parts
9. Separate labia to expose urethral opening: – If using dorsal recumbent position, separate labia with thumb and forefinger by gently lifting upward and outward (Fig. 6.4.2 illustrates this technique and identifies parts of the female perineum). – If using side-lying position, pull upward on upper labia minora as shown in Fig. 6.4.1B).	Allows nurse to identify urethral opening clearly before area is cleansed Subtle variations in location of structures of female genitalia often cause a delay that increases chance of contamination of field
10. Wash genital area with warm water, rinse, and pat dry with towel.	Decreases microorganisms around urethral opening
11. Discard gloves, bath water, washcloth, and towel; then wash hands.	Decreases clutter Reduces microorganisms
12. If inserting an indwelling catheter in which the drainage apparatus is separate from catheter (not preconnected):	

Action   **Rationale**

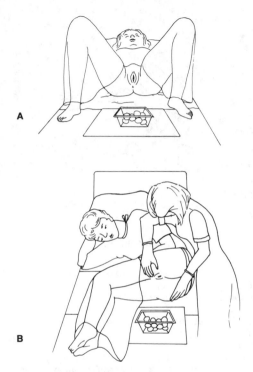

Figure 6.4.1

– Check for closed clamp
  on collection bag.
– Secure drainage collec-   Places drainage tubing within
  tion bag to bed frame.   immediate and easy reach,
– Pull tubing up between   decreasing chance of cath-
  bed and bed rails to top   eter contamination once
  surface of bed.   inserted
– Check to be sure tubing
  will not get caught
  when rails are lowered
  or raised.

Action   **Rationale**

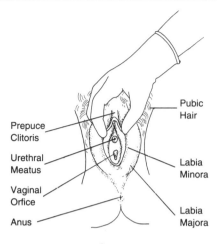

Prepuce
Clitoris
Urethral
Meatus
Vaginal
Orfice
Anus
Pubic
Hair
Labia
Minora
Labia
Majora

Figure 6.4.2

13. Position client in dorsal recumbent or side-lying position with knees flexed (Fig. 6.4.1*A* and *B*); in side-lying position, slide client's hips toward edge of bed.

Exposes labia

14. Drape client so that only perineum is exposed.

Provides privacy
Reduces embarrassment

15. Remove gloves and wash hands; lift side rails and cover client before leaving bedside.

Reduces microorganism transfer
Prevents client from falling
Reduces embarrassment

16. Carefully open catheter set and remove it from plastic outer package.

Removes kit without opening inner folds

17. Tape outer package to bedside table with top edge turned inside.

Provides waste bag

18. Places catheter kit between client's knees and carefully open outer edges (if using side-lying posi-

Places items within easy reach

Action	Rationale
tion, place kit about 1 foot from perineal area near thighs).	
19. Remove full drape from kit with fingertips and place, plastic side down, just under buttocks by having client raise hips; keep other side sterile.	Provides work field
20. Don sterile gloves.	Avoids contaminating other items in kit
21. Prepare items in kit for use during insertion as follows:	
– Pour iodine solution over cotton balls.	Prepares cotton balls for cleaning
– Separate cotton balls with forceps.	Promotes easy manipulation
– Lubricate 3 to 4 inches of catheter tip and place carefully on tray such that tip is secure in tray.	Prevents local irritation of meatus on catheter insertion Promotes ease of insertion
– If inserting indwelling catheter, attach prefilled syringe to balloon port of catheter by twisting syringe in clockwise direction.	Connects syringe needed to inflate balloon to balloon port
– Push plunger in and inject 2 to 3 ml of sterile water from prefilled syringe into balloon and observe balloon for leaks as it fills.	Tests balloon for defects
– Discard and obtain another kit if any leaks are noted.	Prevents catheter dislodgment after insertion
– Deflate balloon and leave syringe connected.	Leaves syringe within reach
– If inserting closed indwelling system with drainage tubing already attached to catheter, move tubing and bag close to other equip-	Facilitates organization while maintaining sterility

Action	Rationale
ment on work field, making certain that drainage system is on the sterile field only. (Check clamp on collection bag to be sure it is closed)	Prevents loss of urine prior to measurement
– Open specimen collection container and place on sterile field.	Places container within easy reach for specimen
22. Remove fenestrated drape from kit and place on perineum such that only labia is exposed (or discard the drape if you prefer).	Expands sterile field
23. Separate labia minora with nondominant hand in same manner as in step 9 and hold this position until catheter is inserted (*Note*: Dominant hand is only hand sterile now; contaminated hand continues to separate labia).	Exposes urethral opening
24. Using forceps, cleanse meatus with cotton balls:	
– Making one downward stroke with each cotton ball, begin at labia on side farthest from you and move towards labia nearest you.	Cleanses meatus without cross-contaminating
– Afterwards, wipe once down center of meatus.	
– Wipe once with each cotton ball and discard (Fig. 6.4.3).	
25. After all cotton balls have been used, remove forceps from field.	Prevents contamination of sterile field
26. Move cleaning tray to end of sterile field and move collection container and catheter closer to client.	Facilitates organization Prevents accidental contamination of system

Action	Rationale

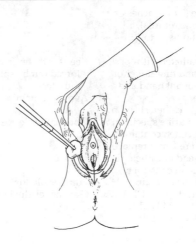

Figure 6.4.3

Action	Rationale
27. With thumb and first finger, pick catheter up about 1.5 to 2 inches from tip.	Gives nurse good control of catheter (which easily bends)
28. Carefully gather additional tubing in hand.	Gives nurse good control of full catheter length
29. Ask client to bear down as if voiding and take slow, deep breaths; encourage her to take deep breaths until catheter is fully inserted.	Opens sphincter Relaxes sphincter muscles of bladder and urethra
30. Insert tip of catheter slowly through urethral opening 3 to 4 inches (or until urine returns), releasing tubing from hand as insertion continues; direct open end of catheter into collection container.	Inserts catheter
31. After catheter has been advanced an appropriate	Ensures catheter advances far enough not to dislodge

Action	Rationale
distance (3 to 4 inches or until urine returns), advance another 1 to 1.5 inches.	
32. Grasp catheter with thumb and first finger of nondominant hand and hold steady.	Keeps catheter from being forced out by sphincter muscles Avoids contamination
33. If straight catheterization: – Obtain urine specimen in specimen container, if ordered, and replace open end of catheter in collection container.	Obtains sterile specimen
– Allow urine to drain until it stops or UNTIL MAXIMUM NUMBER OF MILLILITERS SPECIFIED BY AGENCY (usually 1000 to 1500 ml) have drained into container; use second container, bedpan, or urinal if necessary.	Empties bladder Obtains residual urine amount Prevents temporary hypovolemic shock state
– Remove catheter.	
34. If indwelling catheter is being used, inflate balloon with attached syringe, and gently pull back on catheter until it stops (catches).	Secures catheter placement
35. If the indwelling catheter is separate from bag and tubing, remove protective cap from end of tubing and attach drainage tubing to end of catheter.	Converts system to closed system
36. Secure catheter loosely with tape to thigh on side from which drainage bag will be hanging (preferably away from door); make certain that tubing	Stabilizes catheter Prevents accidental dislodgment

Action	Rationale
is not caught on railing locks or obstructed.	
37. Clear bed of all equipment, reposition client for comfort, and replace linens for warmth and privacy; lift side rails.	Promotes clean environment, comfort, and safety
38. Measure amount of urine in collection container or drainage bag and discard.	Provides assessment data
39. Gather up all additional equipment and discard with gloves.	Promotes clean environment
40. Wash hands.	Reduces microorganism transfer

Evaluation

Goals met, partially met, or unmet?

Desired Outcomes (sample)

A urine output of at least 250 ml per shift is attained and maintained during hospital stay.

Client verbalizes relief of lower abdominal pain within 1 hour of catheter insertion.

Documentation

The following should be noted on the client's chart:

- Assessment of lower abdomen prior to catheterization
- Assessment of genitalia, if abnormalities noted
- Types of catheterization
- Size of catheter
- Amount, color, and consistency of urine returned upon catheterization
- Amount of urine returned prior to catheterization (if residual urine was collected)
- Difficulties encountered, if any, in passing catheter smoothly
- Reports of unusual discomfort during insertion
- Specimen obtained

Sample Documentation

DATE	TIME	
1/5/94	1000	Catheter (#16 French Foley) inserted without resistance or report of discomfort. Procedure yielded 700 ml of straw-colored urine without sediment or foul odor.

Bladder/Catheter Irrigation

☒ Equipment

- Two-way indwelling catheter set
  or
- Three-way indwelling catheter set
- Solution ordered for irrigation
- Catheter irrigation kit
  - Large catheter-tip syringe with protective cap
  - Sterile linen saver
  - Graduated irrigation container
- Medication additives, as ordered
- Medication labels
- IV tubing
- IV pole
- Two pairs of clean gloves
- Basin of warm water
- Soap
- Washcloth
- Towel
- Linen saver
- Betadine (or recommended antiseptic solution for cleansing irrigation port)
- Catheter clamp or rubber band

Purpose

Maintains bladder and catheter patency by removing or minimizing obstructions such as clots and mucus plugs in bladder
Prevents or treats local bladder inflammation or infection
Instills medications for local bladder treatments

Assessment

Assessment should focus on the following:

Type of irrigation order

Characteristics of urine prior to irrigation, such as hematuria

Amount of urine output

Distension, pain, or tenderness of the lower abdomen

Signs of inflammation or infection of bladder and perineal structures

Status of catheter (if already inserted) prior to irrigations

Nursing Diagnoses

The nursing diagnoses may include the following:

Altered comfort: pain related to bladder infection

Decreased urinary elimination related to bladder outlet obstruction from blood clots

Planning

Key Goals and Sample Goal Criteria

The client will

Verbalize a decrease in lower abdominal discomfort within 2 days

Demonstrate an absence of bladder obstruction by passing a minimum of 250 ml of urine every 8 hours

Special Considerations

When calculating urine output for a client receiving bladder irrigations, subtract the amount of irrigation solution infused within a designated period of time from the total amount of fluid accumulated within the bag.

Implementation

Action	Rationale
Bladder Irrigation:	
1. Wash hands.	Reduces microorganism transfer
2. Explain procedure to client.	Decreases anxiety
3. Determine if client is allergic to iodine-based antiseptics or additives to be	Avoids allergic reactions

Action	Rationale
injected into irrigation fluid.	
4. Prepare irrigation fluid: – Remove fluid and IV tubing from outer packages. – Close roller clamp on tubing. – Insert additives, if ordered, into fluid container additive port. – Insert spike of tubing into insertion port of fluid bag. – Place on IV pole.	Prepares irrigation solution
– Pinch fluid chamber until fluid fills chamber halfway. – Remove protective cover from end of tubing line, taking care not to contaminate end of tubing or protective cover.	Prevents infusion of air into bladder
– Slowly open roller clamp and fill tubing with fluid.	Removes air from tubing
– Close roller clamp and replace protective cover.	Maintains sterility of tubing
– Place label on bag of fluid stating type of solution, additives, date, and time solution was opened.	Identifies contents of irrigant
5. Provide for privacy.	Decreases embarrassment
6. If three-way catheter has not already been inserted, don clean gloves, place linen saver under buttocks, and wash and dry perineal area.	Reduces microorganisms in local perineal area before catheter insertion
7. Discard gloves, bath water, washcloth, and towel; then wash hands.	Decreases bedside clutter Reduces microorganism transfer
8. Insert catheter using Procedure 6.3 for men or Procedure 6.4 for women.	Inserts catheter for irrigation

Action	Rationale
9. Don clean gloves.	Reduces nurse's exposure to body secretions
10. Cleanse irrigation port of catheter with antiseptic solution recommended by agency.	Removes microorganisms from port Decreases contamination
11. Connect tubing of irrigation fluid to irrigation port of three-way catheter (Fig. 6.5).	Connects tubing to appropriate catheter port for irrigation
12. Slowly open roller clamp on tubing and adjust drip rate.	Sets fluid at appropriate infusion rate for type of infusion

For intermittent irrigation:
- Clamp catheter drainage tubing (or kink tubing and bind with rubber band).
- Open roller clamp so that 100 ml of irrigation fluid flows into bladder by gravitational flow; close roller clamp.
- Allow fluid to remain for 15 minutes (or

Allows proper exchange of electrolytes and fluid

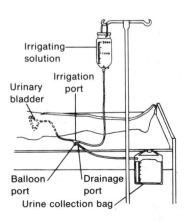

Irrigating solution

Irrigation port

Urinary bladder

Balloon port

Drainage port

Urine collection bag

Figure 6.5

Action	Rationale
amount of time specified by physician's order).	
– Unclamp drainage tubing.	Allows fluid to drain from abdomen into drainage bag
– Repeat irrigation at frequency ordered.	
For continuous irrigation:	
– Leave drainage tubing open.	
– Slowly open roller clamp of irrigation fluid tubing.	
– Adjust irrigation to ordered drip rate (see Procedure 5.5 to review calculation of drip rates).	Provides continuous flushing of bladder
13. Remove linen saver.	Removes soiled linen saver
14. Discard gloves and wash hands.	Prevents spread of microorganisms
15. Record urinary output on intake and output flow sheet.	Provides accurate record of urine output

Catheter Irrigation:
For catheter irrigation using a two-way catheter

Action	Rationale
1. Open catheter irrigation kit.	
2. Remove catheter-tip syringe from sterile container. Remove sterile cap and place syringe back into sterile container. Hold cap between fingers, being careful not to contaminate the open end.	Ensures continued sterility of syringe tip while allowing use of sterile cap to protect drainage tubing tip
3. Fill container with saline or ordered irrigant and fill syringe.	Prepares syringe for irrigation process
4. Disinfect the drainage tubing–catheter connection using an antimicrobial agent recommended by the institution.	Decreases microorganisms at the connection site

Action	Rationale
5. Open sterile linen saver and spread onto bed near catheter.	Provides sterile field
6. Disconnect catheter and drainage tubing. Place cap over drainage tube tip, being careful to keep catheter end sterile. Lie capped tubing onto linen saver.	Maintains sterility of drainage tubing for reconnection
7. Remove syringe from container and insert tip securely into catheter using sterile technique.	Re-establishes closed sterile system for irrigation
8. Slowly infuse irrigant into catheter until full amount of ordered fluid has been infused or patient complains of inability to tolerate additional fluid infusion.	Minimizes discomfort caused by rapid or excessive fluid infusion
9. Clamp catheter by bending end above syringe tip and remove the syringe. Disinfect the catheter end with antimicrobial agent. Remove cap from the drainage tubing and insert it into catheter end.	Prevents leakage of irrigant from catheter Minimizes microorganisms at connection site
10. Repeat irrigation at frequency ordered.	Reestablishes closed bladder drainage system
11. Proceed to steps 13 to 15 of Bladder Irrigation.	

Evaluation

Goals met, partially met, or unmet?

Desired Outcomes (sample)

Client verbalizes decrease in lower abdominal discomfort within 24 hours.
Client maintains urine output of at least 250 ml per shift.

Documentation

The following should be noted on the client's chart:

- Amount, color, and consistency of fluid obtained
- Type and amount of irrigation solution and medication additives administered
- Infusion rate
- Abdominal assessment
- Urine output (total fluid volume measured minus irrigation solution instilled)
- Discomfort verbalized by client

Sample Documentation

DATE	TIME	
7/6/94	1330	Three-way irrigation catheter inserted and continuous bladder irrigation initiated with 1000 ml sterile normal saline irrigant. Drip rate is 50 ml/hour via infusion regulator. Client reports "cramping sensation in lower abdomen as if having spasms." Urine and irrigant clear without sediment or evidence of blood clots.

☝ Hemodialysis Shunt, Graft, and Fistula Care

☒ Equipment

- Nonsterile gloves
- Two pairs of sterile gloves
- Antiseptic cleansing agent or antiseptic swabs
- Topical antiseptic, if ordered
- Sterile 4 × 4-inch gauze pads
- Kling wrap
- Cannula clamps

Purpose

Maintains patency of access for dialysis
Detects complications of a hemodialysis access site related to infection, occlusion, or cannula separation

Assessment

Assessment should focus on the following:

Status of fistula, graft, or cannula site and dressing
Location of shunt, fistula, or graft
Vital signs
Pulses distal to shunt, fistula, or graft
Color and temperature of extremity in which access is located
Presence of pain or numbness in extremity in which access is located
Time of last dressing change

Nursing Diagnoses

The nursing diagnoses may include the following:

Potential altered tissue perfusion related to possible shunt/fistula/graft occlusion or infection

Planning

Key Goals and Sample Goal Criterion

The client will

Maintain a functional access site as evidenced by the presence of a bruit on auscultation and a thrill on palpation and by the absence of edema, redness, pain, drainage, or bleeding

Special Considerations

A potential complication related to the presence of the shunt is cannula separation. Hemorrhage can occur if the shunt is not clamped off until a new cannula is inserted; therefore, a pair of cannula clamps should be kept at the client's bedside at all times.

Home Health

To enable client to change dressings between nursing visits, secure the dressing with a stockinette dressing that the client can roll down over Kerlix and remove old dressing and roll up to secure new dressing.

Implementation

Action	Rationale
1. Wash hands.	Reduces microorganism transfer
2. Explain procedure to client.	Decreases anxiety
3. Open several 4 × 4 packages and soak several gauze pads with antiseptic solution *or* open antiseptic swabs and position for easy access. Keep one package of gauze 4 × 4s dry.	Facilitates cleaning process; provides gauze to cover shunt
4. Don clean gloves.	Reduces nurse's exposure to body secretions
5. Remove old dressing, if present, and check access site.	Exposes access site
6. Discard dressing and gloves.	Removes contaminated items
7. Wash hands and don sterile gloves.	Avoids site contamination

Action	**Rationale**
8. Cleanse access area with antiseptic agent recommended by agency: for shunt care, begin at exit areas and work outward, discarding antiseptic swab or folded gauze pad after each wipe.	Reduces contamination
9. Lightly place two or three fingertips over access site and assess for presence of thrill (a palpable vibration should be present); assess site for extreme warmth or coolness.	Tests for adequate blood flow through shunt
10. Apply topical ointment, if ordered.	Prevents infection
11. Place dry sterile gauze pads over access site.	Reduces site contamination
12. For shunt, apply Kerlix or Kling wrap over gauze pads and around extremity (wrap firmly enough that dressing is secure but not so tight as to occlude blood flow) and tape securely; leave small piece of shunt tubing visible.	Prevents accidental dislodgment of cannula Allows for visualization of continuous blood flow
13. Discard equipment and gloves; then wash hands.	Reduces spread of infection
14. Place call light within reach.	Enables client to communicate
15. Assess status of dressing, access site, and pulses in affected extremity every 2 hours.	Monitors frequently for complications
16. During immediate postoperative period, inform client, family, and staff of the following care instructions: – If shunt is in arm or leg, keep extremity elevated on pillow until instructed otherwise.	Prevents unnecessary loss of access site due to occlusion, infection, or cannula separation

Action	**Rationale**

- Keep extremity as still as possible.
- Do not apply pressure to or lift heavy objects with extremity (If shunt is in leg, crutches will be used for a short while when client becomes ambulatory).
- Do not allow access area to get wet during showering, bathing, or swimming.

17. Inform client, family, and staff of the following care instructions:
    -- Never perform the following procedures on the affected extremity:
       (1) Blood pressure assessment or any procedure that might occlude blood flow
       (2) Venipuncture or any procedure involving a needlestick. PLACE A SIGN OVER BEDSIDE PROHIBITING USE OF AFFECTED EXTREMITY FOR THESE PROCEDURES.
    - Avoid restricting blood flow of affected extremity with tight-fitting clothes, watches, name bands, knee-high stockings, antiembolytic hose, restraints, and so forth.
    - Notify nurse immediately if bleeding or cannula disconnection is noted

Action	Rationale
– Apply cannula clamps if disconnection is noted.	Prevents hemorrhage

Evaluation

Goals met, partially met, or unmet?

Desired Outcomes (sample)

A bruit is present on auscultation, a thrill is palpable, and there is no edema, redness, pain, drainage, or bleeding at the hemodialysis access site.

Documentation

The following should be noted on the client's chart:

- Location of access site
- Status of site and dressing
- Vital signs
- Status of pulses distal to access area
- Color and temperature of extremity in which access is located
- Presence of pain or numbness in extremity in which access is located

Sample Documentation

DATE	TIME	
2/6/94	1115	Left forearm Goretex-graft site care given. Radial pulse normal (3+) in left arm. Left fingers pink with 2-second capillary refill. Client denies pain or numbness of left arm. Thrill palpable at graft site. Site cleaned with Betadine solution and sterile dressing applied.

🖐 Peritoneal Dialysis Management

☒ Equipment

- Dialysate fluid(s) ordered
- Medication additives ordered (usually some combination of potassium chloride, heparin, sodium bicarbonate, and, possibly, antibiotics)
- Syringes for additives
- Medication labels
- Dialysis flow sheet
- Dialysate tubing
- IV pole
- Peroxide or sterile saline
- Antiseptic recommended by agency
- Masks (for each person in room, including client and visitors)
- Clean gown
- Sterile gloves
- Gauze dressing pads (2×2 inches and 4×4 inches)
- Tape
- Graduated container

Purpose

Instills solutions into peritoneal cavity to remove metabolic end products, toxins, and excess fluid from body when kidney function is totally or partially ineffective

Treats electrolyte and acid-base imbalances

Assessment

Assessment should focus on the following:

Changes in mental status

Fluid balance indicators (vital signs, weight, skin turgor, condition of mucous membranes, presence or absence of edema, intake and output)

Abdominal status, including abdominal girth
Cardiopulmonary status
Status of dressing and catheter site
Status of skin surrounding site
Indicators of peritonitis (sharp abdominal pain, cloudy or pink-
tinged dialysate fluid return, increased temperature)
Laboratory data (blood gases, potassium, blood urea nitrogen,
creatinine, hemoglobin, hematocrit)

Nursing Diagnoses

The nursing diagnoses may include the following:

Fluid volume excess related to inability of kidneys to remove
excess fluids
Potential for infection related to peritoneal catheter

Planning

Key Goals and Sample Goal Criteria

The client will be free of

Cardiopulmonary complications of fluid volume excess, such as
jugular vein distension, tachycardia, edema of extremities, or
shortness of breath
Peritonitis, as evidenced by abdominal pain, cloudy or pink-
tinged dialysate return, elevated temperature, and redness,
abnormal drainage, or odor from abdominal catheter site

Special Considerations

Peritonitis is a frequent complication in clients with peritoneal
dialysis; therefore, strict aseptic technique must be maintained
to protect the client from peritonitis.

Pediatric
The pediatric client may be anxious, apathetic, or withdrawn:
offer understanding and support.

Home Health
Many homebound clients dialyze intermittently at home with
use of a cycler. Many also use continuous ambulatory peritoneal dialysis (CAPD) or continuous cycling peritoneal dialysis (CCPD)
Observe return demonstrations until you are certain the client
and family understand the importance of preventing infection.

Implementation

Action	Rationale
1. Wash hands.	Reduces microorganism transfer
2. Explain procedure to client.	Decreases anxiety
3. Weigh client each morning and as ordered for each series of exchanges and record weight.	Provides data needed to determine appropriate concentrations of fluids and additives
4. Place unopened dialysate-fluid bag or bottle in warmer, if solution is not at least room temperature.	Enhances solute and fluid clearance Prevents abdominal cramping
5. Don mask.	Reduces spread of airborne microorganisms
6. Prepare dialysate with medication additives as ordered; prepare each bag according to the five rights of drug administration (see Procedure 11.1); place completed medication label on bag.	Avoids errors that could affect end results of dialysis—concentration affects osmolality, rate of fluid removal, electrolyte balance, solute removal, and cardiovascular stability
7. Insert dialysate infusion tubing spike into insertion port on dialysate-fluid bag/bottle and prime tubing; place fluid bag/bottle on IV pole. *Note*: Some tubing spikes are designed like a screw cap with a spike in the center of the cap. An antiseptic solution should be placed in the cap before spiking bag.	Eliminates air that may contribute to client discomfort
8. Adjust position of bed so that fluid hangs higher than client's abdomen and drainage bag is lower than abdomen (Fig. 6.7).	Enhances gravitational flow as fluid infuses and drains
9. Provide privacy.	Reduces embarrassment
10. Open and arrange cleaning supplies (soak 4 × 4	

Action   **Rationale**

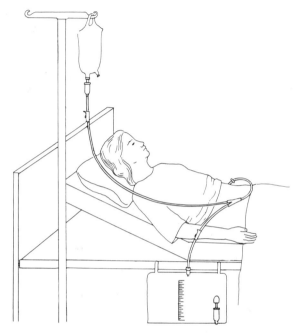

Figure 6.7

gauze pads leaving dry
pads for covering or other
dressing, if ordered.)

Action	Rationale
11. Don clean gown and sterile gloves; instruct each person in room to don appropriate protective wear (masks for all persons in room, sterile gloves for nurse and assistant handling fluid bags).	Decreases nurse's exposure to microorganisms and client's exposure to airborne microorganisms Reduces client's chance of developing peritonitis
12. Remove old peritoneal catheter dressing and examine catheter site for catheter dislodgment or	Assesses catheter intactness Facilitates identification of infectious agent

Action	Rationale
signs of infection; if leakage or abnormal drainage is noted, culture site.	
13. Discard dressing and gloves; then wash hands and don sterile gloves.	Reduces microorganism transfer
14. Beginning at catheter insertion site, cleanse site in a circular motion outward, using peroxide or sterile saline on gauze or swab, and allow to dry; apply antiseptic agent recommended by agency or ordered by doctor (discard each gauze or swab after each wipe when cleansing site and applying antiseptic).	Decreases microorganisms at catheter insertion site Reduces risk of peritonitis
15. Using sterile technique, apply new dressing and secure with tape.	Protects site from microorganisms
16. Discard gloves and wash hands.	Reduces microorganisms
17. Label dressing with date and time of change and your initials.	Provides data needed to determine when next dressing change is due
18. Don sterile gloves.	Reduces microorganisms
19. Connect end of dialysate tubing to abdominal catheter.	Connects tubing to begin dialysate infusion
20. Clamp tubing from abdominal catheter to drainage bag (outflow tubing).	Prevents dialysate from running through
21. Check client's position (abdomen lower than height of fluid, which allows gravity to facilitate flow); check tubing for kinks or bends.	Removes obstructions that could affect infusion rate
22. Open dialysate infusion tubing clamp(s) and allow fluid to drain into peritoneal cavity for 10 to 15	Infuses dialysate for fluid and electrolyte exchange in peritoneal cavity

Action	Rationale
minutes. Observe respiratory status while fluid infuses and while fluid remains in the abdomen (dwell time).	
23. Allow fluid to dwell in abdomen for 20 minutes (or amount of time specified by doctor).	Allows time for proper exchange of fluids and electrolytes
24. Open clamp leading to drain bag and allow fluid to drain for specified amount of time or until drainage has decreased to a slow drip (if all the fluid does not return, reposition client and recheck tubing leading to drainage bag). For CAPD, client may fold dialysis bag and secure bag and tubing to abdomen or clothing and allow fluid to dwell while performing daily activities. To drain dialysate, client would unfold and lower bag and allow fluid to drain from abdominal cavity (same bag is used for infusion and drainage). A new bag is then hung and infusion-dwelling–drainage cycle is repeated continuously.	Allows end products of dialysis to drain
25. Record amount of fluid infused and amount drained after each exchange; add balance of fluids infused and drained on appropriate flowsheet (if net output is greater than amount infused by a large margin—200 ml or more—notify doctor).	Provides accurate record of fluid exchanges for determining fluid balance

Action	Rationale
26. Reassess the following client data every 30 to 60 minutes thereafter throughout exchanges: vital signs, output, respiratory status, mental status, abdominal status, appearance of dialysate return, abdominal dressing (should be kept dry), and signs of lethal electrolyte imbalances.	Alerts nurse to impending complications or need to change fluid and additive concentrations
27. Weigh client at end of appropriate number of fluid exchanges.	Provides data regarding efficiency of exchanges in removing excess fluid
28. Obtain laboratory data, as ordered and as needed (check doctor's orders and agency policy regarding p.r.n. laboratory data).	Provides data about clearance of metabolic wastes as well as electrolyte status
29. When the total series of exchanges is completed, empty drainage bag into graduate container, discard bag and tubing, and cap peritoneal catheter.	Removes fluid waste so other fluid may drain
30. Discard or restore equipment appropriately.	Promotes clean environment
31. Wash hands.	Reduces microorganisms

Evaluation

Goals met, partially met, or unmet?

Desired Outcomes (sample)

Cardiopulmonary complications during dialysis, if any, are detected as they occur.

Client verbalizes no acute abdominal pain. Temperature within normal range. Pulse, 88. Dialysate return clear. No redness, edema, or abnormal drainage at catheter insertion site.

Documentation

The following should be noted on the client's chart:

- Fluid balance indicators (vital signs, weight, skin turgor, condition of mucous membranes, presence or absence of edema, intake and output) before and after dialysis
- Mental status before and after dialysis
- Cardiopulmonary assessment
- Abdominal assessment, including abdominal girth
- Status of dressing and catheter site
- Status of skin surrounding site
- Indicators of peritonitis (sharp abdominal pain, cloudy or pink-tinged dialysate-fluid return, increased temperature)
- Changes in laboratory data (blood gases, potassium, BUN, creatinine, hemoglobin, hematocrit)
- Type and amount of dialysate infused
- Medication additives in dialysate

Sample Documentation

DATE	TIME	
5/9/94	1400	First series of dialysis exchanges begun. Twelve bags of 1.5% dialysate fluid hung to infuse via dialysis cycler. Abdominal dressing clean, dry, and intact. Client denies abdominal pain. Dialysate return clear. Predialysis weight, 88 kg. Postdialysis weight, 87 kg.

✋ Fecal Impaction Removal

❎ Equipment

- Three pairs of nonsterile gloves
- Packet of water-soluble lubricant
- Bedpan
- Linen saver
- Basin of warm water
- Soap
- Washcloth
- Towel
- Air freshener

Purpose

Manually removes hardened stool blocking normal evacuation
   passage in lower part of colon
Relieves pain and discomfort
Facilitates normal peristalsis
Prevents rectal and anal injury

Assessment

Assessment should focus on the following performance of

Agency policy and physician's o... buttocks (*i.e.*, presence of
   procedure   excoriation)
Status of anus and skin surr... abdominal and rectal pain,
   ulcerations, tears, hemorr... bility to pass stool, general
Indicators of impaction ... but being able to do so, nausea
   seepage of liquid s...eath)
   malaise, urge to de...
   and vomiting, sh...nd after removal
Abdominal stat...
Vital signs bef...

Time of last bowel movement and usual bowel evacuation pattern

History of factors that may contraindicate or present complications during impaction removal (such as cardiac instability or spinal cord injury)

Client history regarding dietary habits (*i.e.*, intake of bulk and liquids), changes in activity pattern, frequency of use of laxatives or enemas

Client knowledge regarding promotion of normal bowel elimination

Medications that decrease peristalsis, such as narcotics

Nursing Diagnoses

The nursing diagnoses may include the following:

Altered elimination: fecal impaction related to decreased activity

Altered comfort: abdominal pain related to bowel distension from impaction

Planning

Key Goals and Sample Goal Criteria

The client will

Have bowel movement within 24 hours of impaction removal

Verbalize relief of pain within 1 hour of impaction removal

Special Considerations

Digital removal of impacted stool stretches the anal sphincter causing vagal stimulation. As a result, electrical impulses may be inhibited the S-A node of the heart causing a decrease in pulse rate as dysrhythmias. This procedure is, therefore, contraindes in cardiac clients.

Consult agency and physician's orders regarding the performance of this procedure on any client.

Certain tube feedings (hypertonic) promote constipation and fecal impaction. Check medication record and nutritional supplement list ... tion occurs.

Geriatric

Many elderly clients are es... palpitations related to va... one to dysrhythmias and cardiac problems. Observe ...ion because of chronic ...ure. ...closely during proce-

Many elderly clients are especially prone to fecal impaction because of decreased metabolic rate, decreased activity levels, inadequate dietary intake, and tendency to overuse laxatives and enemas as a routine means of promoting bowel evacuation. A thorough history related to these factors should be obtained.

Pediatric
Use little finger when removing impaction in small children.

Implementation

Action	Rationale
1. Wash hands.	Reduces microorganism transfer
2. Explain procedure to client, admitting that the procedure will cause some discomfort.	Reduces anxiety
3. Assess blood pressure and rate and rhythm of pulse.	Provides baseline data in case of complications
4. Provide privacy; drape client so that only buttocks are exposed.	Reduces embarrassment
5. Don gloves, placing one on nondominant hand and two gloves on dominant hand.	Decreases nurse's exposure to body secretions in case hardened fecal mass tears glove
6. Position client in side-lying position with knees flexed.	Allows good exposure of anal opening
7. Place linen saver under buttocks.	Prevents soiling of linens
8. Place bedpan on bed within easy reach.	Facilitates disposal of fecal mass
9. Raise side rail on side facing client.	Prevents injury due to fall
10. Generously lubricate first two gloved fingers of dominant hand.	Prevents injury to anus and rectum
11. Gently spread buttocks with nondominant hand.	Exposes anal opening
12. Instruct client to take slow, deep breaths through mouth.	Relaxes sphincter muscles facilitating entry

Action	Rationale
13. Insert index finger into rectum (directed towards umbilicus) until fecal mass is palpable (Fig. 6.8).	Prevents rectal trauma
14. Gently break up hardened stool and remove one piece at a time until all of stool is removed; place stool in bedpan as it is removed.	Manually removes impacted stool
15. Observe client for untoward reactions or unusual discomfort during stool removal; obtain pulse and blood pressure if unusual reaction is suspected.	Prevents complications from vagal stimulation
16. Remove finger, wipe excess lubricant from perineal area, and release buttocks.	Promotes comfort
17. Empty bedpan and discard gloves.	Promotes clean environment
18. Wash hands.	Reduces microorganism transfer
19. Don new pair of gloves.	
20. Wash, rinse, and dry buttocks.	
21. Reposition client and raise side rails.	Promotes comfort and safety
22. Leave bedpan within easy reach.	Impaction removal may have stimulated defecation reflex

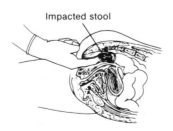

Impacted stool

Figure 6.8

Action	Rationale
23. Discard bathwater and gloves.	Promotes clean environment
24. Spray air freshener at bedside.	Eliminates odor
25. Wash hands.	Reduces microorganism transfer

Evaluation

Goals met, partially met, or unmet?

Desired Outcomes (sample)
Client has normal bowel movement within 24 hours.
Client verbalizes pain relief within 1 hour.

Documentation

The following should be noted on the client's chart:

- Color, consistency, and amount of stool removed
- Condition of anus and surrounding area
- Status of vital signs before and after removal
- Description of adverse reactions during removal
- Abdominal assessment before and after removal
- Presence of discomfort after removal
- Client teaching regarding prevention of fecal impaction

Sample Documentation

DATE	TIME	
6/6/94	1100	Large, dark brown, impacted stool removed manually with no signs of adverse effects. Pulse, 75 and regular before removal and 68 and regular afterwards. Bowel sounds auscultated in four quadrants after removal. Abdomen soft and nondistended. Discussed with client factors preventing constipation and impaction. Factors verbalized by client.

🖐 Enema Administration

⊠ Equipment

- Two pairs of nonsterile gloves
- Enema setup (administration bag or bucket with rectal tubing, castile soap, protective plastic linen saver, packet water soluble lubricant)
- Solution for enema (for adults, 750 to 1000 ml; for children, up to 350 ml; for infants, up to 250 ml)
- Bath thermometer
- Bedpan
- Linen saver
- Basin of warm water
- Soap
- Washcloth
- Towel
- Air freshener

Purpose

Relieves abdominal distension and discomfort
Stimulates peristalsis
Resumes normal bowel evacuation
Cleanses and evacuates colon

Assessment

Assessment should focus on the following:

Physician's order for type of enema
Agency policy and physician's order regarding performance of procedure
Status of anus and skin surrounding buttocks (*i.e.,* presence of ulcerations, tears, hemorrhoids, and excoriation)
Indicators of constipation (*i.e.,* lower abdominal pain or hard, small stools)

Abdominal status

Vital signs before, during, and after enema

Time of last bowel movement and usual bowel evacuation pattern

History of factors that may contraindicate enema or present complications during enema administration (such as cardiac instability)

Client history regarding dietary habits (*e.g.,* intake of bulk and liquids), changes in activity pattern, frequency of use of laxatives or enemas

Client knowledge regarding promotion of normal bowel evacuation

Client medications that decrease peristalsis, such as narcotics

Nursing Diagnoses

The nursing diagnoses may include the following:

Altered elimination: constipation related to decreased activity

Altered comfort: abdominal pain related to bowel distension from constipation

Planning

Key Goals and Sample Goal Criteria

The client will

Evacuate moderate to large amount of stool after enema

Verbalize relief of pain within 1 hour after enema

Special Considerations

Geriatric

Many elderly clients are especially prone to dysrhythmias and palpitations related to vagal stimulation because of chronic cardiac problems. Observe such clients closely during procedure.

Many elderly clients are especially prone to constipation and impaction because of decreased metabolic rate, decreased activity levels, inadequate dietary intake, and tendency to overuse laxatives and enemas as a routine means of promoting bowel evacuation.

A thorough history related to these factors should be obtained.

Pediatric

Minimal elevation of fluid above the anus (4 to 18 inches) is needed to achieve adequate influx of solution.

Implementation

Action	Rationale
1. Wash hands.	Reduces microorganism transfer
2. Explain procedure to client, admitting that the procedure may cause some mild discomfort.	Reduces anxiety
3. Prepare solution, making certain that temperature of solution is lukewarm (about 105°F to 110°F).	Reduces abdominal cramping during procedure
4. Prime tubing with fluid and close tubing clamp; place container on bedside IV pole.	Prevents distension of colon and abdominal discomfort from air
5. Lower pole so that enema solution hangs no more than 18 to 24 inches above buttocks (Fig. 6.9); (for infants and children, solution hangs no more than 4 to 18 inches above the anus).	Slows rate of fluid infusion and prevents cramping

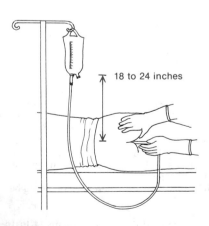

18 to 24 inches

Figure 6.9

Action	Rationale
6. Provide privacy by draping client so that only buttocks are exposed.	Reduces embarrassment
7. Don gloves.	Decreases nurse's exposure to body secretions
8. Place linen saver under buttocks.	Prevents soiling of linens
9. Position client in side-lying position with knees flexed, if not contraindicated.	Allows good exposure of anal opening
10. Lubricate 4 to 5 inches of catheter tip.	Reduces anorectal trauma
11. Place bedpan on bed within easy reach.	Facilitates disposal of enema solution
12. Raise side rail on side facing client.	Prevents injury due to fall
13. Gently spread buttocks with nondominant hand.	Exposes anal opening
14. Instruct client to take slow, deep breaths through mouth.	Relaxes sphincter muscles, facilitating entry
15. With dominant hand, insert rectal tube into rectum (directed towards umbilicus) about 3 to 4 inches and hold in place with dominant hand (1 to 1½ inches for infants; 2 to 3 inches for a child).	Prevents rectal trauma Places tube in far enough to effect cleansing of colon
16. Release tubing clamp.	Allows solution to flow
17. Allow solution to flow into colon slowly, observing client closely.	Avoids cramping
18. If cramping, extreme anxiety, or complaint of inability to retain solution occurs: – Lower solution container. – Clamp or pinch tubing off for a few minutes. – Resume instillation of solution.	Decreases or stops solution flow to allow client to readjust and gain composure
19. Administer all of solution or as much as client can	Delivers enough solution for proper effect

Action	Rationale
tolerate; be sure to clamp tubing just before all of solution clears tubing.	Prevents infusion of air
20. Slowly remove rectal tubing while gently holding buttocks together.	Prevents accidental evacuation of solution
21. Remind client to hold solution for amount of time appropriate for type of enema.	Ensures optimal effect
22. Reposition client.	Facilitates comfort
23. Place call light and bedpan or bedside commode within easy reach.	Provides means of contacting nurse Provides receptacle for enema solution
24. Discard or restore equipment appropriately.	Promotes clean environment
25. Wash hands.	Reduces microorganism transfer
26. Check client every 5 to 10 minutes.	Reassesses client condition and results of enema
27. Assist client on bedpan or toilet after retention time has expired.	Facilitates evacuation of solution
28. Spray air freshener after evacuation.	Eliminates odor
29. Wash hands.	Reduces microorganism transfer

Evaluation

Goals met, partially met, or unmet?

Desired Outcomes (sample)

Client evacuates moderate to large stool.
Client verbalizes pain relief within 1 hour.

Documentation

The following should be noted on the client's chart:

- Type and amount of solution used
- Color, consistency, and amount of stool return

- Condition of anus and surrounding area
- Status of vital signs before and after enema
- Description of adverse reactions during enema
- Abdominal assessment before and after enema
- Presence of discomfort after enema
- Client teaching regarding prevention of constipation

Sample Documentation

DATE	TIME	
2/6/94	2200	Soap suds enema (750 ml) given. Large, dark brown stool returned from enema. No signs of adverse effects. Bowel sounds auscultated in four quadrants. Abdomen soft and nondistended. Discussed factors for promoting normal bowel evacuation with client. Factors verbalized by client.

🖐 Colostomy Stoma Care

☒ Equipment

- Two pairs of nonsterile gloves (add pair for client, if desired)
- Graduated container
- Two linen savers
- Basin of warm water
- Mild soap (without oils, perfumes, or creams)
- Washcloth
- Towel
- Air freshener
- New pouch appliance
- Scissors
- Pen or pencil
- Mirror
- Peristomial skin paste or powder
- Ostomy pouch deodorizer
- Toilet paper

Purpose

Maintains integrity of stoma and *peristomial* skin (skin surrounding stoma)

Prevents lesions, ulcerations, excoriation, and other skin breakdown caused by fecal contaminants

Prevents infection

Promotes general comfort

Promotes positive self-concept

Assessment

Assessment should focus on the following:

Appearance of stoma and peristomial skin (should be pink and shiny)

Characteristics of fecal waste

Abdominal status
Teaching needs, ability, and preference of client for self-care

Nursing Diagnoses

The nursing diagnoses may include the following:

Potential impaired skin integrity related to fecal diversion
Knowledge deficit regarding stoma care

Planning

Key Goals and Sample Goal Criteria

The client will

Maintain intact skin integrity of stoma and peristomial skin, as evidenced by absence of tears, excoriation, ulcerations, redness, edema, and pain
Demonstrate with 100% accuracy self-care of stoma within 2 weeks

Special Considerations

Once client (or family member) shows readiness to begin learning how to perform ostomy care, supervise client performance of procedure until it is accomplished accurately and comfortably.
Ostomy care alters an individual's self-concept significantly; perform care unhurriedly, and discuss care in a positive manner with the client.

Home Health

Homebound clients may dry the skin after cleaning the stoma by using a hair dryer on a low setting.

Pediatric

Minimal pressure should be used when providing stomal care to prevent prolapse of the small stoma.

Implementation

Action	Rationale
1. Wash hands.	Reduces microorganism transfer
2. Explain general procedure to client.	Reduces anxiety

Action	Rationale
3. Explain each step as it is performed, allowing client to ask questions or perform any part of the procedure.	Reinforces detailed instructions client will need to perform self-care
4. Provide privacy.	Reduces embarrassment
5. Position mirror.	Permits client to observe and learn procedure
6. Don gloves.	Avoids nurse's exposure to body secretions
7. Place linen saver on abdomen around and below stoma opening.	Prevents seepage of feces onto skin
8. Carefully remove pouch appliance (bag and skin barrier) and place in plastic waste bag; remove pouch and skin barrier by gently lifting corner with fingers of dominant hand while pressing skin downward with fingers of nondominant hand; remove small sections at a time until entire barrier wafer is removed.	Avoids tearing skin
9. Empty pouch; measure, discard, and record amount of fecal contents (see Procedure 6.12).	Maintains records
10. Wash hands and reglove.	Reduces contamination
11. Gently clean entire stoma and peristomial skin with gauze or washcloth soaked in warm soapy water (if some of fecal matter is difficult to remove, leave wet gauze or cloth on area for a few minutes before gently removing fecal matter); rinse and pat dry.	Removes fecal matter from skin and stoma opening
12. Dry skin thoroughly and apply new pouch device (see Procedure 6.11).	Provides skin protection from fecal contaminants

Action	Rationale
13. Remove gloves and re-store or discard all equip-ment appropriately.	Promotes clean environment
14. Spray room deodorizer, if needed.	Eliminates unpleasant odor
15. Wash hands.	Reduces microorganism transfer

Evaluation

Goals met, partially met, or unmet?

Desired Outcomes (sample)

No redness, edema, swelling, tears, breaks, ulceration, or fistu-las appear at stoma area.
Client performs procedure with 100% accuracy.

Documentation

The following should be noted on the client's chart:

- Color, consistency, and amount of feces in pouch
- Condition of stoma and peristomial skin
- Abdominal assessment
- Emotional status of client
- Verbal and nonverbal indicators of altered self-concept dur-ing procedure
- Verbal and nonverbal indicators of readiness to perform self-care
- Teaching and client participation in performance of procedure
- Additional teaching needs of client

Sample Documentation

DATE	TIME	
2/3/94	1600	Stoma care performed by client with 100% accuracy. Discarded large amount of semiformed brown stool. Stoma pink without excoriation or ab-normal discharge. New pouch applied.

✋ Colostomy Pouch Application

☒ Equipment

- Three pairs of nonsterile gloves
- Graduate container
- Two linen savers
- Basin of warm water
- Mild soap (without oils, perfumes, or creams)
- Washcloth
- Towel
- Air freshener
- New pouch appliance
- Scissors
- Pen or pencil
- Mirror
- Peristomial skin paste or powder
- Ostomy pouch deodorizer

Purpose

Provides clean ostomy pouch for fecal evacuation
Reduces odor from overuse of old pouch
Promotes positive self-image

Assessment

Assessment should focus on the following:

Appearance of stoma and peristomial skin
Characteristics of fecal waste
Type of appliance needed for type of colostomy, nature of
    drainage, and client preference
Teaching needs, ability, and preference of client for self-care

Nursing Diagnoses

The nursing diagnoses may include the following:

Potential altered skin integrity related to incorrect application of pouch

Knowledge deficit regarding application of ostomy pouch

Planning

Key Goals and Sample Goal Criteria

The client will

Show no signs of seepage of fecal contents onto skin
Maintain an intact pouch without accidental disconnection
Demonstrate with 100% accuracy self-application of ostomy pouch

Special Considerations

A wide variety of ostomy appliances is available to meet clients' personal preferences and needs. Minor variations in techniques of application may be needed to ensure adequate skin protection and pouch security. Some ostomy appliances are permanent and should be discarded only every few months. Consult appliance manuals for complete information regarding application and recommended usage time for the pouch.

Once client (or family member) shows readiness to learn how to perform ostomy care, supervise client performance of the procedure until it is accomplished accurately and comfortably.

Ostomy care alters an individual's self-concept significantly. Perform care unhurriedly and discuss care in a positive manner with the client.

Implementation

Action	Rationale
1. Wash hands.	Reduces microorganism transfer
2. Explain general procedure to client.	Reduces anxiety

Action	Rationale
3. Explain each step as it is performed, allowing client to ask questions or perform any part of the procedure.	Reinforces detailed instructions client will need in order to perform self-care
4. Provide privacy.	Reduces embarrassment
5. Don gloves and offer client gloves.	Avoids nurse's exposure to body secretions
6. Place towel or linen saver around stoma pouch close to stoma, remove old pouch, and discard contents; discard gloves.	Removes old pouch for new pouch application Maintains clean environment
7. Wash hands and don fresh gloves.	Reduces microorganism transfer
8. Assess stoma and peristomial skin.	Provides assessment data
9. Perform stoma care (see Procedure 6.10).	
10. Wash hands.	Reduces microorganism transfer
11. Position mirror.	Allows client to observe and learn procedure
12. Reglove.	
13. Place linen saver in client's lap or on bed under client's side where colostomy opening is located.	Protects skin and linens during pouch change
14. Measure stoma with measuring guide.	Provides for accurate fit of pouch appliances
15. Leaving intact adhesive covering of skin-barrier wafer (a flat platelike piece, without pouch attached, that fits on skin around stoma), draw a circle on adhesive liner the same size as stoma; cut out circle.	Cuts barrier to size appropriate for stoma
16. Cut circular adhesive back of ostomy pouch so that it measures about $1/8$ inch larger than actual stoma size.	Allows pouch to be placed over and around stoma without adhering to stoma membrane

Action	Rationale
17. Open bottom of pouch and apply a small amount of pouch deodorizer, if client prefers; reclose pouch securely.	Reduces odor and embarrassment Avoids leakage of feces
18. Remove adhesive covering of skin-barrier wafer and place wafer on skin with hole centered over stoma; HOLD IN PLACE FOR ABOUT 30 SECONDS.	Adheres barrier wafer to skin Warmth of skin and fingers enhances adhesiveness once wafer makes contact with skin
19. Apply stomal paste or powder to any exposed skin between skin-barrier wafer and stoma.	Prevents skin irritation of uncovered peristomial skin
20. Remove adhesive covering of back of pouch and center pouch over stoma, and place on skin-barrier wafer. (If pouch has a flange, snap pouch onto circular flange on barrier wafer as in Fig. 6.11.)	Secures pouch for collection of feces

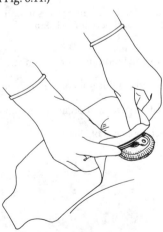

Figure 6.11

Action	Rationale
21. Remove gloves; restore or discard all equipment appropriately.	Promotes clean environment
22. Spray room freshener, if needed.	Eliminates unpleasant odor
23. Wash hands.	Reduces microorganism transfer

Evaluation

Goals met, partially met, or unmet?

Desired Outcomes (sample)

No seepage of fecal material from pouch occurs.
Pouch is secured without dislodgment.
Client demonstrates application of new pouch appliance with 100% accuracy.

Documentation

The following should be noted on the client's chart:

- Color, consistency, and amount of feces in pouch
- Condition of stoma and peristomial skin
- Abdominal assessment
- Emotional status of client
- Verbal and nonverbal indicators of altered self-concept during procedure
- Verbal and nonverbal indicators of readiness to perform self-care
- Teaching and client participation in performance of procedure
- Additional teaching needs of client
- Type of appliance client prefers

Sample Documentation

DATE	TIME	
2/3/94	1100	New colostomy pouch applied by client with 100% accuracy. Discarded large amount of semi-formed brown stool. Stoma pink without excoriation or abnormal discharge. Client verbalized anxiety about how wife will accept assisting with his care and stated preference for pouch appliance with flange rings.

☝ Colostomy Pouch Evacuation and Cleaning

☒ Equipment

- Three pairs of nonsterile gloves
- Bedpan and/or graduate container
- Two linen savers
- Air freshener
- Two washcloths
- Mirror
- Ostomy pouch deodorizer
- Toilet paper
- Paper towels

Purpose

Removes fecal material from ostomy pouch
Cleans pouch for reuse
Maintains integrity of stoma and peristomal skin
Promotes general comfort
Promotes positive self-concept

Assessment

Assessment should focus on the following:

Appearance of stoma and peristomal skin (should be pink and shiny)
Characteristics of fecal waste
Abdominal status
Type of ostomy appliance (permanent or temporary) and condition of appliance
Teaching needs, ability, and preference of client for self-care

Nursing Diagnoses

The nursing diagnoses may include the following:

Potential altered skin integrity related to fecal diversion
Knowledge deficit regarding evacuation and cleaning of pouch
Altered self-concept related to fecal diversion

Planning

Key Goals and Sample Goal Criteria

The client will

Maintain skin integrity of stoma and peristomial area, as evidenced by absence of tears, excoriation, ulcerations, redness, edema, and pain
Demonstrate self-care of stoma within 2 weeks with 100% accuracy
Verbalize feelings about the colostomy

Special Considerations

Once client (or family member) shows readiness to learn how to perform ostomy care, supervise client performance of the procedure until it is accomplished accurately and comfortably.
Ostomy care alters an individual's self-concept significantly. Perform care unhurriedly and discuss care in a positive manner with the client.

Implementation

Action	Rationale
1. Wash hands.	Reduces microorganism transfer
2. Explain general procedure to client.	Reduces anxiety
3. Explain each step as it is performed, allowing client to ask questions or perform any part of the procedure.	Reinforces detailed instructions client will need to perform self-care
4. Provide privacy.	Reduces embarrassment
5. Position mirror.	Allows client to observe and learn procedure

Action	**Rationale**
6. Don gloves.	Avoids nurse's exposure to body secretions
7. Place linen saver on abdomen around and below pouch.	Prevents seepage of feces onto skin
8. If using toilet, seat client on toilet or in a chair facing toilet, with pouch over toilet; if using bedpan, place pouch over bedpan.	Positions client so that feces drain into receptacle
9. Remove clamp on bottom of pouch and place within easy reach.	Promotes efficiency
10. Slowly unfold end of pouch and allow feces to drain into bedpan or toilet (Fig. 6.12.1).	Removes feces from pouch
11. Press sides of lower end of pouch together (Fig. 6.12.2).	Expels additional feces from pouch
12. Open lower end of pouch and wipe out with toilet paper.	Removes excess feces from lower end of pouch
13. Determine if pouch is suitable for reuse; if not, discard and apply new pouch to skin-barrier wafer.	Prevents embarrassment due to pouch odor or leakage
14. Flush toilet or, if using bedpan, take time to resecure end of pouch with rubber band and then empty bedpan. If client has not established good bowel control, go to step 18.	Reduces client embarrassment and room odor
15. If client has established good bowel control: – Carefully remove pouch from skin-barrier wafer and wash entire pouch out with soap and water – Rinse and dry with paper towels	Cleanses pouch collector

Action	Rationale

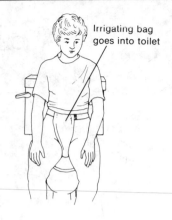

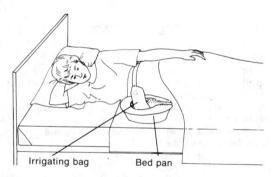

Figure 6.12.1

– Complete steps 16, 17, and 19 through 24.

Action	Rationale
16. Wash hands and reglove.	Reduces microorganism transfer
17. Wash clamp while in bathroom and dry with paper towel. Proceed to step 19.	Cleans exterior clamp
18. Reopen end of pouch and wipe out inside of lower	Cleans bottom of pouch

Action   **Rationale**

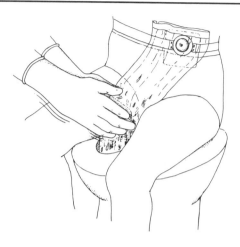

Figure 6.12.2

Action	Rationale
end of pouch with wet washcloth or paper towels.	
19. Apply pouch deodorizer to lower end of pouch.	Reduces unpleasant odor
20. Reclamp pouch with cleaned clamp.	Prevents leakage of feces
21. Wipe outside of pouch with clean, wet washcloth; be sure to wipe around clamp at bottom of pouch.	Completes cleaning of pouch
22. Remove gloves and restore or discard all equipment appropriately.	Promotes clean environment
23. Spray room freshener, if needed.	Eliminates unpleasant odor
24. Wash hands.	Reduces microorganism transfer

Evaluation

Goals met, partially met, or unmet?

Desired Outcomes (sample)

No redness, edema, swelling, tears, breaks, ulceration, or fistulas are present in stoma area.

Client performs procedure with 100% accuracy within 2 weeks.

Client verbalizes feelings about fecal diversion.

Documentation

The following should be noted on the client's chart:

- Color, consistency, and amount of feces in pouch
- Condition of stoma and peristomial skin
- Abdominal assessment
- Emotional status of client
- Verbal and nonverbal indicators of altered self-concept during procedure
- Verbal and nonverbal indicators of readiness to perform self-care
- Teaching and client participation in performance of procedure
- Additional teaching needs of client

Sample Documentation		
DATE	**TIME**	
8/31/94	1430	Ostomy pouch cleaning and evacuation performed by client with 100% accuracy. Discarded large amount of semiformed brown stool. Stoma pink without excoriation or abnormal discharge.

✋ Colostomy Irrigation

❌ Equipment

- IV pole or wall hook
- Irrigation bag and tubing
- Irrigation cone
- Water-soluble lubricant
- Commode or commode chair
- Warm saline or tap water
- Antiseptic (optional)
- Bath thermometer
- Two towels
- Two washcloths
- Linen savers
- Bath basin or sink
- Fresh pouch
- Nonsterile gloves

Purpose

Facilitates emptying of colon

Assessment

Assessment should focus on the following:

Doctor's order for frequency of irrigation and type and amount of solution
Type of colostomy and nature of drainage
Client's ability and preference to perform colostomy care
Client teaching needs

Nursing Diagnoses

The nursing diagnoses may include the following:

Altered bowel elimination: constipation related to decreased roughage and activity
Altered comfort related to constipation
Potential for decreased self-esteem related to odor and altered self-image

Planning

Key Goals and Sample Goal Criteria

The client will

Show unobstructed passage of stool
Demonstrate correct technique for irrigation
Show no adverse physical reactions to irrigation

Special Considerations

If no stool returns and irrigant is retained, reposition client, apply drainable pouch, if needed. You may have client ambulate, if permissible. Notify doctor if there is no return or if abdominal distension is noted.

Pediatric
Routine irrigations are seldom done for the purpose of bowel regulation.
Caution should be exercised because of the small size of the stoma.

Home Health
If homebound client plans to irrigate colostomy while sitting on commode, teach client the proper procedure and have him demonstrate it to you. Correct client's technique, if necessary.

Implementation

Action	Rationale
1. Explain procedure to client.	Reduces anxiety

Action	Rationale
2. Wash hands and organize equipment.	Reduces microorganism transfer and promotes efficiency
3. Obtain extra lighting, if needed.	
4. Provide for warmth and privacy.	Promotes comfort and reduces embarrassment
5. Prepare irrigating solution as follows:	Ensures proper preparation of solution and tubing
– Obtain irrigation bag and solution (usually tepid water); use 250 to 500 ml for initial irrigation, 500 to 1000 ml for subsequent irrigations (minimal amounts are recommended).	Allows bowel to adjust to fluid pressure
– Check temperature of solution (should feel warm to touch but not hot).	Prevents injury from hot solution or cramping from cold solution
– Close tubing clamp.	Allows better fluid control
– Fill bag with tap water or ordered solution at appropriate temperature.	
– Open clamp and expel air from tubing.	Prevents air infusion into bowel
– Close off clamp.	
– Hang bag and tubing on pole or hook.	Permits drainage by gravity
– Lubricate 3 to 4 inches of tubing tip with water-soluble gel and cover end of tubing.	Prevents irritation of stomal tissue
6. Don gloves.	Prevents nurse's contact with body secretions
7. Place client comfortably in any of the following positions (place linen saver under client if performing procedure in bed):	
– On commode	
– Sitting on chair facing toilet	Provides for effective irrigation
– In side-lying position, turned towards side of stomal opening, with	

Action	Rationale
head of bed elevated 30 to 45 degrees	
– In supine position	
8. Gently remove existing pouch from stomal area.	Avoids skin irritation or injury
9. Assess site for redness, swelling, tenderness, and excoriation.	Determines need for other skin care measures
10. Gently wash stomal area with warm soapy water.	Removes secretions
11. Rinse with clear water and dry thoroughly.	
12. Apply irrigation sleeve and belt:	Holds irrigation bag in place to prevent spillage
– Round opening of irrigation sleeve fits over stoma	
– Belt fits around waist	
13. Position irrigation bag (with tubing attached) at a height of 18 inches above stoma (approximately shoulder level).	Avoids undue pressure on mucosal tissues from rushing of fluid
14. Place lower end of sleeve into toilet or large bedpan and unclamp.	Provides receptacle for drainage and begins flow of irrigant
15. Expose stoma through upper opening of sleeve.	
16. Lubricate tip of cone and gently ease into stomal opening (Fig. 6.13.1).	Prevents escape of bowel content onto skin
17. Gently insert 3 to 4 inches of irrigation tubing through cone opening into stoma; if tubing does not ease into opening, do not force (Fig. 6.13.2).	Prevents injury to stomal or bowel tissue
18. Release irrigation tubing clamp and allow solution to infuse over 10 to 15 minutes.	Slow infusion prevents cramping from over-distension
19. Encourage client to take slow, deep breaths as solution is infusing.	Relaxes client and decreases cramping of bowel

Action   **Rationale**

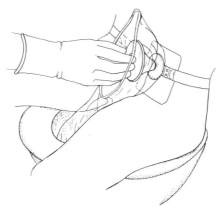

Figure 6.13.1

Action	Rationale
20. If client complains of cramping, stop infusion for several minutes; then resume infusion slowly.	Allows bowel time to adjust to fluid
21. Observe for return of fecal material and solution and assess drainage.	Indicates effectiveness of irrigation
22. Remove bottom of sleeve from drainage receptacle and flush toilet or empty bedpan.	Restores room cleanliness
23. Dry bottom of sleeve and clamp.	Prevents soiling and collects further drainage
24. Allow client to move about for the next 30 to 45 minutes (or assist, as needed, for safety during mobility).	Allows irrigant to loosen remaining bowel contents
25. Repeat steps 14, 21, and 22.	
26. Clean bedpan.	Restores room cleanliness and order
27. Remove irrigation sleeve and belt.	Concludes irrigation procedure
28. Discard or restore equipment.	Promotes clean, organized environment

Action	Rationale

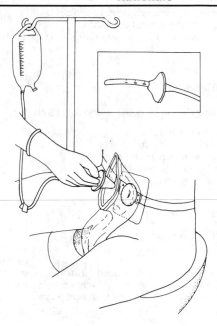

Figure 6.13.2

Action	Rationale
29. Discard old gloves and don new pair.	Reduces contamination
30. Wash, rinse, and dry stoma area.	Cleanses peristomial area
31. Apply antiseptic, if ordered.	Prevents infection
32. Apply new dressing or ostomy pouch, if needed.	
33. Wash hands.	Reduces microorganism transfer

Evaluation

Goals met, partially met or unmet?

Desired Outcomes (sample)

Stool passes freely through stomal opening.
Client demonstrates correct procedure.
Client experiences no excessive cramping or pain during irrigation.

Documentation

The following should be noted on the client's chart:

• Condition of stoma site
• Amount of irrigant infused
• Amount and nature of drainage
• Client tolerance for procedure
• Client teaching accomplished and/or needed

Sample Documentation

DATE	TIME	
3/23/94	1250	Colostomy irrigation done with 600 ml tap water infused. Approximately 800 ml soft and liquid brown drainage noted. Client tolerated procedure without cramping or pain. Client demonstrated correct technique.

✋ Stool Testing for Occult Blood With Hemoccult Slide

✖ Equipment

- Stool specimen
- Hemoccult specimen collection card
- Chemical reagent (developer)
- Tongue blade
- Nonsterile gloves
- Stop watch or watch with second hand
- Specimen container labels
- Pen

Purpose

Obtains stool specimen to detect occult blood related to gastrointestinal bleeding and anemia

Serves as a preliminary screening test for colorectal cancer

Assessment

Assessment should focus on the following:

Specific orders regarding specimen collection
Characteristics of stool
Manifestations associated with gastrointestinal bleeding or anemia
History of gastrointestinal bleeding or anemia
Dietary intake of foods or drugs that could alter test reliability
Intake of medications that cause occult bleeding

Nursing Diagnoses

The nursing diagnoses may include the following:

Potential altered tissue perfusion related to possible gastrointestinal bleeding

Planning

Key Goal and Sample Goal Criterion

The client will

Have no undetected signs and symptoms of gastrointestinal bleeding

Special Considerations

Some vitamins and minerals (such as vitamin C and iron) can cause erratic test results. Consult a pharmacy reference for a complete listing of such preparations and the amounts necessary to alter results.

Many clients are placed on special diagnostic diets 2 to 3 days before hemoccult testing. Emphasize to client the importance of adhering to diet restrictions.

Implementation

Action	Rationale
1. Wash hands.	Reduces microorganism transfer
2. Explain procedure to client.	Decreases anxiety
3. Provide for privacy.	Decreases embarrassment
4. Don clean gloves.	Reduces nurse's exposure to body secretions
5. Obtain stool specimen with tongue blade and smear thin specimen onto guaiac test paper: – Smear specimen onto slot A on front of card.	Prepares specimen for test

Action	Rationale
– Smear a second specimen from another part of stool onto slot B.	
– Close card.	
6. Turn card over and open back window; apply two drops of reagent to slot over each specimen and wait 60 seconds.	Activates chemical components necessary for results (alpha guaiacoconic and hydrogen peroxide)
7. Read results (consult product instructions for visual comparison):	Determines if results are positive or negative
– If either slot has bluish discoloration, test is positive.	
– If there is no bluish discoloration, test is negative.	
8. Restore or discard equipment appropriately (test card may be discarded).	Promotes clean environment
9. Wash hands.	Reduces microorganism transfer

Evaluation

Goals met, partially met, or unmet?

Desired Outcome (sample)

Signs and symptoms of gastrointestinal bleeding (bloody or dark black stools, fatigue, decreased bowel sounds, abdominal discomfort) are detected early.

Documentation

The following should be noted on the client's chart:

- Amount, color, odor, and consistency of stool obtained
- Specimen collection time
- Signs and symptoms consistent with gastrointestinal bleeding

Sample Documentation

DATE	TIME	
3/2/94	1100	Second stool tested for occult blood with hemoccult slide. Results negative. Stool is dark brown, large, and formed. Client reports no discomfort during defecation.

CHAPTER 7

Activity and Mobility

OVERVIEW

- The ability to remain physically active and mobile is essential in maintaining health and well-being.
- Immobility may pose psychological as well as physiological hazards.
- Nurses should be alert for such physical complications of immobility as the following:
  - Hypostatic pneumonia
  - Pulmonary embolism
  - Thrombophlebitis
  - Orthostatic hypotension
  - Decubitus ulcers or pressure areas
  - Decreased peristalsis with constipation and fecal impaction
  - Urinary stasis with renal calculi formation
  - Contractures and muscle atrophy
  - Altered fluid and electrolyte status

Jean Smith-Temple and Joyce Young Johnson:
Nurses' Guide to Clinical Procedures, Second Edition.© 1994
J. B. Lippincott Company

- Psychological hazards of immobility may range from mild anxiety to psychosis.
- Improper use of body mechanics when moving a client could result in injury to client and nurse. Knowledge of principles of body mechanics and proper body alignment is essential to injury prevention.

🖐 Using Principles of Body Mechanics

☒ Equipment

- Equipment needed to move client or lift object (*e.g.,* Hoyer lift, sling scales, trapeze bar)
- Turn sheets
- Chair, stretcher, or bed for client
- Adequate lighting
- Positioning equipment (*e.g.,* trochanter rolls, pillows, footboards)
- Nonsterile gloves
- Visual and hearing aids needed by client

Purpose

Prevents physical injury of care-giver and client

Promotes correct body alignment

Facilitates coordinated, efficient muscle use when moving clients

Conserves energy of care-giver for accomplishment of other tasks

Assessment

Assessment should focus on the following:

Presence of deformities or abnormalities of vertebrae

Physical characteristics of client and care-giver that will influence techniques used (weight, size, height, age, physical limitations and abilities, condition of target muscles to be used in moving client, problems related to equilibrium)

Characteristics of object to be moved during client care (*e.g.,* weight, height, shape)

Immediate environment (amount of space available to work in; distance to be traveled; presence of obstructions in pathway; condition of floor; placement of chairs, stretchers, and other equipment being used; lighting)

Adequacy of function and stability of all equipment to be used

Extent of knowledge of assisting personnel, client, and family regarding proper use of body mechanics and body alignment

Status of equipment attached to client that must be moved (*e.g.,* IV machines, tubes, drains)

Nursing Diagnoses

The nursing diagnoses may include the following:

Potential for physical injury related to improper use of body mechanics

Knowledge deficit regarding proper use of body mechanics

Planning

Key Goals and Sample Goal Criteria

The client will

Experience no physical injury related to improper use of body mechanics during moving, lifting, turning, or repositioning and will reveal no new bruises, tears, or skeletal trauma following these procedures

Demonstrate proper use of body mechanics to be used in performing major lifting and moving tasks at home by the time of discharge

Special Considerations

Secure as much additional assistance as is needed for safe moves. NEVER BECOME SO IMPATIENT THAT UNSAFE RISK IS TAKEN WITH ANY TYPE OF MOVE. As a general rule of thumb, if mechanical equipment is available that will make lifting, turning, pulling, or positioning easier, use it.

Check all equipment to be used, including chairs, for adequate function and stability.

If physical injury of personnel is sustained because of performance of any work-related activity, follow agency policies regarding follow-up medical attention and completion of incident report forms. This provides for proper care and ensures financial assistance as needed.

Geriatric and Pediatric

If client is restless, agitated, confused, or has a condition that causes loss of muscle control, secure assistance to prevent injury during the moving process.

Home Health

The client's home environment should be assessed adequately to determine the need to rearrange furniture and other items and to secure mechanical equipment to ensure the safety of client and family as they perform care.

Implementation

Action	Rationale
1. Wash hands.	Reduces microorganism transfer
2. Determine factors indicating need for additional personnel such as: – Equipment attached to client – Does move require persons of approximately the same height?	Promotes efficiency
3. Restore client's glasses and hearing aids if client is able to assist at all.	Enables client to assist in making a safe move
4. Explain required movement techniques to assisting personnel, family, and client; instruct and allow client to do as much as possible.	Facilitates coordinated movement and prevents physical injury Promotes independence
5. Don gloves as needed if contact with body fluids is likely.	Prevents exposure to body secretions
6. Organize equipment so that it is within easy reach, stabilized, and in proper position: – If moving client to chair, place chair so that back of chair is in same direction as head of bed.	Avoids risks once movement begins Keeps number of actions needed for the move to a minimum

Action	**Rationale**
– If placing client on stretcher, align stretcher with side of bed.	
7. Raise or lower bed and other equipment to comfortable and suitable height.	Prevents use of back muscles in performing tasks
8. Maintain proper body alignment by using the following principles when handling equipment and when moving, lifting, turning, and positioning clients:	
– Stand with back, neck, shoulders, pelvis, and feet in as straight a line as possible; knees should be slightly flexed and toes pointed forward (Fig. 7.1.1).	Maintains proper body alignment
– Keep feet apart to establish broad support base;	Provides greater stability

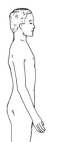

Head up

Neck straight

Back straight

Arms relaxed at sides

Eyes straight ahead

Chest out

Abdomen in

Knees slightly flexed

Figure 7.1.1

Action	Rationale
keep feet flat on floor (Fig. 7.1.2).	
– Flex knees and hips in order to lower center of gravity (heaviest area of body) close to object to be moved (Fig. 7.1.3).	Establishes more stable position Prevents pulling on spine
– Move close to object to be moved or adjusted; do not lean or bend at waist.	Promotes use of muscles of extremities rather than of spine
– Use smooth, rhythmic motions when using bedcranks or any equipment requiring a pumping motion.	Prevents improper alignment and inefficient muscle use
– Use arm muscles for cranking or pumping.	Avoids use of spine and back muscles

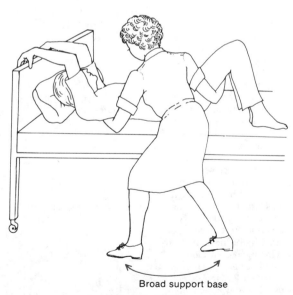

Broad support base

Figure 7.1.2

Action	**Rationale**

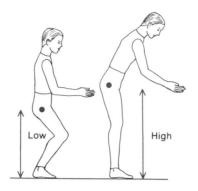

Figure 7.1.3

Action	**Rationale**
and arm and leg muscles for lifting.	
8. Secure all tubes, drains, traction equipment, and so forth by whatever means are needed for proper functioning during moving, lifting, turning, and positioning.	Prevents dislodgment of tubes and reflux of contaminants into body
9. Move client close to edge of bed in one unit, or move client to side of bed at any time during procedure, moving one unit of the body at a time from top to bottom or vice versa (*i.e.*, head and shoulders first, trunk and hips second, and legs last). Coordinate move so that everyone exerts greatest effort on count of "three"; the individual carrying the heaviest load should direct the count.	Maintains correct alignment Facilitates comfort

Prevents physical injury |
| 10. Use the following principles to move a heavy object or client: | |

Action	Rationale
a. Review each move again before move is made.	Reinforces original plan
b. Face client or object to be moved.	Allows full use of arm and leg muscles
c. Place hands or arms fully under client or object; lock hands with assistant on opposite side, if necessary.	Provides extra leverage
d. Prepare for move by taking in a deep breath, tightening abdominal and gluteal muscles, and tucking chin towards chest. (If client is unable to provide assistance, instruct client to cross arms on chest.)	Facilitates use of large muscle groups
e. Allow adequate rest periods, if needed.	Prevents fatigue and subsequent physical injury
f. When performing move, keep heaviest part of body within base of support.	Promotes stability
g. Perform pulling motions by leaning backward and pushing motions by leaning forward, maintaining wide base of support with feet, keeping knees flexed and one foot behind the other; pushing and pulling (use instead of lifting, whenever possible) should be done with muscles of the arms and legs, not back.	Prevents injury to vertebrae and back muscles
h. Always lower head of bed as much as permissible.	Avoids pulling against gravity
i. When moving from a bending to standing position, stop momen-	Allows time to straighten spine and re-establish stability

Action	Rationale

tarily once in standing
position before com-
pleting next move.
When getting clients
into a chair, stop to
allow client and self to
stand to establish sta-
bility before pivoting
into chair.

j. Move in as straight and
direct a path as possi-
ble, avoiding twisting
and turning of spine.

Avoids vertebral and back
injury related to rotating
and twisting spine

k. When turning is un-
avoidable, use a pivot-
ing turn; when
positioning client in
chair or carrying client
to a stretcher, pivot to-
ward chair or stretcher
together.

11. Position props and body
parts for appropriate
body alignment of client
after move is completed:
– When client is sitting,
hips, shoulders, and
neck should be in line
with trunk; knees, hips,
and ankles should be
flexed at a 90-degree
angle and toes should
be pointed forward.
– When client is in bed,
neck, shoulders, pelvis,
and ankles should be in
line with trunk, and
knees and elbows
should be slightly flexed.

12. After move is completed,
provide for comfort and
safety of client with the
following actions, if ap-
plicable:
– Raise protective rails.

Prevents falls

Action	Rationale
– Apply safety belts on stretchers and wheel-chairs.	Promotes safety
– Lower height of bed.	Promotes safety
– Elevate head properly.	Supports airway clearance
– Restore all tubes, drains, and equipment being used by client to proper functioning and placement.	Re-establishes proper functioning of equipment
– Place pillows and position equipment properly.	Promotes proper body alignment and supports airway
– Replace covers.	Provides warmth and privacy
– Place call light within reach.	Provides means of communication
– Place items of frequent use within client reach.	Enhances comfort and general satisfaction
13. Discard gloves and wash hands.	Reduces microorganism transfer

Evaluation

Goals met, partially met, or unmet?

Desired Outcomes (sample)

Client displays no evidence of physical injury, such as new bruises, tears, or skeletal trauma after moving.

Before discharge client demonstrates proper use of body mechanics to be used in performing major lifting and moving tasks at home.

Documentation

The following should be noted on the client's chart:

- Amount of assistance given by client
- Position client was placed in (*e.g.,* in chair, returned to bed, placed on stretcher)
- Reports of discomfort, dizziness, or faintness during or after move
- Re-establishment of proper functioning of equipment

- Safety belts applied
- Status of side rails
- Auxiliary equipment used
- Status of equipment being used to maintain alignment

Sample Documentation

DATE	TIME	
10/19/94	1030	Assisted client into chair. Client able to provide partial assistance; reported slight dizziness when standing. IV remains intact and infusing correctly. Posey vest reapplied. Call light placed within reach.

Body Positioning

☒ Equipment

- Support devices required by client (*e.g.*, trochanter roll, footboard, heel protectors, sandbags, hand rolls, restraints)
- Pillow for head and extra pillows needed for support

Purpose

Positions client for comfort and body alignment
Positions client for a variety of clinical procedures

Assessment

Assessment should focus on the following:

Client's age and medical diagnosis
Physical ability of client to maintain position
Integumentary assessment
Length of time client has maintained present body positioning
Doctor's orders for specific restrictions in positioning client or for special position required by impending procedure

Nursing Diagnoses

The nursing diagnoses may include the following:

Potential altered skin integrity related to prolonged pressure on bony prominences

Planning

Key Goal and Sample Goal Criterion

The client will

Maintain skin integrity without pressure areas or decubitus ulcers during confinement

Special Considerations

To avoid injury when positioning clients, it is important that body alignment of the client and nurse or assistant be supported and that appropriate body mechanics be used. (Procedure 7.1 presents the principles of body mechanics.) Secure as much additional assistance as is needed for the safe repositioning of the client and for protection of your back. NEVER BECOME SO IMPATIENT THAT RISKS ARE TAKEN.

Foot drop, decubitus ulcers, shoulder subluxation, and internal and external rotation of large joint areas are preventable complications if the client is positioned and supported correctly. Be sure that pillows, trochanter rolls, footboards, and other supportive equipment are positioned to maintain body alignment; that joint and ligament pulling is prevented; that head, feet, and hands do not droop; that large joint areas do not rotate internally or externally; and that excess pressure on any body area is avoided.

Geriatric

Bedridden elderly clients are particularly susceptible to impaired skin integrity when they are not repositioned frequently; this is due to a decreased amount of subcutaneous fat and to skin that is less elastic, thinner, drier, and thus more fragile than that of a younger person.

Home Health

In the home, pillows, sofa cushions, or rolled linen may be used for positioning. A recliner may be used to maintain a Fowler's or semi-Fowler's position.

Implementation

Action	Rationale
1. Wash hands.	Reduces microorganism transfer

Action	**Rationale**
2. Explain procedure to client, emphasizing importance of maintaining proper position.	Decreases anxiety Increases compliance
3. Provide for privacy.	Decreases embarrassment
4. Adjust bed to comfortable working height.	Prevents back and muscle strain in nurse
5. Place or assist client into appropriate position (various positions are illustrated in Fig. 7.2 and described in Table 7.2).	
6. Use the following guidelines in repositioning client:	
– Place all equipment, lines, and drains attached to client so that dislodgment will not occur.	Prevents accidental dislodgment and client injury
– Close off drains, if necessary, and remember to reopen them after positioning client.	Prevents reflux of drainage
– Be sure that an assistant is designated to handle extremities bound by heavy stabilizers (such as casts and traction) and heavy equipment that must be moved with client (such as traction apparatus).	Maintains stability of body part to prevent injury and pain
– Maintain head elevation for clients prone to dyspnea when flat; allow brief rest periods, as needed, during procedure.	Facilitates breathing and reduces anxiety Prevents exertion
– When moving client to side of bed, move major portions of the body sequentially, from top to bottom or vice versa (*e.g.*, head and shoulders first, trunk and hips second, legs last).	Maintains body alignment Facilitates comfort

A. High Fowler's

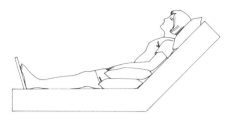

B. Supine

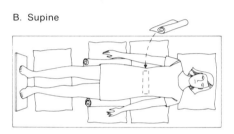

C. Prone

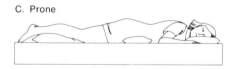

D. Side-lying

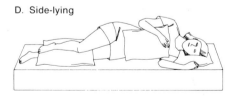

Figure 7.2

E. Sim's

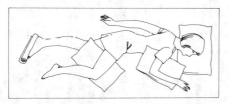

F. Lithotomy

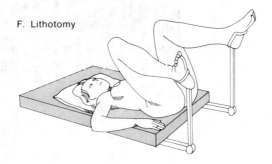

G. Dorsal Recumbent

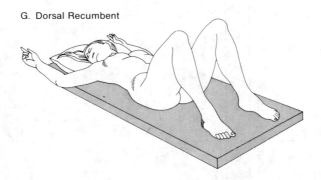

Figure 7.2 (cont.)

TABLE 7.2 Body Positioning

Position	Purpose	Description
Fowler's (low to high)	Improves breathing capacity Prevents aspiration Promotes comfort	Head of bed up 30 to 90 degrees Client in a semisitting position Knees slightly flexed
Supine	Prevents bending at crucial areas, such as groin or spine, after diagnostic procedures	Client flat on back in bed Body straight and in alignment Feet protected with footboard to support 90-degree flexion
Prone	Serves as positioning alternative in turning procedure for immobilized clients	Client flat on abdomen with knees slightly flexed Head turned to side Arms flexed at sides, hands near head Feet over end of mattress or protected with footboard to support normal flexion
Side-lying (lateral)	Serves as position for some procedures and alternative position for turning procedure	Client lying on side with upper leg flexed at hip and knee Top arm flexed Lower arm flexed and shoulder positioned to avoid pulling and excessive weight of body or shoulder

Sim's	Serves as position for some procedures and alternative position for turning procedure	Client halfway between side-lying and prone positions with bottom knee slightly flexed Knee and hip of top leg flexed (about 90 degrees) Lower arm behind back Upper arm flexed, hand near head
Lithotomy	Places client in position for vaginal or anorectal exams	Client on back with legs flexed 90 degrees at hips and knees Feet up in stirrups
Dorsal recumbent	Places client in position for vaginal exams and insertion of catheters	Client on back with legs flexed at hips and knees Feet flat on mattress
Modified Trendelenburg's	Places client in "shock" position to increase blood flow to heart and cerebral tissue	Client flat on back with legs straight and elevated at hips Head and shoulders slightly raised

Pillows and other support equipment are placed to support alignment and normal flexion points, and to prevent pressure on any body area.

Action	Rationale
– Use pillows, trochanter rolls, and special positioning supports as needed to maintain body alignment and normal position of extremities.	Prevents injury and promotes comfort
– Be certain that client's face is not pressed into bed or pillows while turning and that body position does not prevent full expansion of diaphragm.	Maintains adequate respirations
– Use appropriate body mechanics (see Procedure 7.1).	Prevents injury
7. Assess status of client comfort and character of respirations; recheck client periodically.	Prevents injury
8. Lift side rails and place bed in low position. If traction apparatus is being used, be certain weights are not dragging on floor or touching bed.	Prevents falls
9. Place call light within reach.	Facilitates communication
10. Move over-bed table close to bed and place items of frequent use on table.	Places items used frequently within easy reach
11. Wash hands.	Decreases microorganism transfer

Evaluation

Goals met, partially met, or unmet?

Desired Outcomes (sample)

Client's skin is warm, dry, intact, and without discoloration over pressure points.

Documentation

The following should be noted on the client's chart:

- Client's position
- Client reports of pain, dyspnea, discomfort
- Exertion or dyspnea observed during repositioning
- Abnormal findings on integumentary assessment
- Status of equipment needed for stabilization of body parts (*e.g.*, traction, casts)
- Teaching regarding importance of maintaining position

Sample Documentation

DATE	TIME	
10/5/94	1430	Client repositioned into right side-lying position. Slight shortness of breath reported during repositioning. Client given a brief rest period and no further shortness of breath reported. No redness, breaks, or discoloration noted over bony prominences.

Hoyer Lift Usage

☒ Equipment

- Hoyer lift (should include base, canvas mat, two pairs of canvas straps)
- Large chair with arm support for client to sit in

Purpose

Helps move and transfer heavy clients who are unable to assist mover

Prevents undue strain on mover's body

Assessment

Assessment should focus on the following:

Medical diagnosis

Doctor's activity orders (positions contraindicated and number and amount of time client may be up)

Client ability to keep head erect

Chart to determine previous tolerance of client to sitting position (*e.g.*, orthostatic hypotension, amount of time client tolerated sitting up)

Client's need for restraints while sitting up

Room environment (*i.e.*, adequate lighting, presence of clutter and furniture in pathway between chair and bed)

Condition of Hoyer device, hooks, and canvas mats

Nursing Diagnoses

The nursing diagnoses may include the following:

Altered mobility related to weakness and activity intolerance

Planning

Key Goal and Sample Goal Criterion

The client will

Experience no injury during transfer

Special Considerations

It is important for the nurse to be familiar with the Hoyer lift in order to operate it correctly (parts of the lift are labeled in Fig. 7.3). Practice using the lift without a client on the mat if you are unfamiliar with this device.

Organization is crucial when performing numerous moving procedures on heavy clients to avoid client exertion and physical injury to the movers. Plan activities such as changing bed linens while client is out of bed; encourage client to use bedside toilet once out of bed.

Geriatric

Chronic conditions in elderly clients require extra caution when moving them using the Hoyer lift. Clients with chronic cardiopulmonary conditions should be observed closely while

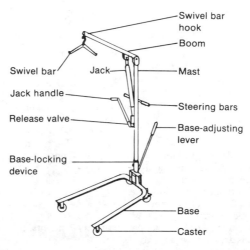

Figure 7.3

sitting up and during transfer for exertion, respiratory difficulty, chest pain, and general discomfort.

Pediatric
Using the Hoyer lift can be frightening to a child. Demonstrate the procedure, using a puppet or game, and allow the child to participate in some way.

Home Health
Help family obtain the equipment, if needed. Educate the family on the use of the equipment and on proper body mechanics.

Implementation

Action	Rationale
1. Wash hands.	Reduces microorganism transfer
2. Explain procedure and assure client that precaution will be taken to prevent falls.	Decreases anxiety
3. Provide for and maintain privacy throughout procedure.	Decreases embarrassment
4. Place chair on side of bed client will be sitting on (lock wheels, if wheelchair).	Places chair at close distance
5. Adjust bed to comfortable working height.	Prevents back and muscle strain in nurse
6. Lock bed.	Prevents bed movement
7. Place client on mat as follows:	Centers heaviest parts of body on mat
– Roll client to one side and place half of mat under client from shoulders to midthigh.	Positions client on mat with minimal movement
– Roll client to other side and finish pulling mat under client.	
– Be sure one or both side rails are up as you move from one side of bed to other.	Prevents accidental falls

Action	Rationale
8. Roll base of Hoyer lift under side of bed nearest to chair with boom in center of client's trunk; lock wheels of lift.	Moves mechanical part of lift to bedside Prevents lift from rolling
9. Using base-adjustment lever, widen stance of base.	Provides greater stability to lift
10. Raise and then push jack handle in towards mast, lowering boom (this is accomplished with appropriate button or control device in the electric Hoyer).	Lowers booms close enough to attach hooks
11. Place the strap or chain hooks through the holes of mat (hooks of short straps go into holes behind back and hooks of long straps into holes at other end), making certain that hooks are not indenting client's skin.	Secures hook placement into mat holes Attaches rest of device to mat
12. Place all equipment, lines, and drains attached to client so that dislodgment will not occur and close off drains, if necessary (remember to reopen them after moving client).	Prevents accidental dislodgment and client injury Prevents reflux of drainage
13. Instruct client to fold arms across chest.	Prevents accidental injury
14. Using jack handle, pump jack enough for mat to clear bed about 6 inches and tighten release valve.	Safely assesses client stability and centering on mat
15. Determine if client is fully supported and can maintain head support. Provide head support as needed throughout the procedure.	Assesses stability in relation to weight and placement
16. Unlock wheels and pull Hoyer lift straight back and away from bed; instruct assistant to provide	

Action	Rationale
support for equipment and client's legs throughout procedure.	Promotes stability
17. Move toward chair with open end of lift's base straddling chair; continue until client's back is almost flush with back of chair.	Moves and guides client into chair
18. Lock wheels of lift.	Provides Hoyer stability
19. Slowly lift up jack handle and lower client into chair until hooks are slightly loosened from mat; guide client into chair with your hands as mat lowers. Avoid lowering client onto chair handles.	Lowers client fully into chair
20. Remove mat (unless difficult to replace or client's first time out of bed).	Facilitates comfort
21. Place tubes, drains, and support equipment for proper functioning, comfort, and safety:	Prevents accidental dislodgment of tubes and drains and maintains necessary functions
– Pillow behind head	Ensures client stability in chair
– Sheet over knees and thighs	
– Restraints, if needed (*e.g.*, Posey vest, sheet, arm restraints)	Facilitates adequate support of other body parts
– Phone and items of frequent use within close range	Places items desired or needed by client within reach
– Catheter hooked to lower portion of chair	
– IV pole close enough to avoid pulling	
– Call light	Facilitates communication
22. Assess client tolerance to sitting up.	Reduces risk of falling
23. Leave door to client's room open when leaving room, unless someone else will be with client.	Allows visual observation of unattended client

Action	Rationale
24. Monitor client at 15- to 60-minute intervals.	Reduces risk of falling
25. Return client to bed using above steps.	Prevents injury and discomfort during transfer
26. Wash hands and restore equipment.	Reduces microorganism transfer
	Promotes clean environment

Evaluation

Goals met, partially met, or unmet?

Desired Outcome (sample)

Client is moved from and returned to bed by Hoyer lift without injury.

Documentation

The following should be noted on the client's chart:

- Status update with indication for continued use of mobility-assist device
- Time of client transfer and type of lift used
- Client tolerance of procedure
- Duration of time in chair

Sample Documentation

DATE	TIME	
7/15/94	1400	Client lifted out of bed using Hoyer lift. Placed in bedside chair. Client tolerated procedure well with respirations regular and nonlabored and is watching television. Call bell within reach. Door left partially open.

Stryker Frame Management

 Equipment

- Stryker frame, wedge or parallel
- Backboard
- Linen
- Arm rests
- Footboard
- Pillows
- Sheepskins
- Safety straps

Purpose

Turns client from supine to prone position without excess
  movement
Maintains good skin care for immobilized clients

Assessment

Assessment should focus on the following:

Client's mobility level and level of sensation
Type and extent of spinal injury
Date of injury
Activity orders and mobility limitations
Client's ability to understand procedure and participate in deci-
  sion making about turning times

Nursing Diagnoses

The nursing diagnoses may include the following:

Impaired physical mobility related to fractured cervical spine
Potential altered skin integrity related to immobility
Anxiety related to turning procedure or fear of injury from fall

Planning

Key Goals and Sample Goal Criteria

The client will

Maintain alignment of spine and body parts

Experience minimum movement of spine during turning, as evidenced by no additional loss of mobility or sensation; no complaint of back pain

Maintain good ventilatory pattern, as evidenced by respiratory rate within normal limits, smooth, and unlabored

Demonstrate no excessive anxiety, as evidenced by calm facial expression, respiratory and heart rates within normal limits 5 minutes after turn is complete

Evidence no skin breakdown or irritation during convalescence

Maintain bowel evacuation without constipation

Special Considerations

Prone position might restrict respirations and cause distress: monitor the client closely after turning.

Encourage the client to indicate when to start turning procedure and what comfort devices are needed. Participation in turning process decreases anxiety during procedure.

Although the turning procedure usually requires only one person, obtain assistance, when available, for the added safety and emotional security of the client.

If the lower extremities are paralyzed, monitor for a possible shift in client weight as the client is turned.

For added safety, apply safety straps before turning the client.

Pediatric

Demonstrate the turning procedure with a doll or use a game. Allow client to select timing of the turning procedure.

Implementation

Action	Rationale
1. Provide explanation of procedure to client, including reason for use, direction of turning, need for safety straps, and client assistance needed.	Decreases anxiety and increases cooperation

Action	Rationale
2. Show anterior frame to client and demonstrate use of entire frame before starting turning process.	Decreases anxiety
3. Test equipment for proper functioning before using on client.	Ensures safety
4. Wash hands and organize equipment.	Reduces contamination Promotes efficiency

Initial Application

Action	Rationale
5. Using a three-person carry method or mechanical lift, place client on posterior frame of Stryker frame in supine position; maintain backboard if present.	Keeps client in alignment during transfer Prevents injury to spine
6. After explanation to client, attach anterior frame, secure safety straps, turn client, remove straps and posterior frame, and remove backboard (see Turning Procedure, steps 9 to 21).	Prevents pressure on bony prominences from backboard
7. Replace posterior frame; turn client to supine position, and remove anterior frame.	Returns client to supine position
8. Adjust linens and pillows.	Promotes client comfort

Turning Procedure

Action	Rationale
9. After explanation to client, position pillows on client and anterior frame over client with its narrow-end face support over client's face.	Decreases pressure and supports face when lying prone
10. Position pillow from client's head across client's legs. Lay sheepskin pad on top of client, if desired. Remove covering linens.	Provides comfort pads Stabilizes legs during turn Decreases pressure on legs while lying prone

Action	Rationale
11. Lock anterior frame onto bolt on posterior frame using provided lock nut and screw down tightly (Fig. 7.4.1); fasten foot of anterior frame by tightening lock nut.	Secures anterior frame to posterior frame to prevent client fall during turning
12. Check client's legs and feet for proper positioning between the frames.	Prevents injury of legs and feet within frame during turning
13. Have client grasp anterior frame (if client is unable to do so secure arms and chest with the safety straps [Fig. 7.4.2] for added security).	Provides added support during turn Decreases anxiety
14. Remove furniture in turning area.	Ensures that turn will be unobstructed by objects

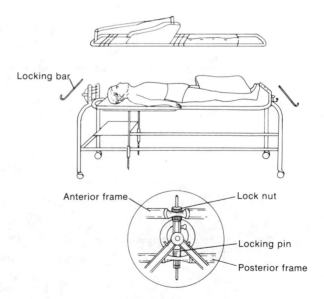

Figure 7.4.1

Action **Rationale**

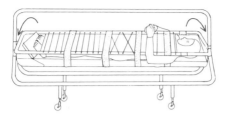

Figure 7.4.2

Action	Rationale
15. Check that both lock nuts are tight before turning client.	Ensures secure support during turn
16. Disengage locking pin and turn bed slightly; then complete the turn (Fig. 7.4.3).	Keeps bed disengaged until full turn can be effected
17. Turn frame until it locks automatically (frame enters locking pin when it is fully horizontal).	Indicates completion of safe turn
18. Unbolt top and bottom lock nuts, remove safety straps, and remove top frame.	Completes turning procedure

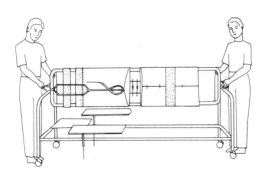

Figure 7.4.3

Action	Rationale
19. Apply cover linens as desired.	Promotes warmth and privacy
20. Assess vital signs immediately after the turning procedure and 15 minutes later.	Determines client tolerance to the prone position
A CHANGE IN THE CLIENT'S LEVEL OF MOBILITY OR ABILITY TO PERCEIVE SENSATIONS AFTER TURNING SHOULD BE REPORTED TO DOCTOR. REPORT ANY COMPLAINTS THAT BACK WAS TWISTED OR TURNED DURING MOVE.	May indicate client injury
21. Position bedside table with reading materials, as desired.	Provides distraction while client is in prone position

Assisting Client on Stryker Frame with Bedpan

Action	Rationale
22. Place client in supine position.	Exposes section of linen on which buttocks rest
23. Release and remove center section of posterior frame by removing the hooks or bands from sides of frame.	
24. Place bedpan on top of plastic bed saver or folded towel; loosen linen and slide bedsaver and bedpan underneath client (on some beds, linen might be a part of the removable section).	Protects bed linens
25. Place bedpan table, if available, under pan or hold pan securely to client.	Supports bedpan
26. If bedpan table is available, step away from bed but remain close by.	Provides privacy for client but also reassures that assistance is near
27. When client is finished, remove bedpan; clean	Promotes cleanliness and comfort

Action	Rationale
client's buttocks and re-move linen saver; reattach center section of frame securely.	Restores support of posterior frame
28. Use room deodorizer, if desired.	
29. Position linens for client comfort or turn client, if it is time.	

Evaluation

Goals met, partially met, or unmet?

Desired Outcomes (sample)

Client is in good alignment, with mobility and sensation at same level as before turn.

Skin is warm with capillary refill less than 5 seconds; skin integrity is maintained, with no bruises or abrasions.

Respirations are even and nonlabored; pulse is within normal range after turn is completed.

Client does not verbalize extreme anxiety, fear of procedure, or refusal to be turned.

Documentation

The following should be noted on the client's chart:

- Condition requiring use of frame
- Client-teaching performed and additional teaching needs, if any
- Vital signs before and after procedure
- Position of client after transfer
- Client comfort level and tolerance of turning procedure and questions or concerns expressed
- Amount of time spent on each side
- Security of locks holding bed in position
- Condition of skin and bony areas
- Bowel or bladder elimination

Sample Documentation

DATE	TIME	
12/3/94	1230	Client transferred to Stryker frame with backboard in place. Teaching done regarding use of anterior frame to turn. Client turned to remove backboard and extra linens, then turned back to supine position. Tolerated procedure with no injury or physical distress and minimal anxiety expressed or noted.
	1430	Client passed soft brown stool and urine; no straining noted. Skin on sacral area without redness. Client tolerated turning process with no significant changes in status assessment.

🖐 Range-of-Motion Exercises

⊠ Equipment

- No equipment needed except gloves, if contact with body fluids is likely

Purpose

Maintains present level of functioning and mobility of extremity involved

Prevents contractures and shortening of musculoskeletal structures

Prevents vascular complications of immobility

Facilitates comfort

Assessment

Assessment should focus on the following:

Medical diagnosis

Doctor's orders for indications of specific restrictions

Present range of motion of each extremity

Physical and mental ability of client to perform the activity

History of factors that contraindicate or limit the type or amount of exercise

Nursing Diagnoses

The nursing diagnoses may include the following:

Altered mobility related to unhealed fracture

Potential for skin breakdown related to prolonged bedrest

Planning

Key Goals and Sample Goal Criteria

The client will

Maintain present level of functioning of joints that are not immobilized by cast

Avoid complications of immobility, such as:
- Decubitus ulcers or pressure areas
- Contractures
- Decreased peristalsis
- Constipation and fecal impaction
- Orthostatic hypotension
- Pulmonary embolism (evidenced by chest pain, dyspnea, wheezing, increased heart rate)
- Thrombophlebitis (evidenced by redness, heat, swelling, or pain in a local area)

Special Considerations

A client able to perform all or part of a range-of-motion exercise program should be allowed to do so and should be properly instructed. Observe the client performing activities of daily living to determine the limitations of movement and the need, if any, for passive range-of-motion exercise to various joints.

When performing a range-of-motion exercise, a joint should be moved only to the point of resistance, pain, or spasm, whichever comes first.

Consult doctor's orders before performing a range-of-motion exercise on a client with acute cardiac, vascular, or pulmonary problems or a client with musculoskeletal trauma and acute flare-ups of arthritis.

Geriatric

The presence of various chronic conditions in elderly clients requires the use of extra caution when performing range-of-motion exercises. Clients with chronic cardiopulmonary conditions should be observed closely during range-of-motion activity for respiratory difficulty, chest pain, and general discomfort.

Pediatric

Demonstrate the procedure using a doll; instruct the child to perform simple techniques on the doll.

Home Health
Instruct family members in performance of range-of-motion techniques to be used during periods between nurse visits.

Implementation

Action	Rationale
1. Wash hands.	Reduces microorganism transfer
2. Explain procedure to client.	Decreases anxiety
3. Provide for privacy.	Decreases embarrassment
4. Adjust bed to comfortable working height.	Prevents back and muscle strain in nurse
5. Move client to side of bed closest to you.	Facilitates use of proper body mechanics

6. Beginning at top and moving downward on one side of body at a time, perform passive (or instruct client through active) range-of-motion exercises of joints in each of the following areas, as applicable for client (Fig. 7.5.1):
  a. head and neck
  b. shoulder
  c. elbow
  d. wrist
	Exercises all joint areas

HEAD–NECK

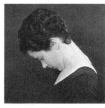 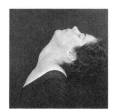

Flexion   Extension

Figure 7.5.1

HEAD–NECK (*continued*)

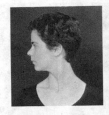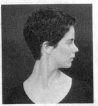

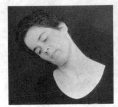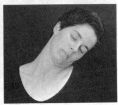

Lateral Flexion

VERTICAL COLUMN

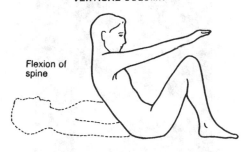

Flexion of spine

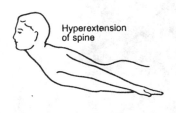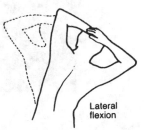

Hyperextension of spine

Lateral flexion

SHOULDER

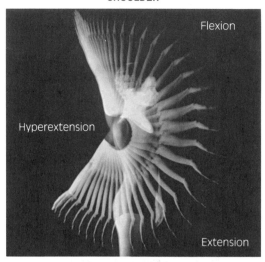

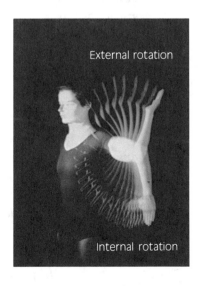

SHOULDER (*continued*)

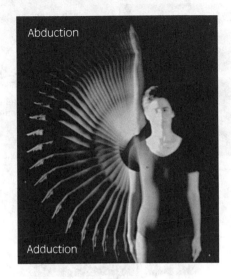

Abduction

Adduction

ELBOW

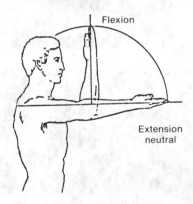

Flexion

Extension
neutral

FOREARM

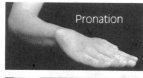

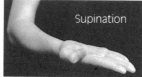

WRIST

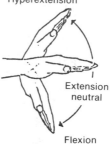

FINGERS

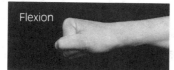

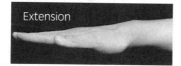

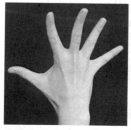

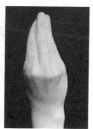

Abduction   Adduction

HIPS

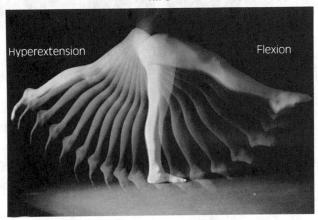

Hyperextension Flexion

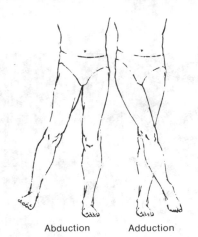

Abduction   Adduction

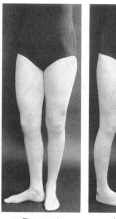 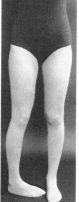

External
rotation

Internal
rotation

KNEE

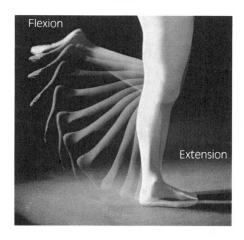

Flexion

Extension

KNEE (*continued*)

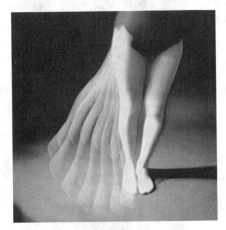

Circumduction

TOES

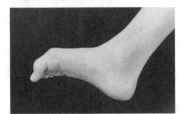

Flexion

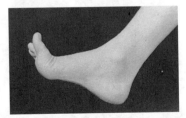

Extension

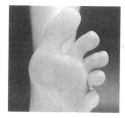
Abduction

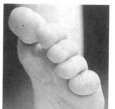
Adduction

ANKLES

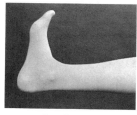
Dorsiflexion

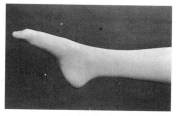
Plantar flexion

Figure 7.5.1 (end)

e. hand
f. fingers
g. hips
h. knees
i. ankles
j. feet
k. toes
l. spine

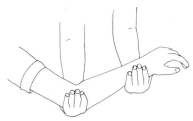

Figure 7.5.2

TABLE 7.5 Descriptions of Range-of-motion Maneuvers

Maneuver	Description	Applicable Areas
Flexion	Bending joint at point of normal anatomical fold	All areas
Extension	Straightening joint into as straight a line as possible	All areas
Hyperextension	Straightening joint into extension, then moving past that point	Neck, fingers, wrists, toes, spine
Abduction	Moving extremity away from midline of body	Arms, legs, fingers, toes
Adduction	Moving extremity toward midline of body	Arms, legs, fingers, toes
Internal rotation	Rotating extremity toward midline of body	Hips, ankles, shoulders
External rotation	Rotating extremity away from midline	Hips, ankles, shoulders
Supination	Turning palm upward	Hands
Pronation	Turning palm downward	Hands
Circumduction	Rotating extremity in a complete circle	Shoulders, hips

Action	Rationale
7. As maneuvers are performed, support body areas being exercised by holding the following in the rounded palms of your hands (Fig. 7.5.2): – Arms at elbow and wrist – Legs at knee and ankle – Head at occipital area and chin	Prevents pulling and careless handling of extremity, which could result in pain or injury
8. Slowly move each extremity through full range of positions 3 to 10 times or as tolerated by client (see Table 7.5 for definition of each motion).	Provides adequate exercise of extremity
9. Observe client for signs of exertion or discomfort while performing range-of-motion exercises.	Alerts nurse for cues to terminate activity
10. Replace covers and position client for comfort and in proper body alignment.	Promotes comfort
11. Assess vital signs.	Provides follow-up data regarding effects of activity on client
12. Lift side rails, and place bed in position.	Prevents falls
13. Place call light within reach.	Facilitates communication
14. Wash hands.	Reduces microorganism transfer

Evaluation

Goals met, partially met, or unmet?

Desired Outcomes (sample)

Client's present range of motion is being maintained.
Range of motion of left elbow increased from 30- to 40-degree flexion.
No signs or symptoms of complications of immobility are present.

Documentation

The following should be noted on the client's chart:

- Areas on which range-of-motion exercises are performed
- Areas of limited range of motion and the degree of limitation
- Areas of passive versus active range of motion
- Reports of pain or discomfort
- Observations of physiologic intolerance to activity

Sample Documentation

DATE	TIME	
11/12/94	1400	Passive range-of-motion exercises performed on all extremities. Client has full range of motion of all joints and reports no pain or discomfort during exercises. No signs of intolerance of activity.

Crutch Walking

☒ Equipment

- Appropriate-size crutches
- Safety belt (gait belt)
- Shoes
- House coat
- Eyeglasses or contacts, if worn

Purpose

Facilitates mobility and activity for client

Increases self-esteem by decreasing dependence

Decreases physical stress on weight-bearing joints and unhealed skeletal injuries

Assessment

Assessment should focus on the following:

Medical diagnosis

Doctor's orders for activity restrictions

Type of crutch–gait movement indicated

Neuromuscular status (muscle tone, strength, and range of motion of arms, legs, and trunk; gait pattern; body alignment when walking; ability to maintain balance)

Focal point of injury and reason for crutches

Measurement parameters of crutches

Ability of client to comprehend instructions regarding use of crutches

Additional learning needs of client

Nature of walking area (*i.e.*, presence of clutter, scatter rugs, adequacy of floor for good traction, proximity of adequate rest area)

Nursing Diagnoses

The nursing diagnoses may include the following:

Potential for physical injury related to unsteady gait pattern
Knowledge deficit regarding crutch-walking principles and
technique

Planning

Key Goals and Sample Goal Criteria

The client will

Experience no falls during crutch walking
Demonstrate correct crutch-walking techniques

Special Considerations

Crutch walking on slippery, cluttered surfaces and on stairs can
be hazardous. Clients should use railing of staircase (or walk
close to walls) during crutch walking.
Clients with visual deficits should always wear visual aids
when crutch walking.

Geriatric and Pediatric

Geriatric and pediatric clients are especially prone to injuries
from falls because of brittle or underdeveloped bones. Safety
belts should always be used when assisting these clients with
crutch walking.

Home Health

The client's home environment should be assessed carefully for
hazards and adequate space. Assist client with arrangement of
furniture and decorative items to eliminate hazards in the
home while client is on crutches.

Implementation

Action	Rationale
1. Wash hands.	Reduces microorganism transfer
2. Explain procedure to client, emphasizing that it	Decreases anxiety and frustration

Action	Rationale
will take time to learn techniques; stress safety and the importance of moving slowly initially; when providing explanations, include demonstrations.	Increases compliance Prevents injury
3. Assist client into shoes that are comfortable, nonskid, hard soled, and low heeled.	Prevents falls
4. Assist client into housecoat or loose, comfortable clothes.	Maintains privacy Facilitates comfort
5. Measure client for correct crutch fit: – Have client lie flat in bed with proper shoes on. – Measure from axillary pit outward 6 to 8 inches and from axillary pit to side of heel (Fig. 7.6.1). – Have client stand with elbows slightly flexed; measure distance between axillary pit and top of crutch to be sure a space at least the width of 2 or 3 fingers exists.	Prevents damage to brachial and radial nerves Prevents fall by measuring crutch height using shoes person usually wears Promotes correct body alignment Avoids damage to brachial plexus, which can result in paralysis of extremity
6. Lower height of bed, then lock wheels.	Prevents falls

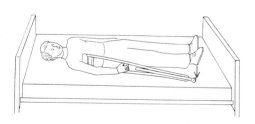

Figure 7.6.1

Action	**Rationale**
7. Slowly help client into sitting position; assess for dizziness, faintness, or decrease in orientation.	Prevents injury from sudden change in blood pressure when sitting up
8. Apply safety belt.	Prevents client injury
9. Assist client with maneuvers appropriate for type of gait and with other general crutch-walking techniques (steps 10 and 11). Initially, always have someone with client but allow greater independence as techniques are performed more proficiently and client demonstrates ability to crutch walk in all areas safely (encourage client to use rails and walk close to walls when climbing stairs).	Provides assistance and ensures client safety
10. In general, demonstrate correct technique for type of gait to be used before client gets out of bed; have client demonstrate these techniques to you; reinforce instructions and make corrections as client performs crutch walking.	Permits concentration on maneuvers before client attempts them.
11. Begin demonstrating gait technique from tripod position with crutches 6 inches to side and 6 inches to front of seat (Fig. 7.6.2).	Promotes stability and balance
a. Four-point gait: Advance right crutch, then left foot, then left crutch, then right foot (Fig. 7.6.3).	Places weight on legs while crutches provide stability
b. Three-point gait: Advance both crutches and affected extremity at same time; advance	Places weight on unaffected leg and crutches, with light weight on affected leg

Action   **Rationale**

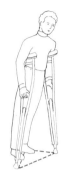

Figure 7.6.2

unaffected extremity
(Fig. 7.6.4).

c. Two-point gait: Places partial weight on both
    Advance right crutch   legs
    and left foot together,
    then left crutch and
    right foot together
    (Fig. 7.6.5).

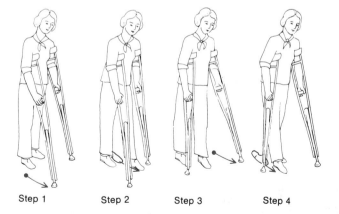

Step 1   Step 2   Step 3   Step 4

Figure 7.6.3

Action	**Rationale**

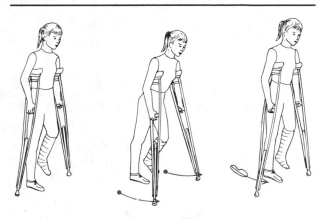

Figure 7.6.4

d. Swing-to or swing-through gait: Advance both crutches at same time and swing body forward to crutches or past them (Fig. 7.6.6).	Provides additional stability for clients with bilateral leg disability

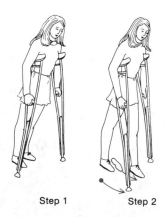

Step 1   Step 2

Figure 7.6.5

Action	Rationale

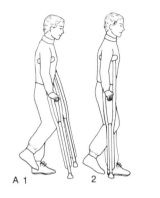 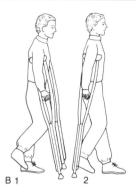

A 1   2   B 1   2

Figure 7.6.6

12. Demonstrate correct techniques for sitting, standing, and stair walking with crutches (Display 7.6), Figures 7.6.7 and 7.6.8.

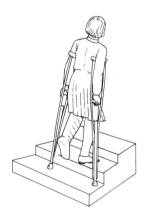 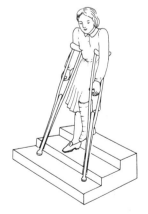

Figure 7.6.7   **Figure 7.6.8**

Action	Rationale
illustrate stair walking with crutches.	

Display 7.6 Techniques for General Crutch-walking Maneuvers

Moving From Sitting to Standing	*Moving From Standing to Sitting*
– Place both crutches in hand on affected side (holding crutches together and even).	– Inch back until backs of lower legs touch bed or center of chair.
– Push down on stable support base (locked bed, arm or seat of chair) with free hand, put weight on stronger leg, and lift body.	– Hold crutches together in hand on unaffected side.
– Stand with a straight back, bearing weight on stronger leg and crutches.	– Begin easing down onto chair or bed with back straight, using crutches and stronger leg as support.
– Place both crutches on same level as feet.	– When close enough, gently hold onto arm of chair and complete the move.
– Advance unaffected leg to next step while bearing down on crutch handles.	
– Pull affected leg and crutches up to step while bearing weight on stronger leg.	

Walking Up Stairs (see Fig. 7.6.7)	*Walking Down Stairs (see Fig. 7.6.8)*
– Place both crutches on same level as feet.	– Place both crutches on same level as feet.
– Advance unaffected leg to next step while bearing down on crutch handles.	– Shift weight to stronger leg.
– Pull affected leg and crutches up to step while bearing weight on stronger leg.	– Lower affected leg and crutches to next step while bearing down on crutch handles.
	– Advance unaffected leg last.

Action	Rationale
13. Observe return demonstrations and help client practice until proficiency in crutch walking is attained (provide intermittent praise and encouragement); encourage rest between activity periods, assisting client, as needed, to a comfortable position.	Ensures procedure has been learned Provides avenue for feedback
14. Wash hands and properly store equipment.	Reduces microorganism transfer Maintains order

Evaluation

Goals met, partially met, or unmet?

Desired Outcomes (sample)

Client does not fall while on crutches.
Client demonstrates correct techniques for crutch-walking maneuvers.

Documentation

The following should be noted on the client's chart:

• Gait pattern used
• Crutch height
• Steadiness of gait and amount of assistance needed
• Distance walked by client
• Client tolerance to procedure
• Teaching done and additional learning needs of client

Sample Documentation

DATE	TIME	
4/28/94	1200	Client completed first week of crutch walking. Efficient with use of four-point gait pattern. Steady with good body alignment while on crutches. Walking entire hall length three times per day without fatigue or reports of discomfort. Has not begun stair walking.

Cast Care

✖ Equipment

- Washcloth
- Towel
- Soap
- Basin of warm water
- Linen savers for bed
- Pen
- Roll of 1- or 2-inch tape
- Pillows wrapped in linen saver or plastic bag
- Bed linens with pull/turn sheet
- Sterile gloves

Purpose

Prevents neurovascular impairment of areas encircled by cast
Maintains cast for immobilization of treatment area
Prevents infection

Assessment

Assessment should focus on the following:

Medical diagnosis
Doctor's orders for special care of treatment area
Client's report of pain or discomfort
Integumentary status
Neurovascular indicators of health of extremities, particularly
of areas distal to cast: color, temperature, capillary refill, sensation, pulse quality, ability to move toes or fingers
Indicators of infection (foul odor from cast, pain, fever, edema,
extreme warmth over a particular area of cast)
Indicators of complications of immobility: decubitus ulcers or
pressure areas; reduced joint movement; decreased peristalsis,
constipation, and fecal impaction; signs of pulmonary em-

bolism (chest pain, dyspnea, wheezing, increased heart rate); signs of thrombophlebitis (redness, heat, swelling, or pain in local area)

Nursing Diagnoses

The nursing diagnoses may include the following:

Potential for neurovascular complications related to edema, bleeding, nerve compression, or vascular compression
Lack of knowledge regarding general cast care

Planning

Key Goals and Sample Goal Criteria
The client will

Have no undetected signs of developing neurovascular complications
Verbalize actions necessary for cast maintenance by discharge

Special Considerations
If client experienced traumatic injury to the extremity in the cast, watch for a sudden decrease in capillary refill and loss of pulse during first 24 to 48 hours due to development of compartment syndrome.

Geriatric
Watch client closely during initial gait retraining: additional weight of cast could cause lack of balance and result in stress and fracture of fragile bones.

Home Health
Inform the homebound client that a wet cast may be dried with a hair dryer on the LOW setting.

Implementation

Action	Rationale
1. Wash hands.	Reduces microorganism transfer

Action	Rationale
2. Place pull/turn sheet and linen savers on bed before client returns from casting area (place these items on bed with each linen change).	Promotes ease of positioning client Prevents unnecessary pain when moving client
3. Explain procedure to client, emphasizing importance of maintaining elevation of extremity, of not handling wet cast, and of frequent assessment; instruct client not to insert anything between cast and extremity.	Decreases anxiety Increases compliance Prevents injury and infection
4. Don gloves.	Avoids contact with body fluids
5. Provide for privacy.	Decreases embarrassment
6. Handle casted extremity or body area with *palms* of hands for first 24 to 36 hours, until cast is fully dry.	Avoids dents that could ultimately result in edema and pressure areas
7. If cast is slow to dry, place small fan directly facing cast (about 24 inches away). DO NOT PLACE LINEN OVER CAST UNTIL CAST IS DRY.	Enhances speed of drying Allows air to circulate and assist in drying cast
8. If cast is on extremity, elevate on pillows (cover pillow with linen savers or plastic bags) so that normal curvatures created with casting are maintained.	Prevents edema Enhances venous return Prevents soiling of pillows Prevents flattened areas on cast as it dries and prevents pressure areas
9. Wash excess antimicrobial agents (such as povidone) from skin. Rinse, and pat dry.	Allows for clear skin and vascular assessment
10. Perform skin and neurovascular assessment (every ½ to 1 hour for first 24 hours, every 2 hours	Detects signs of abnormal neurovascular function, such as vascular or nerve compression

Action	Rationale
for next 24 hours, then every 4 hours thereafter); if cast is on extremity, compare to opposite extremity.	Suggests possible nature of neurovascular deficit
11. If breakthrough bleeding is noted on cast, circle area, then write date and time on cast; if moderate to large amount of bleeding, notify doctor (otherwise, follow orders as written for bleeding).	Provides baseline data for amount of bleeding Facilitates early intervention and prevention of complications
12. Assess for signs of infection under cast; obtain temperature.	Detects infectious process at early stage
13. Reposition client every 2 hours; if client has body or spica cast, secure three assistants to help turn client.	Prevents client discomfort Makes turning quick, efficient, and safe
14. Provide back and skin care frequently.	Prevents skin breakdown
15. If flaking of cast around edges is noted, remove flakes, pull stockinette over cast edges, and tape down.	Prevents accumulation of particles inside cast, which cause infection
16. Place client with leg or body cast on fracture pan for elimination: for clients with good bowel and bladder control, temporarily line edge of cast close to perineal area with plastic; if client has little or no elimination control (*e.g.*, some pediatric and elderly clients), maintain plastic lining on cast edges and change once a shift.	Provides for elimination needs Prevents soiling of cast
17. Perform range-of-motion exercises on all joint areas every 4 hours (except where contraindicated).	

Action	Rationale
18. Instruct client to cough and deep breathe and reposition client (within guidelines for orders) every 2 hours.	Prevents pneumonia, decubitus ulcers, and other complications of immobility
19. Lift side rails and lower height of bed.	Prevents falls
20. Place call light within reach.	Facilitates communication
21. Restore or discard equipment properly.	Removes waste and clutter
22. Wash hands.	Removes microorganisms

Evaluation

Goals met, partially met, or unmet?

Desired Outcomes (sample)

Signs of neurovascular deficits are detected early.
Client verbalizes actions necessary for cast maintenance by discharge.

Documentation

The following should be noted on the client's chart:

- Data from neurovascular assessment
- Abnormal data indicating inflammation or infection
- Indicators of complications of immobility
- Frequency of body alignment and repositioning and positions into which client is placed
- Frequency and nature of skin care given
- Frequency of coughing and deep breathing exercises performed
- Frequency and nature of range-of-motion exercises performed
- Teaching completed and additional teaching needs of client

Sample Documentation

DATE	TIME	
12/19/94	1030	Fourth hour since return of client from casting room. Left leg full-length cast remains cold and wet. Toes of both left and right feet are pink, warm, and dry. Client able to wiggle toes and identify which toe is being touched. Cough and deep breathing done. Repositioned every 2 hours. Active range-of-motion exercise performed to all extremities except left leg.

☝ Traction Maintenance

☒ Equipment

- Alcohol wipes
- Antimicrobial agent for cleaning pins (skeletal tractions)
- One sterile gauze pad (2×2 or 4×3) for each traction pin
- Sterile gloves
- Sterile dressings, if needed
- Equipment for supporting body positioning *e.g.*, trochanter roll, pillows, sandbag, footboard)
- Traction setup

Purpose

Maintains traction apparatus with appropriate counterbalance
Prevents infection at site of insertion of traction pins

Assessment

Assessment should focus on the following:

Medical diagnosis
Doctor's orders for traction weight and pin care
Type of skin traction or skeletal traction
Status of weights, ropes, and pulleys
Reports of pain or discomfort
Integumentary status
Neurovascular indicators distal to pin sites (skin color and temperature, capillary refill, sensation, presence of pulse, ability to move toes or fingers)
Indicators of complications of immobility: decubitus ulcers or pressure areas; contractures; decreased peristalsis, constipation, and fecal impaction; signs of pulmonary embolism (chest pain, dyspnea, wheezing, increased heart rate); signs of thrombophlebitis (redness, heat, swelling, or pain in local area)

Nursing Diagnoses

The nursing diagnoses may include the following:

Potential for infection-related disrupted skin integrity at insertion site of metal pin of skeletal traction

Potential for complications of immobility related to bedrest associated with spinal fracture

Planning

Key Goals and Sample Goal Criteria

The client will

Not develop infection from pin site, as evidenced by absence of redness, swelling, pain, discharge, and odor at site

Not develop complications of immobility, as evidenced by absence of signs and symptoms of complications such as decubitus ulcers, thrombophlebitis, and so forth

Special Considerations

If weights do not swing freely, traction can be counterproductive.

Assess status of weights every 1 to 2 hours and after moving client.

Geriatric

Elderly clients are particularly prone to the development of broken skin integrity when they are bedridden and not repositioned frequently; this tendency is due to a decreased amount of subcutaneous fat and to skin that is less elastic, thinner, drier, and more fragile than that of a younger person.

Pediatric

Arrange for quiet play activities, of appropriate developmental level, to occupy child during confinement. Include child in moving procedure (*e.g.,* by letting child count aloud to time movement).

Home Health

When the homebound client is mobile, with intermittent traction on an extremity, install traction setup over a door with a measured source of weight (*e.g.,* flour bag with sand, rocks, bricks).

Implementation

Action	Rationale
1. Wash hands.	Reduces microorganism transfer
2. Explain procedure to client, emphasizing importance of maintaining counterbalance and position.	Decreases anxiety
3. Provide for privacy.	Decreases embarrassment
4. Assess traction setup (Fig. 7.8): – Weights hanging freely and not touching bed or floor – Ordered amount of weight applied – Ropes moving freely through pulleys – All knots tight in ropes and away from pulleys – Pulleys free of linens	Ensures accurate counterbalance and function of traction

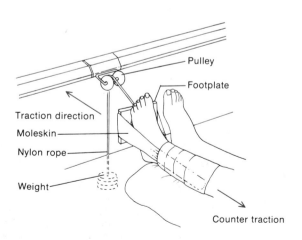

Figure 7.8

Action	Rationale
5. Check client position (client's head should be near head of bed and properly aligned).	Maintains proper counter-balance
6. Assess skin for signs of pressure areas or friction under skin traction belts.	Detects early signs of skin breakdown
7. Assess neurovascular status of extremity distal to traction.	Detects neurovascular complications
8. Assess site at and around pin for redness, edema, discharge, or odor.	Determines presence of infection
9. Wash hands.	Reduces microorganism transfer
10. Don gloves.	Prevents exposure to body fluids
11. Wash, rinse, and dry skin thoroughly; if permissible, remove skin traction periodically to wash under skin (check doctor's order and agency policy).	Promotes circulation to skin
12. Discard gloves, wash hands, and don sterile gloves.	Prevents contamination
13. Cleanse pin site and complete site care using sterile technique.	Prevents infection
14. Discard gloves and wash hands.	Removes microorganisms
15. Perform range-of-motion exercises on all joint areas, except those contraindicated, every 4 hours.	Prevents pneumonia, decubitus ulcers, and complications of immobility
16. Instruct client to cough and deep breathe and reposition client (within guidelines for orders) every 2 hours; use trochanter rolls and footboard to prevent internal and external hip rotation and footdrop.	Prevents complications related to improper positioning
17. Lift side rails.	Prevents falls

Action	Rationale
18. Place call light within reach.	Facilitates communication
19. Wash hands.	Reduces microorganism transfer

Evaluation

Goals met, partially met, or unmet?

Desired Outcomes (sample)

No redness, swelling, pain, discharge, or odor occurs at pin site. There is no evidence of complications of immobility.

Documentation

The following should be noted on the client's chart:

- Type of traction and amount of weight used
- Status of ropes, pulleys, and weights
- Body alignment of client
- Repositioning (frequency and last position)
- Pin care given
- Skin care given
- Coughing and deep breathing exercises performed
- Range-of-motion exercises performed
- Client teaching completed and additional teaching needs of client

Sample Documentation

DATE	TIME	
10/19/94	1030	Maintains intermittent pelvic traction with 20 pounds of weight. Traction removed twice this shift for client to go to restroom. Skin in pelvic area clean, warm, pink, and dry. Range-of-motion exercises of upper and lower extremities performed by client every 4 hours. Doing own coughing and deep breathing every 2 hours; breath sounds clear bilaterally.

Antiembolism Hose/Pneumatic Compression Device Application

☒ Equipment

- Pneumatic compression equipment with comfort stockings or hose

or

- Antiembolic hose
- Washcloth
- Towel
- Soap
- Basin of warm water
- Tape measure (if not included in package)

Purpose

Promotes venous blood return to heart by maintaining pressure on capillaries and veins

Prevents development of venous thrombosis secondary to stagnant circulation

Assessment

Assessment should focus on the following:

Medical diagnosis

Doctor's orders for hose length and frequency of application

Reports of pain or discomfort of lower extremities

Skin status of legs and feet

Neurovascular indicators of lower extremities (skin color and temperature, capillary refill, sensation, pulse presence and quality)

Indicators of venous disorders of lower extremities (redness, heat, swelling, or pain in local area)

Nursing Diagnoses

The nursing diagnoses may include the following:

Potential for decreased venous return related to prolonged immobility

Potential for decreased circulation related to lack of knowledge regarding application of hose

Planning

Key Goals and Sample Goal Criteria

The client will

Demonstrate no signs of venous thrombosis, as evidenced by absence of pain, redness, edema, and heat of lower extremities, prior to discharge

Demonstrate correct procedure for application and maintenance of hose within 48 hours of surgery

State two ways to reduce chances of developing venous thrombosis

Special Considerations

Clients with known or suspected peripheral vascular disorders should not wear hose because thrombus dislodgment may occur.

Poor maintenance of hose could result in circulatory restriction; hose must remain free of wrinkles, rolls, or kinks.

Geriatric

Elderly clients are particularly prone to development of venous disorders of lower extremities because of age-related physiological changes that occur in the tissue of veins. In addition, chronic cardiac and peripheral vascular dysfunctions also reduce venous return.

Implementation

Action	Rationale
1. Wash hands.	Reduces microorganism transfer
2. Explain procedure to client, emphasizing importance of	Decreases anxiety Increases compliance

Action	Rationale
maintaining hose on extremity for specified amount of time and of wearing hose properly.	
3. Provide for privacy.	Decreases embarrassment
4. Measure for appropriate-size hose according to package directions (large, medium, or small). *or* obtain vinyl sleeves and comfort stockings/hose.	Promotes proper functioning of hose Prevents reduced circulation to legs
5. Wash, rinse, and dry legs; apply light talcum powder, if desired.	Promotes comfort Promotes clean, dry skin
6. Turn hose (except foot portion) inside out.	Promotes proper application of hose
7. Place foot of hose over client's toes and foot; using both hands, slide hose up leg until completely on (smooth and straighten hose as it is pulled up); do not turn top of hose down.	Applies hose, making certain that kinks and wrinkles are smoothed out Prevents tourniquet effect
8. Apply second hose in same manner.	

Pneumatic Compression Device

9. Slide vinyl surgical sleeve over each calf (Fig. 7.9) *or* apply Velcro-secured vinyl compression hose by placing open hose under thigh and leg with knee-opening site under the popliteal area.	Places source of intermittent compression over the veins of the extremities
10. Establish the vinyl hose by overlapping the edges and securing the Velcro connectors.	Establishes air pump source; prepares unit for function
11. Turn the power on to the unit.	

Action   **Rationale**

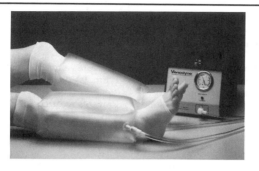

Figure 7.9

Action	Rationale
12. Monitor several inflation/deflation compression cycles.	Permits early detection of excessive compression
13. Replace covers.	Provides privacy and warmth
14. Observe extremities every 2 to 3 hours to assess circulation and hose placement.	Prevents complications
15. Remove hose twice a day for 20 minutes (ideally during morning and evening care).	Allows for skin aeration and reassessment
16. Wash hands and restore equipment.	Reduces microorganism transfer Maintains organized environment

Evaluation

Goals met, partially met, or unmet?

Desired Outcomes (sample)

By end of day

Client states two ways to reduce risk of developing venous thrombosis.

Client remains free of signs of venous thrombosis throughout confinement.

Documentation

The following should be noted on the client's chart:

- Size and length of hose applied
- Lower extremity skin color, temperature, sensation, capillary refill
- Status of pulses in lower extremities
- Presence of pain or discomfort in lower extremities
- Removal of hose twice daily
- Client teaching completed and additional teaching needs of client

Sample Documentation

DATE	TIME	
4/29/94	0830	Full-length embolic hose applied to lower legs—size, large/long. Skin of both lower extremities warm. No tears or abrasions noted. Toes pink with 2-second capillary refill. Bilateral pedal pulses 2+. Client stated purpose of hose and correctly related care measures.

Continuous Passive
Motion Device

☒ Equipment

- Continuous passive motion (CPM) device
- Softgoods kit (single patient use)
- Tape measure
- Goniometer

Purpose

Increases range of motion
Decreases effects of immobility
Stimulates healing of the articular cartilage
Reduces adhesions and swelling

Assessment

Assessment should focus on the following:

Doctor's orders for degrees of flexion and extension
Neurovascular status of extremity prior to start of CPM
Presence of pulses and capillary refill in affected extremity
Skin color and temperature, sensation, and movement of extremity
Reports of pain or discomfort

Nursing Diagnoses

The nursing diagnoses may include the following:

Alteration in physical mobility related to surgical intervention
Potential alteration in peripheral tissue perfusion related to surgical intervention and immobility

Planning

Key Goals and Sample Goal Criteria

The client will

Remain free of contractures
Maintain maximum mobility of extremities
Demonstrate increased tolerance to CPM device until prescribed
  goal is attained

Special Considerations

Geriatric

Elderly clients are particularly prone to the development of broken skin when they are immobilized.

Pediatric

Explain the CPM device clearly, demonstrating with a doll or stuffed animal.
Arrange for quiet play activities that are developmentally appropriate.

Implementation

Action	Rationale
1. Wash hands.	Reduces microorganism transfer
Organize equipment.	Promotes efficiency
Apply softgoods to CPM device (Fig. 7.10.1).	Prevents friction to extremity during motion
2. Check doctor's order for degrees of flexion and extension. Speed will be determined by patient comfort. Begin with a midpoint setting.	May change on a daily or per shift basis as the patient progresses
3. Explain procedure to client.	Decreases anxiety and facilitates cooperation
4. Using the tape measure, determine the distance between the gluteal crease and the popliteal space.	Determines the distance to adjust the Thigh Length Adjustment knobs on the CPM device
5. Measure the length of client's leg from the knee to ¼ inch beyond the bottom of the foot.	Determines the distance to adjust the position of the footplate

Action   **Rationale**

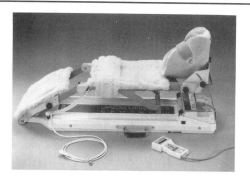

Figure 7.10.1

6. Position the client in the middle of the bed with the extremity in a slightly abducted position.

    Promotes proper body alignment
Prevents CPM device from exerting pressure on opposite extremity
Prepares client for therapy

7. Elevate client's leg and place in padded CPM device (Fig. 7.10.2).

8. Note proper anatomical placement of device: Client's knee should be at the hinged joint of the machine.

    Improper positioning of the device may cause injury

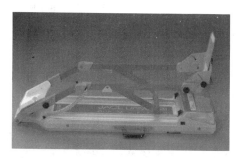

Figure 7.10.2

Action	Rationale
9. Adjust the footplate to maintain the client's foot in a neutral position. Make certain that the leg is neither internally nor externally rotated.	Improper positioning of the device may cause injury
10. Apply the soft restraining straps under CPM device and around extremity loosely enough to fit several fingers under it.	The soft restraints maintain the extremity in position. Allowing several fingers to fit under the restraint prevents pressure from restraint strap on affected extremity
11. Turn unit on at main power switch. Set controls to levels prescribed by physician.	Cannot adjust controls and setting unless power is on; prepares client for onset of therapeutic intervention
12. Instruct the client in the use of the GO/STOP button.	Client participates in care, thus decreasing anxiety
13. Set CPM device in the ON stage and press GO button (Fig. 7.10.3).	Initiates therapeutic intervention

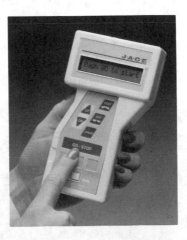

Figure 7.10.3

14. Determine angle of flexion when device has reached its greatest height using the goniometer. *Note*: If unit is not anatomical, there might be a slight difference between reading on the device and the actual angle of the patient's knee.

Evaluation

Goals met, partially met, or unmet?

Desired Outcomes (sample)

Client tolerates progressive increase in flexion and extension with CPM device.

Client demonstrates increasing mobility of affected extremity.

Documentation

The following should be noted on the client's chart:

• Onset of therapy
• Tolerance of procedure
• Degree of extension and flexion and speed of machine
• Amount of time client used device
• Neurovascular status of extremity
• Successive therapeutic aids, immobilizer, etc.

Sample Documentation

DATE	TIME	
8/4/94	1100	CPM device applied to left leg at 0 degrees of extension and 35 degrees of flexion started at slow speed. Verified by goniometer. Patient instructed in use of GO/STOP button. Denies need for pain medication at this time. Padding to all soft tissue near CPM device. Call bell within reach.

(continued)

Sample Documentation   (continued)

DATE	TIME	
	1400	CPM device removed from left leg. Left lower extremity warm and dry to touch. Distal pulses are present, client denies numbness or tingling, no edema noted. Immobilizer applied.

Rest and Comfort

OVERVIEW

- Each individual's perception of pain is unique.
- Cultural background may have a great impact on a client's pain threshold and pain tolerance, as well as on the client's expression of pain. The nurse must consider cultural impacts on the pain experience when planning care.
- Heat and cold may have special cultural significance for some clients, (Asians or Hispanics, for example), who classify conditions accordingly and expect corresponding treatments. (see Table 8.1)
- Nurses must be sensitive to alternative pain relief measures used by clients and the cultural significance of those measures. Efforts should be made to reconcile religious rituals, herbal remedies, or other alternate treatments with the established medical plan to facilitate culturally sensitive care.

Jean Smith-Temple and Joyce Young Johnson:
Nurses' Guide to Clinical Procedures, Second Edition.© 1994
J. B. Lippincott Company

- The assessment of pain should include its location, duration, intensity and its precipitating, alleviating, and associated factors.
- Appropriate duration of treatment is essential for the therapeutic use of heat and cold.
- Cold therapy causes vasoconstriction; reduces local metabolism, edema, and inflammation; and induces local anesthetic effects.
- Heat therapy causes vasodilatation, relieves muscle tension, stimulates circulation, and promotes healing.
- **DANGER—ADDITIONAL TISSUE DAMAGE CAN RESULT IF:**
  - Excessive temperature is used (hot or cold)
  - Overexposure of site to treatment occurs
  - Electrical equipment is not checked for safety

TABLE 8.1 Hot–Cold Conditions*

Hot Conditions	Cold Conditions
Fever	Arthritis
Infections	Colds
Diarrhea	Indigestion
Constipation	Joint pain
Rashes	Menstrual period
Tenesmus	Ear ache
Ulcers	Cancer
Kidney problems	Tuberculosis
Skin ailments	Headache
Sore throat	Paralysis
Liver problems	Teething
	Rheumatism
	Pneumonia
	Malaria

*The usual treatment for hot–cold condition is thought to be use of a food or substance of the opposite temperature.

Aquathermia Pad

✖ Equipment

- Aquathermia module (K-module) with pad (K-pad)
- Overbed or bedside table
- Disposable gloves
- Pillowcase
- Distilled water
- Tape

Purpose

Stimulates circulation, thus providing nutrients to tissues
Reduces muscle tension

Assessment

Assessment should focus on the following:

Treatment order
Client's tolerance to last treatment
Status of treatment area (redness, tenderness, cleanliness, and
 dryness)
Temperature and pulse rate and rhythm
Degree of pain and position of comfort, if any
Mental status of client
Adequate functioning of heating device for proper functioning

Nursing Diagnoses

The nursing diagnoses may include the following:

Altered comfort related to joint pain

Planning

Key Goal and Sample Goal Criterion

The client will

State increased comfort after treatment

Special Considerations

Make sure lamp functions accurately and safely. DO NOT USE IF CORD IS FRAYED OR CRACKS ARE NOTED.

Schedule procedure when client can be assessed frequently.

IF A CLIENT IS CONFUSED OR UNABLE TO REMAIN ALONE WITH A HEATING DEVICE ON, REMAIN WITH THE CLIENT OR FIND SOMEONE TO DO SO.

Clients with decreased peripheral sensory perception, such as diabetics, must be monitored closely for heat overexposure.

Geriatric and Pediatric

Elderly and pediatric clients may be extremely sensitive to heat therapy. Assess more frequently because their skin is fragile.

Home Health

If a homebound client will be using a K-module when a nurse is not present, teach the client or family how to use the module safely.

 Transcultural

Determine cultural perspective regarding use of heat to treat the condition.

Discuss objections and incorporate hot/cold perception of illness and treatment.

Omit treatment if client objects, and consult physician.

Implementation

Action	Rationale
1. Wash hands and organize equipment.	Reduces microorganism transfer
	Promotes efficiency
2. Explain procedure to client.	Decreases anxiety and promotes cooperation
3. Place heating module on bedside or overbed table at	Facilitates flow of fluid

Action	Rationale
a level above the client's body level (Fig. 8.1).	
4. Fill module two thirds full with distilled water.	Enables unit to function properly
5. Turn module on low setting and allow water to begin circulating throughout the pad and tubing.	Detects leakage of fluid or improper functioning before initiating therapy
6. After water is fully circulating through the pad and tubing, check the pad with your hands to ascertain that it is warming.	Checks for proper functioning and heating of unit
7. Don disposable gloves, if indicated.	Decreases exposure to secretions
8. Place pillowcase over the heating pad and position pad on or (if an extremity) around treatment area.	Prevents direct skin contact with pad, minimizing danger of burn injury
9. If placement of pad needs to be secured, use tape. DO NOT USE PINS.	Prevents water leakage from possible puncture to pad

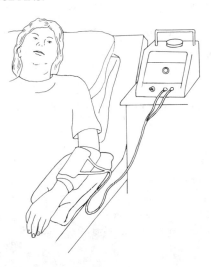

Figure 8.1

Action	Rationale
10. After 60 seconds, assess for heat intolerance by: – Observing client's facial gestures – Asking if heat is too warm – Noting any dizziness, faintness, or palpitations – Removing pad and assessing for redness or tenderness; readjust temperature if necessary	Prevents burn injury and complications of heat therapy
11. Replace pad and secure with tape, if needed.	Resumes treatment
12. Instruct client NOT to alter placement of pad or heating module and to call if heat becomes too warm.	Promotes client cooperation and continued optimum function of unit Prevents burn injury
13. Leave call light within reach.	Permits client communication
14. Recheck client every 5 minutes.	Prevents burn injury
15. After 20 minutes, turn module off and place pad on table with module.	Terminates treatment
16. Reposition client.	Facilitates comfort
17. Return equipment.	Maintains organized environment
18. Remove gloves and wash hands.	Reduces microorganism transfer

Evaluation

Goals met, partially met, or unmet?

Desired Outcome (sample)
Client verbalizes increased comfort after treatment.

Documentation

The following should be noted on the client's chart:

- Appearance of treatment area
- General response of client (weakness, faintness, palpitations, diaphoresis, extreme tenderness, if any)
- Duration of treatment
- Status of pain

Sample Documentation

DATE	TIME	
12/3/94	1400	K-module applied to right calf for 20 minutes. No redness, warmth, or tenderness to touch at treatment area. Vital signs stable during and after treatment.

✋ Cold Pack (Commercial) (8.2)

✋ Hot Pack (Commercial) (8.3)

❎ Equipment

- Prepackaged ice/heat pack
- Tape
- Disposable gloves, if indicated

Purpose

Promotes comfort: heat stimulates circulation; cold decreases edema and helps control minor bleeding

Assessment

Assessment should focus on the following:

Doctor's order and client's response to previous treatment, if used

Appearance of treatment area (edema, local bleeding)

Status of pain

Sensitivity of skin to cold/heat treatment

Nursing Diagnoses

The nursing diagnoses may include the following:

Altered comfort related to ankle sprain

Decreased tissue perfusion related to edema

Planning

Key Goals and Sample Goal Criteria

The client will

Verbalize decreased pain after treatment
Show no bleeding or hematoma at treatment site within 24
hours

Special Considerations

Schedule the treatment when the client can be checked every 5
to 10 minutes.
Do not use on clients with peripheral sensory deficits.

Geriatric and Pediatric
Elderly and young pediatric clients may require more frequent
checks because skin may be more fragile.

Home Health
At home, the client can use a self-sealing plastic bag as an ice
pack.

 Transcultural
Determine cultural perspective regarding hot/cold perception
of illness and appropriateness of treatment.
Incorporate client preference when possible.
Omit treatment if client objects and consult physician.

Implementation

Action	Rationale
1. Explain procedure to client.	Decreases anxiety and promotes cooperation
2. Wash hands and organize equipment.	Decreases microorganism transfer Promotes efficiency
3. Remove ice/heat pack from outer package, if present.	Provides access to pack
4. Break the inner seal: hold pack tightly in the center in upright position and squeeze. DO NOT USE	Activates chemical ingredients to form "cold–heat" pack

Action	Rationale
PACK IF LEAKING IS NOTED (CHEMICAL BURN MAY OCCUR).	
5. Lightly shake pack until the inner contents are lying in the lower portion of the pack.	Localizes activated chemicals
6. Place the pack lightly against treatment area.	Allows for gradual initiation of vasoconstrictive/dilatory effect
7. Remove pack and assess client for redness of skin or complaint of burning after 30 seconds.	Prevents burn injury
8. Replace pack snugly against the area if no problems are noted, and secure placement with tape.	Resumes treatment Stabilizes cold–heat pack
9. Reassess treatment area every 5 to 10 minutes by lifting the corners of the pack.	Monitors effects of treatment over time
10. After 15 to 20 minutes, remove the pack.	Terminates treatment Prevents burn injury from overexposure to heat/cold
11. Reposition client and raise side rails.	Facilitates comfort and safety

Evaluation

Goals met, partially met, or unmet?

Desired Outcomes (sample)

Client states that pain is decreased or relieved after treatment. Skin is intact without bleeding or hematoma after 24 hours.

Documentation

The following should be noted on the client's chart:

- Condition and appearance of treatment area before and after treatment

- Duration and kind of treatment
- Client tolerance to treatment

Sample Documentation

DATE   **TIME**

12/3/94   1000   Cold pack applied to edematous left knee for 20 min. Edema decreased from 2 to 1 cm. Left knee remains slightly bruised, pale, and cool to touch. Client tolerated procedure with minimal discomfort. States knee pain decreased.

✋ Ice Bag/Collar/Glove

✖ Equipment

- Ice bag/collar/glove
- Tape
- Disposable gloves
- Small towel or washcloth
- Ice chips

Purpose

Reduces local edema, bleeding, and hematoma formation
Decreases local pain sensation

Assessment

Assessment should focus on the following:

Treatment order and client's response to previous treatment, if used
Condition and appearance of treatment area (edema, local bleeding)
Status of pain

Nursing Diagnoses

The nursing diagnoses may include the following:

Decreased tissue perfusion related to edema
Altered comfort related to sprained right wrist
Potential tissue damage related to overexposure to cold

Planning

Key Goals and Sample Goal Criteria

The client will

Verbalize decreased discomfort after treatment
Show decreased or no bleeding/hematoma at site
Show decreased edema from 2+ to 0 cm within 36 hours

Special Consideration

Schedule the procedure when the client can be checked frequently.

Geriatric and Pediatric
Elderly and young pediatric clients may require more frequent checks because skin may be fragile.

Home Health
In the home, a self-sealing plastic bag may be used as an ice bag, if necessary.

 Transcultural
Consider cultural perspective and preference for hot/cold therapy.
Consult physician if client objects to planned therapy.

Implementation

Action	Rationale
1. Explain procedure to client.	Decreases anxiety
2. Wash hands and organize equipment.	Reduces microorganism transfer Promotes efficiency
3. Fill bag/collar/glove about three-fourths full with ice chips.	Provides cold surface area
4. Remove excess air from bag/collar/glove: – Place bag/collar/glove on flat surface. – Gently press until ice reaches the opening.	Improves functioning of pack

Action	Rationale
5. Contain ice securely by fastening end of the bag or collar; for plastic glove, tie end of glove itself.	Prevents water seepage
6. Cover with small towel or washcloth (if bag is made of a soft cloth exterior, this is not necessary).	Promotes comfort
7. Don disposable gloves, if needed.	Protects nurse from body fluids
8. Place bag/collar/glove on affected area and secure with tape.	Initiates vasoconstrictive treatment
9. Assess treatment area after several seconds for initial skin response to treatment and reassess every 5 to 10 minutes thereafter.	Prevents injury Monitors effect of treatment over time
10. Terminate treatment after 20 to 30 minutes.	Prevents local injury due to overexposure to treatment
11. Empty ice and water from bag or collar and place at bedside (dispose of glove).	Prevents unnecessary water spillage
12. Remove disposable gloves and wash hands.	Prevents spread of contaminants

Evaluation

Goals met, partially met, or unmet?

Desired Outcomes (sample)

Client states that pain is reduced or relieved after treatment.
Edema decreased from 2 cm to none.
No bleeding or hematoma is noted at treatment site.

Documentation

The following should be noted on the client's chart:

• Size, location, and appearance of treatment area
• Status of pain

- Duration of treatment
- Client tolerance to treatment

Sample Documentation

DATE	TIME	
12/3/94	1300	Ice bag applied to right wrist for 20 minutes. Edema decreased from 2 to 1 cm. Site slightly cool to touch after treatment, capillary refill 3 secs. Client reports relief of pain.

Heat Cradle and Heat Lamp

Equipment

- Heat lamp (with adjustable neck and 60-watt bulb)

or

- Heat cradle (25-watt bulb)
- Disposable gloves
- Washcloth
- Towels
- Soap
- Warm water

Purpose

Increases circulation
Promotes wound healing
Promotes general comfort
Assists with drying of wet cast

Assessment

Assessment should focus on the following:

Treatment order and response of client to previous treatment
Skin and appearance of wound (presence of edema, redness, heat, drainage)
Pulse and temperature
Mental status of client
Ability of client to maintain appropriate position without assistance
Degree of pain
Proper functioning and safety of heating device

Nursing Diagnoses

The nursing diagnoses may include the following:

Altered skin integrity related to episiotomy
Altered comfort: Related to disruption of skin integrity
Decreased tissue perfusion related to edema

Planning

Key Goals and Sample Goal Criteria

The client will

Show no redness, heat, edema, or discharge from site within 48 hours
Verbalize increased comfort or relief of pain within 24 hours after beginning treatment

Special Considerations

Make sure lamp functions accurately and safely. DO NOT USE IF CORD IS FRAYED OR CRACKS ARE NOTED.
Schedule timing of procedure so that client can be checked every 5 minutes. Do not leave confused clients unattended with heating apparatus.
Be sure hands are THOROUGHLY DRY when handling electrical equipment.

Geriatric and Pediatric

Assess elderly and pediatric clients frequently because of the fragile nature of their skin.
If client must be attended (as with many elderly clients) during treatment, FIND SOMEONE TO STAY WITH CLIENT DURING TREATMENT.

Home Health

At home, a mechanic's "trouble light" with appropriate wattage bulb may be used as a heat lamp. Teach client/family safety precautions for using light.

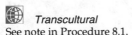 *Transcultural*

See note in Procedure 8.1.

Implementation

Action	Rationale
1. Explain procedure to client.	Reduces anxiety and promotes cooperation
2. Wash hands and organize equipment.	Reduces microorganism transfer Promotes efficiency
3. Don disposable gloves.	Prevents contamination from secretions
4. Position client for comfort and for optimum exposure of treatment area.	Facilitates optimum treatment results
5. With lamp turned off, place lamp 18 to 24 inches from wound to be treated.	Prevents accidental burns from placing lamp too close
6. Turn lamp on and observe client's response to the heat for 1 minute: – Observe facial and body gestures. – Observe wound area for redness. – Ask client if heat is too warm.	Determines initial response to treatment
7. Replace covers while keeping treatment area well exposed to the lamp; for heat cradle, place top sheet over cradle and client (Fig. 8.5). BE SURE THAT NEITHER CLOTHING NOR COVERS ARE TOUCHING THE BULB OF THE LAMP.	Provides privacy Reduces electrical hazard
8. Remove disposable gloves and wash hands; don gloves again, as needed (i.e., when in direct contact with possible body secretions).	Prevents microorganism transfer
9. Place call light within reach.	Permits communication Promotes prompt response to client needs

Action	**Rationale**

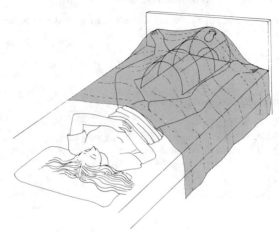

Figure 8.5

10. Assess client response to heat every 5 minutes.	Prevents complications to treatment
11. Remove lamp after 20 minutes.	Terminates treatment Prevents local burn injury from overexposure to heat
12. Reposition client and replace covers.	Promotes comfort and safety
13. Remove equipment from bedside and wash hands.	Prevents hazards and microorganism transfer

Evaluation

Goals met, partially met, or unmet?

Desired Outcomes (sample)

Site is clean, with no redness, edema, or drainage, within 48 hours.

Within 24 hours after beginning treatment, client verbalizes that pain is relieved or decreased.

Documentation

The following should be noted on the client's chart:

- Condition and appearance of wound or treatment area before and after treatment
- Pulse and temperature
- Duration and kind of treatment
- Status of pain

Sample Documentation

DATE	TIME	
12/3/94	1600	Heat lamp applied to perineal area for 20 minutes. Episiotomy site intact and dry with slight redness and 1-cm edema. Client reports no perineal pain.

🖐 Moist Clean Compresses (Warm/Cold)

☒ Equipment

- Towel
- Plastic-lined underpad
- Clean basin
- Bath thermometer
- Pack of 4 × 4-inch gauze pads
- Bath blanket
- Two forceps (optional)
- Two pairs of nonsterile gloves

Additional Equipment

- Warm compress
  - warmed solution, 43°C (110°F)
  - petroleum jelly
  - heating pad or aquathermia pad (optional)
  - distilled water (for aquathermia pad)
- Cold compress
  - solution cooled with ice, 15°C (59°F)
  - cotton-swab stick

Purpose

Promotes comfort
Decreases edema
Hot compress stimulates circulation and promotes localization of purulent matter in tissues
Cold compress reduces inflammation process and decreases local bleeding and hematoma formation

Assessment

Assessment should focus on the following:

Treatment order, type of solution to be used, and response of client to previous treatments

Appearance of skin and treatment area before and after treatment

Status of pain, bleeding, or edema

Nursing Diagnoses

The nursing diagnoses may include the following:

Altered comfort related to inflammation
Altered skin integrity related to abrasion
Decreased tissue perfusion related to hematoma

Planning

Key Goals and Sample Goal Criteria

The client will

Verbalize increased comfort within 1 hour after treatment
Show decreased redness at site within 3 days

Special Considerations

Schedule application of compresses when the client can be assessed at frequent intervals.

Determine with client the best body position for comfort and alignment.

If applying warm compresses, check heating device for safety and proper functioning.

If using aquathermia pad for warm compress, set up heating device according to the guidelines in Procedure 8.1.

Home Health

Warn client that a clothing iron should never be used as a heat source for a warm compress.

 Transcultural

See overview note about hot/cold and note Procedure 8.2.

Implementation

Action	Rationale
1. Explain procedure to client.	Decreases anxiety and promotes cooperation
2. Wash hands and organize equipment.	Reduces microorganism transfer
	Promotes efficiency
3. Place gauze into basin half-filled with ordered solution.	Saturates gauze with solution
4. Assist client into position.	Facilitates compress placement
5. Place plastic pad under treatment area.	Prevents soiling of linens
6. Drape client.	Provides privacy
7. Don gloves.	Reduces microorganism transfer
8. Remove and discard old dressings, if present.	Provides access to treatment site
9. Remove and discard old gloves and don new gloves.	Reduces microorganism transfer
10. If necessary, clean and dry treatment area.	Facilitates effectiveness of treatment
11. For warm compress, use swab stick to apply petroleum jelly to skin around the wound area.	Provides protection from burns
12. Wring one layer of wet gauze until it is dripless (may need forceps to wring warm compress).	Removes excess solution
13. Place compress on the wound for several seconds.	Initiates vasoconstrictive or vasodilatation therapy
14. Pick up edge of compress to observe initial skin response to therapy.	Allows assessment of skin for adverse responses to therapy
15. If no local skin reaction is noted, proceed to step 16; if local skin irritation is noted, allow solution to sit for a few minutes, then repeat steps 12 to 14.	Promotes cooling/warming of solution

Action	Rationale
16. For heat treatment, place towel over compress (a heating device, if available, may be placed over towel); instruct client not to alter settings of heating device.	Maintains heat of warm compress Promotes safety
17. Place call light within reach and raise side rails.	Facilitates client–nurse communication Promotes safety
18. Replace gauze every 5 minutes, or as needed, to maintain coolness or warmth, assessing treatment area each time.	Provides for reassessment of treatment area
19. After 20 minutes, terminate treatment and dry skin.	Prevents local injury due to overexposure to treatment
20. Apply new dressing over wound, if necessary.	Promotes wound healing
21. Reposition client and raise side rails.	Facilitates comfort and safety
22. Remove all equipment from bedside and wash hands.	Maintains clean environment and facilitates asepsis

Evaluation

Goals met, partially met, or unmet?

Desired Outcomes (sample)

Client verbalizes increased comfort within 1 hour after treatment.
Redness at site decreases within 3 days.

Documentation

The following should be noted on the client's chart:

• Appearance of treatment area before and after treatment
• Duration and kind of treatment

- Status of old dressing and application of new, if applicable
- Client response to treatment
- Status of pain

Sample Documentation

DATE	TIME	
12/3/94	1450	Warm moist compress applied to open sore on right thigh for 20 minutes. Treatment tolerated well with no irritation to site. Healing and granulation noted. No drainage from site.

🖐 Sitz Bath

☒ Equipment

- Clean bathtub filled with enough warm water to cover buttocks (or portable sitz tub, if available)
- Bath towel
- Bath thermometer, if available
- Rubber tub ring
- Bathroom mat
- Gown
- Small footstool
- Nonsterile gloves

Purpose

Promotes perineal and anorectal healing
Reduces local inflammation and discomfort

Assessment

Assessment should focus on the following:

Baseline vital signs
Appearance and condition of treatment area
Client knowledge of benefits of sitz bath
Client inability to remain unattended in bathtub (*e.g.,* confusion, weakness)
Status of pain

Nursing Diagnoses

The nursing diagnoses may include the following:

Altered skin integrity related to episiotomy
Altered comfort related to disruption of skin integrity
Decreased tissue perfusion related to edema

Planning

Key Goals and Sample Goal Criteria

The client will

Verbalize increased comfort or relief of pain after treatment
Evidence no redness, edema, or discharge from site within 48
   hours

Special Considerations

Schedule the procedure when the client can be checked frequently.
If client is confused or unable to remain alone, plan to remain
   with client or find someone to do so.

Geriatric

Vasodilatation from exposure to warm water could cause severe
   changes in blood pressure and cardiac function in elderly
   clients with compromised cardiovascular status. Duration and
   temperature of sitz bath might need to be decreased, and
   clients must be watched closely for adverse reactions.

Home Health

Instruct client and family regarding the procedure. Emphasize
   the importance of a family member's checking on the client
   frequently if a potential safety hazard (such as falling in tub or
   on floor) exists.

 Transcultural

See overview regarding hot/cold conditions.
Discuss therapy with client and relate objections to physician.

Implementation

Action	**Rationale**
1. Explain procedure to client.	Promotes relaxation and compliance
2. Wash hands, organize equipment, and don gloves.	Reduces microorganism transfer to client or nurse
	Promotes efficiency
3. Check temperature of water with thermometer (105°F to 110°F [40.5°C to 43°C]); if thermometer is	Prevents skin damage from high water temperature

Action	Rationale
unavailable, test water with your wrist (water should be warm).	
4. Place rubber ring at bottom of tub and bathmat on floor.	Prevents accidental falls
5. Assist client to bathroom.	
6. Close door and assist client with undressing.	Provides privacy
7. Assist client into tub, using footstool if necessary.	Prevents accidental injury
8. Seat client on the rubber ring.	
9. Ascertain client stability in the tub alone and assess reaction to the engulfing heat: – Observe facial expressions and body motions for signs of discomfort. – Ask if heat is too warm. – Watch for dizziness, faintness, profuse diaphoresis. – Note any rapid increase in or irregularity of pulse.	Prevents complications from falling or unusual reaction to therapy
10. Instruct client on use of call light and place light within reach.	Facilitates client–nurse communication and immediate response to emergency
11. Recheck client every 5 to 10 minutes.	Allows assessment of unusual reactions
12. After 15 to 20 minutes, help client out of the tub.	Terminates treatment
13. Assist client with drying and dressing; then place linens in hamper.	Prevents chilling
14. Return client to room or bed.	Promotes comfort
15. Remove equipment and clean tub.	Reduces microorganism transfer to others using tub
16. Remove gloves and wash hands.	Reduces microorganism transfer

Evaluation

Goals met, partially met, or unmet?

Desired Outcomes (sample)

Client verbalizes relieved or decreased pain after treatment. Within 48 hours, site is clean without redness, edema, or drainage.

Documentation

The following should be noted on the client's chart:

- Appearance of treatment area before and after treatment
- Any unusual reactions to treatment, such as profuse diaphoresis, faintness, dizziness, palpitations, or pulse changes
- Duration of sitz bath
- Status of pain

Sample Documentation

DATE	TIME	
12/3/94	1500	Sitz bath to perineal area for 20 minutes. Client states pain decreased after treatment. No drainage from open perineal wound. No complaints of dizziness.

☝ Tepid Sponge Bath

☒ Equipment

- Thermometer (oral or rectal)
- Basin of cold water
- Gown
- Plastic-lined pads
- Bath blanket
- Six or seven washcloths
- Two towels
- Nonsterile gloves

Purpose

Provides controlled reduction of body temperature

Assessment

Assessment should focus on the following:

Doctor's order and client's response to previous treatment
Condition and appearance of skin
Pulse and temperature
Level of consciousness

Nursing Diagnoses

The nursing diagnoses may include the following:

Altered body temperature: elevation, related to sepsis
Potential for injury related to elevated temperature

Planning

Key Goals and Sample Goal Criteria

The client will

Show temperature within normal or acceptable limits for client
Show no untoward reactions to treatment

Special Considerations

If an alcohol bath is ordered, use equal parts of alcohol and water and assess client more frequently. Body temperature is decreased more rapidly by alcohol than by water.

Geriatric and Pediatric

The body temperature of pediatric and elderly clients is less stable than adult clients and may require more frequent assessment.

To lower a child's temperature, try placing the child in a cool bath and splashing water over the body, or place the child on a wet towel and cover groin and axillary areas with wet washcloths for 20 minutes. This technique may effectively reduce the temperature by 1°F.

Home Health

Instruct client and family on the procedure and precautions of the tepid sponge bath and recommend that a thermometer be secured for the home.

 Transcultural

Note overview regarding hot/cold conditions.

Adhere to cultural idiosyncracies regarding same-sex or opposite-sex care providers; family member should be instructed on procedure for sponge bath if preferred by client.

Implementation

Action	Rationale
1. Explain procedure to client.	Reduces anxiety and promotes compliance
2. Close windows and doors.	Eliminates drafts, thus preventing chilling
3. Wash hands and organize equipment.	Reduces microorganism transfer Promotes efficiency

Action	Rationale
4. Undress client, covering body with bath blanket and rolling topsheet to the bottom of bed.	Prevents chilling and protects privacy
5. Place washcloths and one towel in basin of water.	Cools cloths and towel
6. Place plastic pads under client.	Prevents linen soilage

7. Wring washcloths and place one in each of the following areas:
  – Over forehead
  – Under armpits
  – Over groin
	Promotes rapid cooling due to increased vascularity of these regions

8. Rewet and replace washcloths as they become warm.	Maintains coolness of cloths
9. Wring the wet towel and place around client's arm (Fig. 8.8).	Promotes decreased temperature in extremity
10. Wring a washcloth and sponge the other arm for 3 or 4 minutes.	Facilitates gradual cooling of extremity
11. Remove towel from arm and place in basin, dry both arms thoroughly, and replace blanket.	Prepares towel for future use
	Prevents chilling

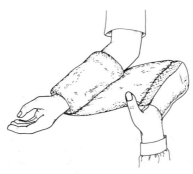

Figure 8.8

Action	Rationale
12. Check client's temperature and pulse: – *if temperature is above 100°F (37.7°C)*, proceed with bath. – *If temperature is at or below 100°F (37.7°C)*, terminate the procedure by skipping to step 17. – *If pulse is significantly increased*, terminate procedure for 5 minutes and recheck; if it remains significantly elevated, terminate procedure and notify physician.	Prevents complications related to overcooling
13. Continue bath by repeating steps 9 to 11 on opposite arm.	Facilitates maximum core-temperature reduction by treating greater body surface area
14. Repeat temperature and pulse check.	Assesses effectiveness of treatment
15. Continue by sponging and drying the following areas for 3 to 5 minutes: • chest • left leg • back • abdomen • right leg • buttocks You may use steps 9 to 11 when sponging legs.	Facilitates cooling by expanding the body surface area being treated
16. STOP EVERY 10 MINUTES TO REASSESS TEMPERATURE AND PULSE.	Assesses effectiveness Prevents overcooling
17. Remove all cloths and towels and dry client thoroughly.	Terminates treatment Promotes comfort
18. Replace gown.	Restores privacy
19. Reposition client and raise side rails.	Promotes comfort and safety
20. Remove and properly discard all washcloths,	Maintains cleanliness of environment

Action	Rationale
towels, plastic pads, and wet linens. (If necessary, obtain dry linens and remake bed.)	
21. Remove and discard gloves.	Reduces microorganism transfer

Evaluation

Goals met, partially met, unmet?

Desired Outcomes (sample)

Client maintains temperature within normal or acceptable limits (specified by physician).

Client tolerates treatment with no adverse changes in status or vital signs.

Documentation

The following should be noted on the client's chart:

- Pulse and temperature before and after bath
- Client mentation and general tolerance of the bath
- Untoward reactions to the treatment
- Length of the treatment and percentage of body sponged

Sample Documentation

DATE	TIME	
12/25/94	0100	Tepid sponge bath administered for 20-minute duration because of client's temperature of 104.7°F. Temperature after bath, 102.6°F; pulse, 118 and regular; respirations, 28 and regular; blood pressure, 110/62. Client dozing quietly in bed. Doctor notified of status. Tylenol suppository grains XX given.

Transcutaneous Electrical Nerve Stimulation Unit

 Equipment

- Transcutaneous electrical nerve stimulation (TENS) unit
- Leads wires
- Electrodes
- Water (optional)
- Fresh 9-volt battery

Purpose

Controls pain by delivering electrical impulse to nerve endings, which blocks pain message along pathway and prevents brain reception

Reduces amount of pain medication required to maintain comfort

Allows client to remain mentally alert, active, and pain free

Assessment

Assessment should focus on the following:

Status of pain (location and degree; alleviating and aggravating factors)

Type and location of incision, if applicable

Previous use of and knowledge level regarding TENS unit

Presence of skin irritation, abrasions, or breakage

Nursing Diagnoses

The nursing diagnoses may include the following:

Altered comfort related to incisional pain

Planning

Key Goal and Sample Goal Criterion

The client will

Cough and deep breathe 10 times every 1 to 2 hours with minimal or no pain medication.

Special Considerations

Apply electrodes to clean unbroken skin only.

If sensitivity to electrode adhesive is noted, notify doctor before application. If skin irritation is noted during TENS usage, remove electrodes and notify doctor.

Client should be informed that TENS unit may not totally relieve pain but should reduce discomfort.

Geriatric

Check skin frequently for tenderness and sensitivity.

If client is confused and electrical stimulation increases irritation, decrease or stop stimulation and notify doctor.

Implementation

Action	Rationale
1. Wash hands and organize equipment.	Reduces microorganism transfer Promotes efficiency
2. Explain procedure to client.	Promotes relaxation and compliance
3. Wash, rinse, and dry skin thoroughly.	Facilitates electrode adhesion
4. Prepare electrodes as described in package insert.	
5. Place electrodes on body areas directed by doctor or physical therapist (often along incision site or spinal column or both, depending on location of pain).	Places electrodes in position for optimal results
6. Plug lead wires into TENS unit (Fig. 8.9).	
7. Turn unit on and regulate for comfort: – Work with one lead (set) at a time.	Ensures proper stimulation of each area addressed

Action	Rationale

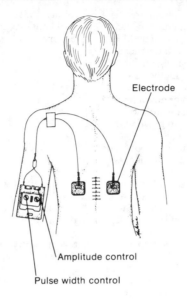

Figure 8.9

- Before beginning, ask client to indicate when stimulation is felt.
- Beginning at 0, increase level of stimulation until client indicates feeling of discomfort (muscle contraction under electrode area).

Achieves maximum stimulation to block pain sensation

- When client indicates discomfort, reduce volume slightly.

Prevents continued contraction of muscles at pain site or around incision

- Try to maintain highest tolerable level of stimulation.

Promotes maximum blockage of pain sensations

Repeat above steps with other lead (set).

Action	Rationale
– Note color of blinking light on unit and change battery, as needed.	Indicates unit is functional (red light may indicate low battery)
8. Stabilize unit for client mobility using one of the following methods:	
– Clamp unit to pajama bottom or gown (may place tape around unit and pin to gown with safety pin).	
– Place in pants pocket or clip to belt, if client is ambulatory.	
9. Monitor client for comfort level with vital signs assessment; check for increased respiratory rate, pulse, or blood pressure.	Indicates effectiveness of unit Indicates need to adjust stimulation due to increased discomfort
* 10. Be alert for malfunctions and correct them; the following guidelines should be used for general management of the TENS unit:	Prevents injury to client and damage to TENS unit
– Client should remove unit before a shower or bath.	Prevents shock to client
– If client complains of increased or sudden pain sensation, check TENS connections and perform general assessment of incision, dressing, and client.	Verifies function of unit and detects possible causes of increased discomfort
– TENS unit should be off whenever removing or applying leads; If lead becomes disconnected, TURN UNIT OFF, RECONNECT LEAD, THEN INCREASE STIMULATION LEVEL FROM 0.	Prevents shocking sensation
– NEVER turn unit on when set at	Prevents client discomfort at shocking sensation

Action	Rationale
maximum stimulation: always start at 0 and gradually increase level.	
– If client complains of "shocking sensation" or muscle contraction, decrease stimulation level.	Prevents excessive stimulation
– Check battery status frequently.	

Evaluation

Goals met, partially met, or unmet?

Desired Outcomes (sample)

Client ambulates in hallway with minimal complaint of pain.
Client requests pain medication less frequently.
Decreased dosages of medication are needed.

Documentation

The following should be noted on the client's chart:

- Type and location of incision, if applicable
- Time and date of TENS application
- Level of stimulation of each lead (set)
- Area stimulated by each lead (set)
- Pain location, level, aggravating and alleviating factors
- Client teaching done and accuracy with which client repeats instructions

Sample Documentation

DATE	TIME	
1/2/94	1200	TENs unit applied for lumbar back pain. Electrodes applied to lumbar area with setting of 5.5 on lead 1 and 6.0 on lead 2. Client verbalized understanding of unit function and state minimum pain felt at present.

Patient-Controlled
Analgesia Pump

☒ Equipment

- Patient-controlled analgesia (PCA) infuser
- PCA administration set (pump tubing)
- IV tubing
- Primary IV fluid
- PCA infuser key
- PCA flow sheet or appropriate form
- Ordered narcotic analgesic vial or syringe (mixed by pharmacy)
- Vial injector (accompanies vial)
- Client information booklet
- IV start kit (unless venous access is already available)

Purpose

Allows client to control delivery of pain medication in a safe, reliable manner

Assessment

Assessment should focus on the following:

Doctor's orders for type of analgesic, loading dosage, concentration of analgesic mixture, *lock-out interval* (minimum time allowed between doses)
Type of illness or surgery
Pain (type, location, character, intensity, aggravating and alleviating factors)
Level of consciousness and orientation
Venous access (patency of IV line, if present; skin status if IV is to be started)
Ability to learn and comprehend
Reading ability

Nursing Diagnoses

The nursing diagnoses may include the following:

Altered comfort: pain, related to thoracic incision site
Anxiety related to lack of pain control

Planning

Key Goals and Sample Goal Criteria

The client will

Verbalize increased comfort within 2 hours of PCA initiation
Correctly demonstrate PCA pump usage

Special Considerations

Geriatric
The analgesic may have an adverse effect on some elderly
clients (*e.g.*, change in level of orientation).

Pediatric
PCA therapy is usually used in adolescents or adults. When it is
used with a pediatric client, instruct the parents as well as the
child.

Home Health
Teach family members how to recognize signs of overdosage in
the homebound client.

Implementation

Action	Rationale
1. Wash hands and organize equipment.	Reduces microorganism transfer
	Promotes efficiency
2. Explain use of system to client and provide written literature; assess accuracy of client's understanding.	Decreases anxiety
	Promotes compliance
3. Prepare analgesic for administration: – Check five rights of drug administration: client,	Ensures delivery of appropriate medication and dosage

Action	Rationale

  drug, dosage (concentration), route, room.
- Connect injector to prefilled vial or syringe (Fig. 8.10).
- Hold vial vertically and push injector to remove air.
- Connect PCA administration set to vial, prime tubing, and close tubing clamp.
- Plug machine into electrical outlet and use PCA infuser key to open pump door.
- Load vial into machine according to equipment operation booklet.

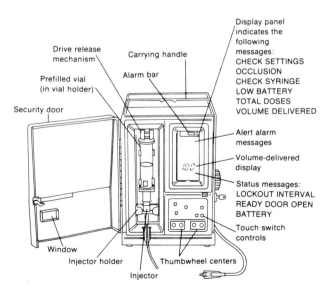

Drive release mechanism

Carrying handle

Prefilled vial (in vial holder)

Alarm bar

Security door

Display panel indicates the following messages:
CHECK SETTINGS
OCCLUSION
CHECK SYRINGE
LOW BATTERY
TOTAL DOSES
VOLUME DELIVERED

Alert alarm messages

Volume-delivered display

Status messages:
LOCKOUT INTERVAL
READY DOOR OPEN
BATTERY

Touch switch controls

Window

Injector holder

Thumbwheel centers

Injector

Figure 8.10

Action	Rationale
4. Prepare primary IV fluid and tubing (see Procedure 5.3).	
5. Attach primary IV tubing to Y-connector line of PCA tubing.	Provides fluid to keep vein open between medication doses
6. Open primary tubing clamp and prime lower portion of PCA tubing.	Removes air from tubing
7. Close clamp on primary IV.	
8. Prepare venous access: – Insert IV catheter (see Procedures 5.2 and 5.4); or if venous access (heparin lock or central line) is already present, verify patency, and connect PCA tubing directly to IV catheter. – Release clamps on PCA and primary tubing. – Regulate primary IV to infuse at keep-vein-open (or ordered) rate (see Procedures 5.5 and 5.6).	Maintains patency of vein between medication doses
9. Administer loading dose, if ordered: – Verify ordered dosage. – Set lock-out interval on pump at 00 minutes. – Set volume to be delivered, using dose-volume thumbwheel control. – Press and release loading-dose control switch.	Delivers dose of analgesic to initiate pain relief
10. Set parameters for dosage control: – Calculate volume of medication needed to deliver ordered dose (available dose per volume divided by ordered dose equals volume); often vials	Determines volume that will deliver ordered dose Delivers 10 mg per 1-ml dose

Action	Rationale
contain 200 mg per 20-ml vial of Demerol or 30 mg morphine per 30-ml vial.	Delivers 1 mg per 1-ml dose
– Set *dose volume,* using thumbwheel control for desired volume for each dose.	Sets amount of fluid and medication to be delivered for each dose
– Set *lock-out interval,* using thumbwheel control to set the desired time interval.	Sets minimum time between allotted doses Prevents medication overdose
– To set 4-hour limit, push control switch to display current limit; if different limit is desired, depress again and hold switch until desired limit is reached, then release switch.	Limits total volume to be infused over any consecutive 4-hour period
– Close and lock security door using infuser key; READY message should appear indicating PCA infuser is in client-control mode and first dose can be administered.	
– Place key with narcotic keys (or per agency policy).	Secures narcotic and parameters set into machine
11. Instruct client on administration of dose; inform client of the following information:	
– When pain is experienced, press and release control button.	Delivers set dose of analgesic
– Medication will be delivered and infuser will enter a lock-out period during which no additional medication can be delivered.	

Action	Rationale
– A ready message will appear when next dose can be delivered	
12. For maintenance of PCA therapy, *every 1 to 2 hours:*	Allows for monitoring of dosages received by client
– Press TOTAL DOSE switch and note number of client doses administered during past period.	
– Monitor client's respiratory rate, level of sedation (alert to sleeping), and pain level (pain-free to severe pain).	Monitors for oversedation
– Document above volumes and observations on flow sheet and calculate total volume on appropriate column.	Identifies total volume infused and remaining in vial
Every 8 hours (at end of shift):	Complies with federal narcotic administration laws
– Check volume of medication delivered; if agency policy, open pump door with infuser key and verify volume remaining in analgesic vial (volume should equal initial volume minus total volume infused).	
13. If you are oncoming shift nurse, check drug infusing, dose volume, and lock-out interval with doctor's order.	Verifies accuracy of infusion
14. Change vial and injector (when empty or at end of 24-hour period, if agency policy):	Provides fresh medication
– Assemble new vial and injector.	
– Clear air and close tubing clamp.	

Action	Rationale
– Use infuser key to unlock and open PCA pump door.	
– Press on/off switch.	
– Close clamp to old vial and primary fluid tubing.	
– Remove empty vial (or old vial) and administration set from pump (see equipment-operation booklet).	
– Attach new vial and injector to PCA administration set and prime to remove air.	
– Attach primary IV to Y-connector of new PCA administration set.	
– Insert administration set into pump (see equipment operation booklet).	
– Close and lock pump door.	
– Release tubing clamps.	
– Press on/off switch.	Initiates client-control mode
– Record vial change on PCA flow sheet.	Identifies current volume of analgesic in PCA pump
– Send previous vial and tubing to pharmacy (per agency protocol).	
15. To discontinue PCA therapy, follow step 14, omitting preparation of new vial; remove PCA tubing from IV catheter and replace with primary fluid tubing or infusion plug.	
16. Send vial and tubing to pharmacy (check agency policy).	Adheres to federal regulations for narcotic control

Evaluation

Goals met, partially met, or unmet?

Desired Outcome (sample)

Client states pain is relieved within 2 hours of PCA initiation

Documentation

The following should be noted on the client's chart:

- Name and dosage of medication being infused
- PCA parameters (hourly dose, lock-out interval, and 4-hour limit)
- Level of consciousness (on scale of 1 to 5)
- Pain level (on scale of 1 to 5)
- Status of respirations
- Amount of medication (analgesic) used each hour
- Number of client attempts to obtain dose (if agency policy)

Sample Documentation

DATE	TIME	
1/2/94	1200	Client received from recovery room after total hip replacement. PCA therapy initiated with 5 mg morphine given IV as loading dose. Dose volume set at 2 ml (2 mg), lock-out interval set at 60 minutes, and 4-hour limit set at 8 mg. Client alert and oriented. States pain measures 2 on a scale of 1 to 5, with 5 indicating severe pain. Return-demonstrated procedure for obtaining dose with 100% accuracy.

CHAPTER 9

Hygienic Care

OVERVIEW

- Personal interest in hygiene is a key symbol of mental and physical well-being.
- Hygiene is usually a private matter; consider the client's preference in timing, family assistance, and toiletries.
- Clients should be encouraged to perform as much of hygienic care as they can, within prescribed limitations.
- Maintaining good hygiene can promote the following:
  - Healthy skin, by preventing infections and skin breakdown
  - Improved circulation
  - Comfort and rest
  - Nutrition, by improving the appetite
  - Self-esteem, by improving the appearance
  - Sense of well-being

Jean Smith-Temple and Joyce Young Johnson:
Nurses' Guide to Clinical Procedures, Second Edition.© 1994
J. B. Lippincott Company

Back Care

☒ Equipment

- Lotion
- Soap
- Towel
- Washcloth
- Warm water

Purpose

Promotes comfort
Stimulates circulation
Relieves muscle tension
Facilitates therapeutic interaction

Assessment

Assessment should focus on the following:

Client's desire for back rub
Client knowledge of purpose of back rub
Blood pressure and pulse rate/rhythm, if history of cardiac or
  vascular problems
Skin and bony prominences
Client's ability to tolerate prone or lateral position
Client allergy to ingredients of lotion

Nursing Diagnoses

The nursing diagnoses may include the following:

Altered comfort related to (muscle tension, decreased mobility,
  impaired circulation)

Potential impaired skin integrity related to immobility, decreased circulation

Anxiety related to fear of the unknown (tests, back rub)

Planning

Key Goals and Sample Goal Criteria

The client will

Verbalize comfort, fall asleep, or show a calm, relaxed facial expression after back rub

Verbalize concerns during the procedure

Special Considerations

Many clients may prefer baby oil or powder, rather than lotion.

Caution should be taken to use only light pressure for clients with back disorders; a doctor's order is required for a back rub for these clients.

Geriatric

Baby oil or oil-based lotion may be best for the skin of elderly clients.

Pediatric

Total body massage with gentle conversation may be soothing and calming for a child and may serve to reduce the stress of hospitalization.

Home Health

Teach the procedure to a family member as a possible method of potentiating the effects of, or decreasing the need for, pain or sleeping medication.

Implementation

Action	Rationale
1. Explain procedure to client.	Promotes relaxation and compliance
2. Maintain a quiet, relaxing atmosphere (temperature at a comfortable setting, lighting dim, room neat, noise eliminated, door closed).	Promotes relaxation

Action	Rationale
3. Wash hands and organize equipment.	Reduces microorganism transfer Promotes efficiency
4. Warm lotion bottle and hands with warm water.	Cold lotion and hands increase discomfort and cause muscle spasms
5. Position client into prone or side-lying position.	Comfortable, relaxing position provides easy access to back
6. Drape with sheet or bath blanket.	Provides warmth and privacy
7. Wash back with soap and water; rinse and dry thoroughly.	Removes dirt and/or perspiration
8. Pour lotion into hands and rub hands together.	Facilitates even lotion distribution
9. Encourage client to take slow, deep breaths as you begin.	Facilitates relaxation
10. Place palms of hands on sacrococcygeal area. ONCE HANDS HAVE BEEN PLACED, DO NOT REMOVE HANDS FROM CLIENT'S BACK UNTIL BACK RUB IS COMPLETED.	Upward massage facilitates circulation Continuous contact with skin is essential for maximum soothing effect
11. Make long, firm strokes up center of back moving towards shoulders, and back down towards buttocks, covering the lateral areas of the back; repeat this step several times.	Stimulates circulation and release of muscle tension (It may be helpful to imagine a large heart on the client's back in accomplishing this step)
12. Move hands up center of the back towards the neck and rub nape of neck with fingers; continue rubbing outward across the shoulders.	Releases tension in neck muscles and promotes relaxation
13. Move hands downward to scapula areas and massage in a circular motion over both scapulae for several seconds.	Stimulates circulation around pressure points

Action	Rationale
14. Move hands downward to the buttocks and massage in a figure-eight motion over the buttocks; continue this step for several seconds (Fig. 9.1).	Stimulates circulation around pressure points
15. Lightly rub towards the neck and shoulders, then back down toward the buttocks for several strokes (using lighter pressure and moving laterally with each stroke).	Ends back rub with a calming, therapeutic effect
16. Remove excessive lotion with towel.	Excessive moisture leads to skin breakdown and bacterial growth
17. Reposition client and replace covers.	Promotes comfort and provides warmth
18. Raise side rails and place call light within reach.	Facilitates client–nurse communication
	Promotes safety

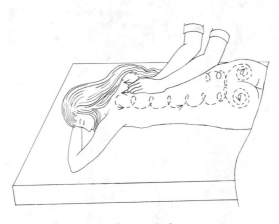

Figure 9.1

Evaluation

Goals met, partially met, or unmet?

Desired Outcomes (sample)

Client expresses feelings of comfort and falls asleep or has calm, relaxed facial expression.
Client verbalizes concerns during back rub.

Documentation

The following should be noted on the client's chart:

- Client's response to back rub
- Condition of skin and bony prominences
- Blood pressure and pulse before and after procedure, if applicable

---

Sample Documentation

DATE	TIME	
12/3/94	2200	Back rub given; activity tolerated without excessive fatigue, shortness of breath, or changes in vital signs. Client now in lateral-recumbent position with call light within reach. Bilateral side rails up. Stated "back rub was relaxing."

☝ Bed Preparation Techniques

☒ Equipment

- Bottom sheet (fitted, if available)
- Top sheet (regular sheet)
- Draw sheet (may use second regular sheet)
- Pillow case for each pillow in the room
- Gloves to remove old linens
- Gown and gloves, if client has draining wound or is in isolation

Purpose

Prepares bed covers to promote client's comfort

Assessment

Assessment should focus on the following:

Doctors' order for activity, impending surgery, or procedure
Need, if any, for assistance in turning client
Bladder and bowel continence
Presence of surgical wound or drains
Plans for client absence from room for a day or anticipation of new admission

Planning

Key Goals and Sample Goal Criteria

The client will

Verbalize comfort
Demonstrate no skin breakdown related to soiled linens

Special Considerations

A bed should be made after the client's bath is completed. You may need assistance to turn the client if you are making an occupied bed.

Implementation

Action	Rationale
1. Assist client to chair for meal or to use bedside commode.	Provides easy access to bed for changing
2. Don gloves, remove old linen, and place in pillowcase or a linen bag; if bed is soiled or new client is due, spray or wash mattress with germicidal agent. If an egg crate mattress is used, place it on bed. Remove gloves and wash hands.	Reduces microorganism transfer
3. Apply bottom sheet:	
– Place bottom sheet over mattress as evenly as possible leaving 1 inch or less hanging over bottom edge.	
– Tuck sheet at top and miter corners.	
– Move along the side of the bed, tucking the sheets securely and pulling tightly to remove wrinkles.	Ensures snug fit on mattress
– If fitted sheets are supplied, pull each corner of the mattress up slightly and slip it into a corner of the fitted sheet (pin the last two corners of sheet to undersides of mattress to keep sheets smooth).	
4. Place a draw sheet or pull sheet on bed:	Assists in repositioning client

Action	Rationale
– Fold full-sized sheet into thirds (Fig. 9.2.1).	
– Place sheet across bed two feet from the top, tucking it in or not, depending on activity level of client, agency policy, or preference.	Places sheet under shoulders and the hips of the client
5. The top sheet should be placed over bed with top edge two inches over top of the mattress; if blanket is used, place on top of sheet, tuck and miter bottom corners of both but make small fold or pleat at bottom edge of top linen.	Provides room for feet
6. Place a clean pillowcase on each pillow in room.	
7. Assist client to bed and position for comfort or finish bed in appropriate manner for circumstances:	
Closed bed – Place the pillow on the bed with open end facing the wall or place pillow on the bedside table.	Preserves bed when client is out of room for extended period or new client is expected
Open bed – Pull top of sheet (and blanket) to the head of bed.	Prepares bed for client when return is expected momentarily

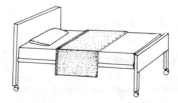

Figure 9.2.1

Action	Rationale

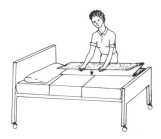

Figure 9.2.2

– Fanfold both back neatly
   to bottom third of bed

Surgical bed

– Make an open bed but
   do not tuck top sheet and
   blanket.

Facilitates moving client from
stretcher to bed without prolonged exposure or draft

– Leave bottom sheet and
   blanket fanfolded to the
   side of bed opposite door
   (Fig. 9.2.2).

Prevents interference of client
   transfer to bed by bed linens

– After client is transferred
   to bed, pull covers across
   bed and tuck and miter
   at bottom.

Covers client easily
Secures linen on bed

8. Discard or restore linen
   appropriately.

Promotes clean environment

Evaluation

Goals met, partially met, or unmet?

Desired Outcomes (sample)

Client verbalizes comfort when assisted into bed.
Client experiences minimum discomfort during turning.

Documentation

The following should be noted on the client's chart:

- Bed linens changed
- Status of client (expected from surgery, discharged, or in bed)

Sample Documentation

A bed change is not usually documented in note form.

DATE	TIME	
12/3/94	1000	Discharged home on one-day pass. Room cleaned and linens changed. Bed in closed position.

✋ Shampoo for the Bedridden Client

✖ Equipment

- Shampoo
- Wash cloth
- Shampoo board
- Two towels
- Nonsterile gloves
- Wash basin or plastic-lined trash can
- Water pitcher
- Linen saver or plastic trash bag
- Hair dryer (safety-approved)

Purpose

Improves appearance and self-esteem
Facilitates comfort and relaxation
Stimulates circulation to scalp
Relaxes client

Assessment

Assessment should focus on the following:

Client need or desire for shampoo
Client knowledge of procedure of bed shampoo
Blood pressure and pulse rate/rhythm, if history of cardiac or
vascular problems
Neurostatus (*e.g.,* increased intercranial pressure or other con-
traindications to manipulation of head)
Client's ability to tolerate prone or side-lying position
Client allergy to ingredients of shampoo or need for medicated
shampoo

Nursing Diagnoses

The nursing diagnoses may include the following:

Altered comfort related to unclean scalp

Altered skin integrity related to inadequate circulation at scalp
  area

Planning

Key Goals and Sample Goal Criteria

The client will

Verbalize increased comfort

Demonstrate adequate circulation to scalp, as evidenced by
  warmth and capillary refill time of less than 10 seconds at
  scalp

Demonstrate an increase in self-esteem by expressing interest in
  grooming

Special Considerations

Some clients require more frequent shampooing than others;
  treat each case individually. See basic hair care techniques in
  Procedure 9.4 for considerations based on racial diversity.

Geriatric

In the elderly client, skin is often thin and hair brittle.

Check scalp for irritation before shampooing.

Pediatric

Shampoo may be obtained for children that is less harsh and
  less irritating to the eyes than regular shampoo.

Assistance may be needed when shampooing the hair of infants
  and children to avoid excessive movement and wetting of
  covers.

Home Health

Teach proper hair-care techniques to family members for continued care. If client has lice, instruct family on need to treat
  all family members for lice as well as need for cleaning of
  home, linens, and personal items to prevent further spread.

Implementation

Action	Rationale
1. Prepare room environment (warm temperature and draft free).	Avoids discomfort from chills
2. Obtain doctor's orders for medicated shampoo, if needed.	Provides scalp treatment
3. Explain procedure to client and family members.	Facilitates cooperation
4. Wash hands and organize equipment.	Reduces microorganism transfer Promotes efficiency
5. Remove pillow from under client's head.	Prevents soiling of pillow
6. Place linen saver or plastic bag under shoulders and head of client.	Avoids wetting of linens
7. Place towel on top of linen saver.	Absorbs water overflow
8. Place the shampoo board under client's neck and head.	Facilitates drainage of water
9. Position wash basin or trash can in direct line with spout of shampoo board (Fig. 9.3).	Provides reservoir for water
10. Fill the pitcher with warm water (105°F to 110°F [40.5°C to 43.3°C]); check with thermometer or test for comfortable temperature with your inner wrist.	Promotes scalp circulation Prevents chilling or skin injury from excess heat
11. Ask client to hold washcloth over eyes during procedure.	Prevents pain from shampoo in eyes
12. Lower head of bed (infants may be held in lap with shampoo board under head); place supplies and sufficient water within easy reach.	Facilitates downward flow of water Prevents delays in procedure
13. Pour warm water over hair and moisten thoroughly.	Facilitates action of shampoo

Action   **Rationale**

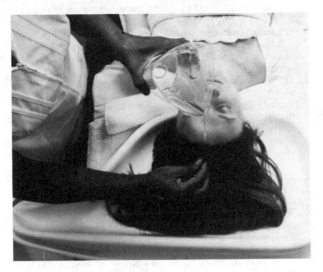

Figure 9.3

14. Don gloves and place small amount of shampoo in palms; massage shampoo into hair at front and back of head, working shampoo into a lather.

Provides lather for removal of dirt and oils

15. Massage lather over entire head in a slow, kneading motion.

Cleans hair and scalp
Promotes scalp circulation

16. Rinse hair by pouring warm water over head several times.

Removes shampoo and debris

17. Repeat application of shampoo and massage hair and scalp vigorously with fingers for a longer period of time.

Promotes thorough cleaning of hair and scalp

18. Rinse thoroughly using several pitchers of water.

Removes remaining residue of shampoo

Action	Rationale
19. Support client's head in hand and remove shampoo board from bed.	Clears area for completion of procedure Prevents inadvertent injury
20. Position client's head on the towel and cover head with it.	Absorbs water from hair
21. Briskly massage hair with towel.	Removes water
22. Replace wet towel with dry one and continue to rub hair.	Promotes drying of hair
23. Leave hair covered with towel until ready to use dryer.	Provides for continued absorption of moisture and prevents chilling
24. *Thoroughly dry hands.*	Promotes safety in next steps
25. Elevate head of bed to desired or prescribed angle.	Promotes access to hair
26. Turn on dryer to warm setting; feel heat to be sure it is not excessively hot.	Prevents injury from dryer heat
27. Blow hair until thoroughly dry; concentrate on one section of hair at a time, moving fingers or comb through hair while drying.	Facilitates thorough drying of hair Removes tangles and ensures drying of all parts of hair
28. Brush or comb hair to remove all tangles.	
29. Oil or spray hair, as desired, and style.	Facilitates styling
30. Remove linen saver, linens, and other equipment from bedside.	Provides clean environment
31. Assist client to position of comfort with side rails raised and call light within reach.	Promotes safety Facilitates communication

Evaluation

Goals met, partially met, or unmet?

Desired Outcomes (sample)

Client verbalizes increased comfort and expresses interest in further grooming.
Scalp is warm with brisk capillary refill and no irritation.

Documentation

The following should be noted on the client's chart:

- When shampoo was done and if completed
- Client response to activity
- Condition of hair and scalp
- Blood pressure, pulse, and neurostatus before and after procedure, if applicable

Sample Documentation

DATE	TIME	
12/3/94	0900	Shampoo performed in bed. Client tolerated supine position and procedure without distress. No scalp irritation noted. Client resting quietly lying on left side.

♣ Hair Care Techniques

✖ Equipment (varies with hair style desired)

- Comb (teeth size varies with coarseness of hair)
- Setting gel and rollers with rolling papers (optional)
- Hair dryer with dome or heat cap (optional)
- Brush
- Hair net (optional)
- Moisturizers, oils (optional)
- Rubber bands, hair pins, clamps
- Nonsterile gloves

Purpose

Improves client's appearance and self-esteem
Increases client's sense of well-being
Stimulates circulation to hair and scalp
Relaxes client
Provides opportunity for therapeutic communication

Assessment

Assessment should focus on the following:

Contraindications to excessive movement and lowering or elevating head (*e.g.*, skull fractures, neck injury)
Knowledge of procedure for care
Type of hair care needed or style desired
Activity level and positions of comfort
Allergy to ingredients of hair-care products
Status of hair and scalp (presence of tangles, dandruff, lice, or need for shampoo)

Nursing Diagnoses

The nursing diagnoses may include the following:

Scalp irritation due to inadequate or excessive hair oils

Potential loss of self-esteem due to inability to perform grooming procedures

Potential infection related to scratching of scalp and head-lice infestation

Planning

Key Goals and Sample Goal Criteria

The client will

Demonstrate good circulation to the scalp, as evidenced by warm scalp with brisk capillary refill

Verbalize no discomfort during hair care

Evidence no scalp irritation or pressure sores

Demonstrate an increase in self-esteem, as evidenced by initiation of or participation in one or more self-care and grooming activities

Special Considerations

DO NOT place braids or knots from rubber bands or hair nets under the head. Check for pressure spots or irritation to the scalp and loosen or release braids in irritated areas.

Geriatric

The elderly client's skin is often thin, dry, and fragile and the hair is brittle. Use a gentle technique when performing care, avoid tightly binding hair, and assess scalp for irritation frequently.

Pediatric

Pediatric clients can't always express the discomfort caused by hair that is too tightly bound or braided. Bind hair loosely and assess frequently for irritation or discomfort.

 Transcultural

Clients of different ethnic and cultural origins require shampoos with different frequencies and use different forms of basic hair care. Black clients usually shampoo every one to two weeks

and often add oils or moisturizers; white clients may shampoo daily or every other day to avoid buildup of hair oils. WHEN IN DOUBT REGARDING HAIR PRACTICES, CONSULT CLIENT OR FAMILY MEMBERS.

Implementation

Action	Rationale
1. Explain procedure to client.	Increases cooperation and assistance
2. Allow 15 to 30 minutes uninterrupted time for hair care.	Avoids rush and possible injury to client
3. Check and clean comb and brush before beginning (particularly if not client's personal property).	Prevents passing of head lice or infection to client
4. Wash hands and organize equipment.	Reduces microorganism transfer Promotes efficiency
5. Lower side rail.	Allows easier access
6. Assist client into position: – Supine position with head of bed elevated and pillows under back – Bedside chair, if able, with towel on shoulders – Side-lying position with towel under head or – Prone position	Allows head to move freely and provides access to hair and towel under head
7. Don gloves (if broken skin present) and comb hair through with fingers.	Prevents body-fluid contact Assesses degree of tangling
8. Massage scalp and observe status.	Increases circulation
9. Shampoo and dry hair, if needed and allowed (see Procedure 9.3).	Improves appearance of hair Promotes scalp circulation
10. Brush hair to remove as many tangles as possible: – Hold hair with one hand and brush with the other (Fig. 9.4).	Decreases discomfort of hair care

Action   **Rationale**

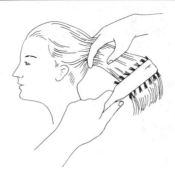

Figure 9.4

– If hair is coarse and kinky, processed for curls, or naturally curly, a comb may be more effective for removing tangles.	
11. Divide hair into sections with comb and fingers.	Provides for easier handling
12. Comb one section through at a time:	Removes tangles
– Gently and slowly comb tangles loose from scalp.	
– Hold hair section stable (near the scalp) with one hand.	Prevents pulling during combing
	Decreases pain to client
– Comb through hair, with other hand (as when brushing).	
13. Keep hair loose at the scalp.	Counteracts pulling from comb

Evaluation

Goals met, partially met, or unmet?

Desired Outcomes (sample)

Client requests mirror to observe appearance of hair and suggests other self-care activities.
Scalp is warm with good capillary refill and no irritation.
Hair is clean and comfortable, without tangles.

Documentation

The following should be noted on the client's chart:

- Response to hair care
- Condition of hair and scalp
- Blood pressure, pulse, and neurostatus before and after procedure, if applicable

---

Sample Documentation

DATE	TIME	
12/3/94	1300	Hair combed with assistance of client. Client took active interest in grooming. Makeup applied by client. Scalp warm with brisk capillary refill.

🖐 Oral Care Techniques (9.5)

🖐 Denture Care Techniques (9.6)

☒ Equipment

- Toothbrush (denture brush)
- Toothpaste
- Toothettes or swabs
- Emesis basin
- Nonsterile gloves
- Towel or linen saver and washcloth
- Cup of warm water
- Mouthwash
- Denture cream
- Denture cup
- Denture cleanser
- Dental floss (optional)
- Suction and catheter (if client is unconscious)

Purpose

Decreases microorganisms in mouth and on teeth or dentures
Decreases cavities and mouth disease
Decreases buildup of food residue on teeth or dentures
Improves appetite and taste of food
Facilitates comfort
Stimulates circulation to oral tissues, tongue, and gums
Improves appearance and self-esteem

Assessment

Assessment should focus on the following:

Client desire and need for oral care
Client knowledge of purpose and procedure
Client's ability to understand and follow instructions (*e.g.,* to expectorate instead of swallowing mouthwash and toothpaste)
Presence of dentures
Status of mouth, tongue, and teeth (*e.g.,* presence of lesions, cavities)

Nursing Diagnoses

The nursing diagnoses may include the following:

Altered oral mucous membranes related to inadequate denture cleaning

Planning

Key Goals and Sample Goal Criterion

The client will

Demonstrate the correct technique for cleaning dentures within 3 days

Special Considerations

Clients on anticoagulation therapy will require use of a soft toothbrush or Toothette only.
Clients with oral lesions or sensitive oral tissues may require dilution of mouthwash.
Encourage client to perform as much oral care as possible and encourage family members to assist, when necessary.

Implementation

Action	Rationale

PROCEDURE 9.5 ORAL CARE TECHNIQUES

Action	Rationale
1. Wash hands and organize equipment.	Reduces microorganism transfer Promotes efficiency

Action	Rationale
2. Provide explanation of procedure to client.	Reduces anxiety Promotes compliance
3. Lower side rail and position client in one of the following positions:	Promotes drainage of mouth-wash from mouth
– Supine at an angle greater than 45 degrees, if possible	Decreases risk of aspiration
– Side-lying	
– Prone with head turned to side	
4. Don gloves.	Prevents exposure to body fluids
5. Drape towel under client's neck and assist client to rinse mouth with water.	Catches secretions Facilitates removal of secretions
6. Assist client in brushing teeth:	Facilitates self-care
– Provide a glass of water, toothbrush, and toothpaste.	
– Moisten toothbrush with water.	
– Apply toothpaste to brush.	
– Allow client to brush teeth, if able.	
7. **If client is unable to perform own care:**	
– Prepare toothbrush as in step 6.	Permits cleaning back and sides of teeth
– Apply brush to back teeth and brush inside, top, and outside of teeth (brush from back to front, using an up-and-down motion) (Fig. 9.5).	
– Repeat these steps brushing teeth on opposite side of mouth.	
– Allow client to expectorate or suction excess secretions.	Removes toothpaste and oral secretions
– Instruct client to clench teeth together, or grasp	Exposes front teeth for brushing

Action	Rationale

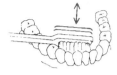 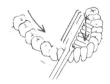

Figure 9.5

the mandible and press
lower teeth to upper
teeth; brush outside of
front teeth.
- Open mouth and brush
top and insides of teeth.
- Rinse toothbrush.
- Brush teeth again.   Removes residual toothpaste
- If use of dental floss is
desired, provide care at
this time.
8. Assist client in cleansing
oral cavity:
- Provide mouthwash-   Freshens mouth
soaked Toothette.
- Encourage client to swab   Decreases microorganism
inner cheeks, lips, tongue   growth in mouth
and gums, or perform
these actions for client, if
needed.
- Instruct client to rinse
with mouthwash and
expectorate, or irrigate
mouth with mouthwash
and suction excess fluid.
- Rinse with water.
- Have client expectorate
or suction excess.
9. **If working with an unconscious client**:
- Don gloves.   Reduces microorganism
transfer

Action	Rationale

– Brush teeth with tooth-
     brush and toothpaste,
     as in step 7.	

– Irrigate mouth with
     small amounts of water,
     suctioning constantly.
	Removes water and avoids
	  pooling

– Swab mouth with too-
     thette moistened with
     mouthwash.	

– Beginning with inside
     of cheeks and lips, pro-
     ceed to swab tongue
     and gums.	

– Suction excess tooth-
     paste, mouthwash, and
     secretions.	

– Wipe lips with wet washcloth.	
– Apply petroleum jelly or mineral oil to lips.	

10. Discard gloves and soiled
     materials; restore supplies
     in proper place.
	Promotes clean environment

11. Position client for comfort
     with call button within
     reach.
	Promotes safety, comfort, and
	  communication

PROCEDURE 9.6 DENTURE CARE TECHNIQUES

1. Wash hands and organize
   supplies.
	Reduces microorganism
	  transfer
	Promotes efficiency

2. Explain procedure to
   client and encourage par-
   ticipation, if able.
	Promotes compliance

3. Don gloves.	Prevents contact with saliva

4. Assist client with denture
   removal:
   – Half-fill denture cup
     with cool water.
   – Put denture cleanser into
     water per instructions.	

– Instruct client to hold
     water in mouth and
     "float" dentures loose.
	Prevents breaking of dentures
	  when removing

Action	Rationale
– Allow client to remove dentures, or gently rock dentures back and forth until free from gums.	Breaks seal created with dentures
– Lift bottom dentures up to remove, pull top dentures downward.	Prevents undue pressure and injury to oral membranes
– Place dentures in denture cup to soak.	Facilitates removal of micro-organisms
5. Assist client with cleansing of oral cavity:	Facilitates removal of micro-organisms
– Provide mouthwash-soaked Toothette.	
– Encourage client to swab inner cheeks, lips, tongue, and gums.	
– Instruct client to swirl mouthwash in mouth and expectorate.	
– Follow with water, as desired.	
6. Cleanse dentures:	
– Use same procedure as when brushing teeth (see Procedure 9.5).	
– Thoroughly rinse paste from dentures with cool water.	
7. Reinsert dentures:	Facilitates intake of solid foods
– Apply denture cream to gum side of denture plate.	
– Insert upper plate and press firmly to gums.	
– Repeat with lower plate.	
– Instruct client to swirl mouthwash in mouth, expectorate, and rinse with water.	
8. Apply petroleum jelly or mineral oil to client's lips.	Maintains skin integrity of lips
9. Remove towel from client's chest.	
10. Discard gloves and soiled materials.	Maintains clean environment

Action	Rationale
11. Position client for comfort with side rails raised and call button within reach.	Promotes comfort, safety, and communication
12. Place personal hygiene items in client's drawer or on bedside table.	Provides an orderly environment

Evaluation

Goals met, partially met, or unmet?

Desired Outcomes (sample)

Oral intake increased from 10% to 50%.
Mucous membranes and lips are intact.
Oral passage and teeth or dentures are clean.

Documentation

The following should be noted on the client's chart:

- Amount of care done by client
- Client's response to activity
- Condition of oral cavity and lips

Sample Documentation

DATE	TIME	
12/3/94	2000	Care of dentures performed with assistance of client. Client fatigued after brushing back teeth but expressed interest in grooming activity. Makeup applied by client after rest period. Mucous membranes moist. Lips moist, skin intact.

Biological Safety Needs

OVERVIEW

- The chain of infection requires that six links be present:
  - An infectious agent in sufficient amount to cause an infection
  - A place for the agent to multiply and grow
  - A point at which the agent can exit the growth area
  - A method of transportation from growth area to other sites
  - An available access or entrance into another site
  - A susceptible host or medium for agent growth
- The aim of all isolation procedures (universal precautions as well as disease-specific, category-specific, or body-substance isolation) is to decrease exposure to and the spread of microorganisms and disease; all actions are

Jean Smith-Temple and Joyce Young Johnson:
Nurses' Guide to Clinical Procedures, Second Edition.© 1994
J. B. Lippincott Company

aimed at breaking the chain of infection by eliminating the links.

- Gloves should be worn whenever exposure to body secretions is likely: ALWAYS WEAR GLOVES WHEN EMPTYING DRAINAGE CONTAINERS.
- If the sterility of materials, gloves, or gowns is in doubt, treat them as nonsterile.

Venipuncture for Blood Specimen

☒ Equipment

- Nonsterile gloves
- Alcohol pads
- Tourniquet (or blood-pressure cuff)
- Povidone-iodine (Betadine) pad (optional)

Vacutainer Method
- Blood-collecting device or vacutainer holder with double-point needle
- Appropriately colored test tube or vacutainer (consult agency laboratory manual):
  - striped (red/black, green/black, or other), used for chemical or drug studies and containing a preservative
  - solid red, used for blood bank
  - purple, used for complete blood count
  - blue or lavender, used for coagulation
- Blood culture bottle(s) (optional)

Syringe Method
- Sterile needles
  - 20 or 21 gauge
  or
  - scalp vein (butterfly) catheter
- Sterile syringe of appropriate size

Purpose

Provides blood specimen for analysis

Assessment

Assessment should focus on the following:

Type of lab test ordered
Time for which test is ordered
Adequacy of client preparation (*e.g.,* fasting state, medication
    withheld or given)
Client's ability to cooperate

Nursing Diagnoses

The nursing diagnoses may include the following:

Altered level of consciousness: lethargy related to drug over-
    dose
Potential for infection related to incision site

Planning

Key Goals and Sample Goal Criteria

The client will

Experience no injury to vein or extreme pain during procedure
Receive therapy based on correct test results

Special Considerations

Geriatric
The elderly often have veins that appear large and dilated. Use
    a blood pressure cuff instead of a tourniquet to prevent exces-
    sive stress on the vessel and subsequent collapse or rupture.

Pediatric
Enlist an assistant to restrain a child during venipuncture to
    prevent injury from resistance.
Use a butterfly catheter with syringe to avoid excessive suction
    on the vein.

Home Health
A blood pressure cuff may be used instead of a tourniquet (main-
    tain a pressure greater than the client's diastolic pressure).

Implementation

Action	Rationale
1. Wash hands and organize equipment; explain procedure and cooperation required to client.	Reduces microorganism transfer Promotes efficiency Promotes relaxation and compliance
2. Lower side rail and assist client into a semi-Fowler's position; raise bed to high position.	Provides easier access to veins Promotes comfort during procedure Facilitates good body mechanics
3. Open several alcohol and Betadine pads.	Provides fast access to cleaning supplies
4. Screw needle into blood collection device, if used (Fig. 10.1).	
5. Place towel under extremity.	Prevents soiling of linens
6. Locate largest, most distal vein (see Procedure 5.2); place tourniquet on extremity 2 to 6 inches (5 to 15 cm) above venipuncture site or inflate blood pressure cuff.	If insertion attempt fails, vein can be entered at a higher point Restricts blood flow, distending vein
7. Don gloves.	Reduces microorganism transfer

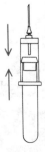

Figure 10.1

Action	Rationale
8. Clean vein area, beginning at the vein and circling outward to a 2-inch diameter.	Maintains asepsis
9. Encourage client to take slow, deep breaths as you begin.	Facilitates relaxation
10. Remove cap from needle and hold skin taut with one hand while holding syringe or vacutainer holder with other hand (with butterfly catheter, pinch "wings" together).	Stabilizes vein and prevents skin from moving during insertion Decreases pain during needle insertion
11. Maintaining needle sterility, insert needle, bevel up, into the straightest section of vein; puncture skin at a 15- to 30-degree angle.	Provides clear area for puncture Provides for downward movement toward vein
12. When needle has entered skin, lower needle until almost parallel with skin.	Decreases risk of penetration of both walls of the vein
13. Following path of vein, insert needle into wall of vein.	
14. Watch for backflow of blood (not noted with vacutainer); push needle slightly further into vein.	Indicates needle has pierced vein wall
15. Gently pull back syringe plunger until adequate amount of blood is obtained.	
16. If using blood collection device, put tube or blood culture bottle into device and push in until needle punctures rubber stopper and blood is pulled into tube by vacuum; keep tube in device until it is three fourths full or until	Connects needle with tube Allows suction in tube to pull blood into tube

Action	Rationale
culture medium is blood-colored; remove tube and replace with new tube, if additional specimens are needed.	
17. Place alcohol pad or cotton ball over needle insertion site and remove needle from vein while applying pressure with pad or cotton ball.	Facilitates sealing of vein Decreases bleeding from site
18. Hold pressure for 2 to 3 minutes (5 to 10 minutes if client is on anticoagulant therapy); check for bleeding and apply pressure until bleeding has stopped.	Facilitates clotting
19. Position client for comfort with call light within reach.	Promotes comfort and communication
20. Attach properly completed identification label to each tube, affix requisition, and send to lab.	Tests should be performed properly Incorrect labeling can cause diagnostic error
20. Dispose of and store equipment properly (unscrew needle from device and save tube holder portion).	Maintains clean and organized environment
21. Remove gloves and wash hands.	Reduces microorganism transfer

Evaluation

Goals met, partially met, or unmet?

Desired Outcomes (sample)

Blood is drawn with minimal discomfort to client.
Blood is placed in appropriate tubes and sent to lab.

Documentation

The following should be noted on the client's chart:

- Time blood is drawn
- Test to be run on specimen
- Client's tolerance to procedure
- Status of skin (*e.g.,* bruising, excessive bleeding)

Sample Documentation		
DATE	**TIME**	
1/2/94	1500	Blood drawn for complete blood count and electrolytes. Specimen sent to laboratory. Needle insertion site intact. Procedure tolerated well.

✋ Dressing Change

✖ Equipment

- Sterile dressing tray (forceps, scissors, gauze pads [optional])
- Sterile gauze dressing pads (2 × 2-inch, 4 × 4-inch, or surgical [ABD] pads, depending on drainage and size of area to be covered), or transparent dressing
- Sterile bowl
- 2-inch tape or Montgomery straps (paper tape, if allergic to others)
- Sterile gloves
- Nonsterile gloves
- Towel or linen-saver pad
- Cotton balls and cotton-tip swabs (optional)
- Sterile irrigation saline or sterile water
- Povidone-iodine (Betadine) solution or peroxide, as ordered
- Povidone-iodine (Betadine) swabs
- Bacteriostatic ointment
- Overbed table or bedside stand
- Paper bag, trash bag

Purpose

Removes accumulated secretions and dead tissue from wound or incision site
Decreases microorganism growth on wound or incision site
Promotes wound healing

Assessment

Assessment should focus on the following:

Doctor's orders regarding type of dressing change, procedure, and frequency of change
Type and location of wound or incision
Time of last pain medication
Allergies to iodine (shellfish or seafood) or tape

Nursing Diagnoses

The nursing diagnoses may include the following:

Impaired tissue integrity related to pressure sore
Potential infection related to decreased skin integrity

Planning

Key Goals and Sample Goal Criteria

The client will

Regain skin integrity
Demonstrate no signs of infection

Special Considerations

Dressing changes are often painful: assess pain needs and medicate client 30 minutes before beginning the procedure.

Geriatric and Pediatric
Clients are often immunosuppressed and have decreased resistance; strict asepsis is needed to minimize exposure to microorganisms.

Home Health
Newspaper should be used to cover the table surface before arranging the work field. Animals in the home should be restricted from the area during the procedure.

Implementation

Action	Rationale
1. Wash hands and organize equipment.	Reduces microorganism transfer
	Promotes efficiency
2. Explain procedure and assistance needed to client.	Decreases anxiety
	Promotes cooperation
3. Assess client's pain level and wait for medication to take effect before beginning.	Decreases discomfort of dressing change
3. Place bedside table close to area being dressed.	Facilitates management of sterile field and supplies

Action	**Rationale**
4. Prepare supplies:	
– Place supplies on bedside table.	Promotes swift dressing change
– Tape paper bag or trash bag to side of table.	Facilitates easy disposal of contaminated waste
– Open sterile gloves and use inside of glove package as sterile field.	Facilitates use of supplies without contamination
– Open gauze-pad packages and drop several onto sterile field; leave some pads in open packages if in plastic container (if not, place some pads into sterile bowl).	Permits wetting of some pads
– Open dressing tray and bowl.	
– Open liquids and pour saline on two gauze pads and povidone on four gauze pads (more if wet-to-dry dressing).	Prevents transmission of organisms from table to supplies
– Open povidone swabs, if used, to expose plastic stick end.	
– Place several sterile cotton-tip swabs and cotton balls on sterile field (use gauze instead if staples are present because cotton may catch on edges of staples).	
5. Don nonsterile gloves.	
6. Place towel or pad under wound area.	
7. Loosen tape by pulling toward the wound and remove soiled dressing (note appearance of dressing and wound). SOAK DRESSING WITH SALINE IF IT ADHERES TO WOUND, THEN GENTLY PULL FREE.	Permits observation of site and exposes site for cleaning

Action	Rationale
8. Place dressing in paper bag.	
9. Discard gloves and wash hands.	

Sterile Dressing Change

Action	Rationale
10. Don sterile gloves and face mask (optional).	
11. Pick up saline-soaked dressing pad with forceps and form a large swab.	
12. Cleanse away debris and drainage from wound, moving from center outward and using a new pad for each area cleaned (Fig. 10.2.1); discard old pads away from sterile supplies.	Prevents contamination of wound from organisms on skin surface Maintains sterility of supplies
13. Wipe wound with povidone-soaked pads, moving from center of wound outward; discard forceps.	Reduces microorganism transfer Avoids cross contamination
14. Assess need for frequent (every 4 to 6 hours) dressing changes and effect of tape on skin, and apply Montgomery straps to hold dressing:	Prevents infection due to soiled dressings Prevents skin injury

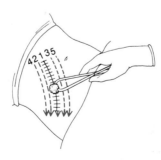

Figure 10.2.1

Action	**Rationale**

- Place 8-inch strip of tape on table with sticky side up and cover with 4-inch strip of tape, sticky side down.
- Place sticky side of tape on client with nonsticky end reaching across half of wound area.
- Repeat process on other side of wound; if wound is long, apply straps to upper and lower portion.
- Place dressings (step 15) over wound and secure by pinning, banding or tying Montgomery straps together (The tying method may be used when frequent dressing changes are anticipated.) (Fig. 10.2.2).

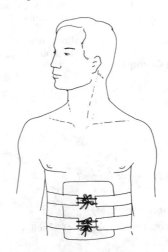

Figure 10.2.2

Action	Rationale
15. Dress the wound or incision in the following manner:	Prevents contamination of dressing or wound
– Pick up dressing pads by edge (Betadine- or saline-soaked, if wet-to-dry dressing).	
– Place pads over wound or incision site until site is totally covered.	Allows air to reach wound
– Cover with surgical pad (if wet-to-dry).	
– Secure dressing with tape along edges or use Montgomery straps.	Indicates last dressing change and need for next change within 24 to 48 hours
16. Write the date and time of dressing change on a strip of tape and place tape across dressing.	Decreases spread of microorganisms
17. Dispose of gloves and materials and store supplies appropriately.	Maintains organized environment
18. Position client for comfort with call bell within reach.	Facilitates comfort and communication
19. Wash hands.	Decreases spread of microorganisms
	Allows handling of dressing without sterile instruments

Clean Dressing Change

20. Follow steps 11 to 18 but forceps and gloves need not be sterile.

Evaluation

Goals met, partially met, or unmet?

Desired Outcome (sample)

Wound healing noted with no signs of infection.

Documentation

The following should be noted in the client's chart:

- Location and type of wound or incision
- Status of previous dressing
- Status of the wound/incision site
- Solution and medications applied to wound
- Client teaching done
- Client's tolerance of procedure

Sample Documentation

DATE	TIME	
1/12/94	0600	Abdominal wound dressing saturated with serous drainage. Area surrounding wound is red. Site cleansed with saline and wiped with Betadine swabs. Gauze pads (4 × 4 inches) moistened with saline applied and covered with dry dressings. Client turned to side with pillow at back. Tolerated dressing change with minimal discomfort.

🖐 Blood Glucose Testing

✖ Equipment

- Blood glucose machine (optional)
- Chemical strips for blood glucose with color chart (on container or insert)
- Nonsterile gloves
- Lancets (or 19- or 21-gauge needle)
- Autoclix or lancet injector (optional)
- Cotton balls
- Alcohol pads (or bottle of alcohol)
- Watch with second hand or stop watch
- Needle disposal unit

Purpose

Determines level of glucose in blood
Promotes stricter blood glucose regulation

Assessment

Assessment should focus on the following:

Doctor's orders for frequency and type of glucose testing and sliding scale for insulin coverage
Client's knowledge of procedure and of diabetic self-care
Response to previous testing

Nursing Diagnoses

The nursing diagnoses may include the following:

Self-care knowledge deficit related to newly diagnosed diabetes

Planning

Key Goals and Sample Goal Criteria

The client will

Demonstrate early detection of blood glucose elevations
Demonstrate correct procedure for blood-glucose testing before
  discharge

Special Considerations

An ideal time for client teaching is during the blood glucose
  testing procedure.

Geriatric
If vision disturbances are present, use of a glucose-monitoring
  machine may be preferable to a visual-comparison chart.

Pediatric
Consider developmental stage and assess the child's ability to
  understand and perform the procedure. For reinforcement of
  teaching, include family members in teaching.

Home Health
An egg timer may be used to time the reaction of the blood-
  glucose testing procedure.

Implementation

Action	Rationale
1. Wash hands and organize equipment.	Reduces microorganism transfer Promotes efficiency
2. Explain procedure to client and inquire as to preference of finger and use of lancet injector.	Facilitates cooperation and promotes sense of involvement in and control of own care
3. Calibrate glucose machine, if used: – Turn machine on. – Compare number on machine or strip in machine with number on bottle of chemical strips (Fig. 10.3.1).	

Action	Rationale

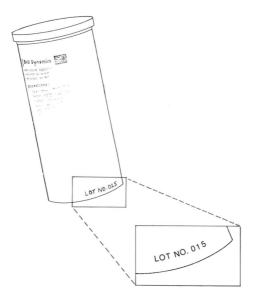

Figure 10.3.1

- Perform procedures to ready machine for operation; consult user's manual for steps and readiness indicator.
- Machine accuracy should be validated daily, or per laboratory policy, with sample low- and high-glucose solutions to ensure accuracy.

4. Remove chemical strip from container and place it face up near client.

Prevents delay
Prevents damage to indicator

5. Load lancet in injector, if used, and set trigger.

Prepares injector to push lancet into finger

Action	Rationale
6. Don gloves.	Prevents exposure to blood
7. Hold chosen finger downward and squeeze gently from lower digits to fingertip, or wrap finger in warm, wet cloth for 30 seconds or longer.	Facilitates flow of blood to finger for easy sampling
8. Wipe intended puncture site with alcohol pad.	Removes dirt and skin oils Decreases microorganisms
9. Place injector against side of finger (where there are fewer nerve endings), and release trigger; or stick side of finger with lancet or needle using a darting motion.	Obtains a large drop of blood with minimal pain stimulation
10. Hold chemical strip under puncture site and squeeze gently until drop of blood is large enough to drop onto strip and cover indicator squares.	Ensures that indicator squares are covered with blood Prevents uneven exposure of indicators
11. Push timer button on machine as soon as blood has covered indicator squares, or note position of second hand on watch.	Determines time to remove excess blood from strip and when to read color change
12. Apply pressure to puncture site until bleeding stops (or have client do so) and place lancet in needle disposal unit.	
13. When timer or watch indicates 60 seconds have passed, wipe excess blood from strip.	Removes blood cells
14. Place into machine, if used, with indicator patch facing reading window (see user's manual). After an additional 60 seconds have passed, read results from the machine.	Determines blood glucose level after timed chemical reaction
15. Or, compare colors on strip with those in chart	

Action	Rationale

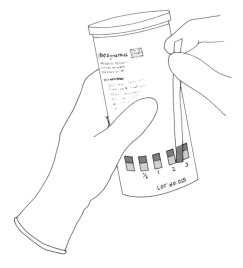

Figure 10.3.2

on chemical-strip container or insert (Fig. 10.3.2) after the additional 60 seconds.

16. Discard soiled materials and gloves in proper container.

Prevents exposure to blood-soiled materials

17. Record results on glucose flow sheet and administer insulin, if indicated.

Maintains record of glucose levels and insulin coverage

18. Position client for comfort, with call light within reach.

Promotes comfort and communication

Evaluation

Goals met, partially met, or unmet?

Desired Outcomes (sample)

Blood glucose elevation is noted and treated promptly per sliding scale.
Blood glucose is maintained within acceptable range.

Documentation

The following should be noted on the client's chart:

* Method of glucose testing
* Level of glucose
* Insulin coverage provided and route
* Teaching done and demonstration of client understanding if necessary

Sample Documentation

DATE	TIME	
1/2/94	1200	Fingerstick blood glucose testing performed by client after teaching and demonstration by nurse. Client's technique good with good asepsis noted. Results showed 256 mg glucose/dl. Five units regular human insulin given in abdominal area by client with good technique.

🖐 Sterile Gown Application (10.4)

🖐 Sterile Glove Application (10.5)

❎ Equipment

- Sterile gown
- Sterile gloves
- Bedside table

Purpose

Preserves sterile field during sterile procedure

Assessment

Assessment should focus on the following:

Client's ability to cooperate and not contaminate sterile gown or gloves

Nursing Diagnoses

The nursing diagnoses may include the following:

Potential for infection related to incision site

Planning

Key Goal and Sample Goal Criterion
The client will

Demonstrate no signs of infection (or additional infection).

Special Considerations

Pediatric

If a child is restless or too young to understand the importance of maintaining a sterile field, restrain the child's arms and legs with linen or soft restraints during the medical procedure. Encourage a parent to sit at child's bedside during the procedure, if possible.

Implementation

Action	Rationale

PROCEDURE 10.4 STERILE GOWN APPLICATION

1. Wash hands and organize equipment; apply mask, if needed; enlist assistant to tie gown.

   Reduces microorganism transfer
   Promotes efficiency

2. Remove sterile gown package from outer cover and open inner covering to expose sterile gown; place on bedside table, touching only outsides of covering, and spread covering over table; open outer glove package and slide inside glove cover onto sterile field.

   Maintains sterility of gown

   Provides sterile field
   Places gloves in convenient location and on sterile field

3. Remove gown from field, grasping inside of gown and gently shaking to loosen folds; hold gown with inside facing you (Fig. 10.4).

   Prepares gown for application

4. Place both arms inside gown at the same time and stretch outward until hands reach edge of sleeves; don sterile gloves (see Procedure 10.5).

   Preserves sterility of gown

5. Have assistant pull tie from back of gown and fasten to inside tie; have assistant pull outside tie around with sterile tongs or sterile gloves. Grasp tie, pull

   Secures gown without contamination of outer portion.

Action	Rationale

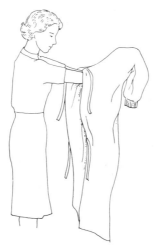

Figure 10.4

around to front of gown, and secure to front tie.	Secures gown

PROCEDURE 10.5 STERILE GLOVE APPLICATION

1. Don gown, if needed; otherwise, open glove package, place on bedside table, and remove inner glove covering; open inner package, using sterile technique, and expose gloves.
2. Pick up one glove by cuff and slip fingers of other hand into glove (keep gown sleeve inside glove if applicable); pull glove over hand and sleeve.
3. Place gloved hand inside cuff of remaining glove

Action	Rationale

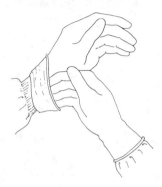

Figure 10.5

and lift slightly; slide other hand into glove and pull cuff over hand and wrist and sleeve of gown, if applicable (Fig. 10.5). DO NOT TOUCH SKIN WITH GLOVED HAND.

Facilitates placing glove on hand without contaminating glove or gloved hand

Stabilizes gown sleeve and creates continuous sterile hand-to-arm connection

4. Pull gloves securely over fingers and adjust for fit using one hand to fix the other.

Places fingers deeply into gloves while maintaining sterility

5. Proceed to sterile field, maintaining hands above waist; do not touch non-sterile items. IF GLOVE OR GOWN BECOMES CONTAMINATED, DISCARD AND REPLACE WITH STERILE GARB.

Prevents contamination of gloves

Evaluation

Goals met, partially met, or unmet?

Desired Outcome (sample)

Procedure is performed with no apparent exposure to micro-organisms.

Documentation

The following should be noted on the client's chart:

- Sterile procedure performed
- Sterile garments used

Sample Documentation		
DATE	TIME	
1/2/94	1200	Temporary pacemaker inserted by Dr. Jones with sterile technique used. Client tolerated procedure with no reports of unusual discomfort.

Principles of Medical Asepsis

 Equipment

- Soap and warm running water
- Nonsterile gloves
- Sterile gloves
- Sterile gown
- Mask
- Waste disposal materials: trash can, bags (isolation bags optional)
- Isolation stickers
- Linen bags
- Specimen bags, if agency policy (see Procedure 10.8, Isolation Techniques)

Purpose

Prevents the growth and spread of pathogenic microorganisms to one individual from another individual or the environment

Assessment

Assessment should focus on the following:

Data from medical history and physical or diagnostic studies indicating susceptibility to, or presence of, infection (fever, cloudy urine, positive culture, decreased white blood count, history of immunosuppression or steroid intake)
Doctor's orders or agency policy regarding isolation procedures
Client or nurse's allergy to soap or bacteriostatic solutions
Client's assignment (ward, double or single room)
Client knowledge of principles of asepsis
Ability of client to cooperate and not contaminate sterile field

Nursing Diagnoses

The nursing diagnoses may include the following:

Altered biological safety: infection related to abdominal abscess
Potential for infection related to immunosuppressive therapy
 for renal transplant

Planning

Key Goals and Sample Goal Criteria

The client will

Demonstrate no signs of infection within 1 week of therapy
Demonstrate no signs of infection during postoperative recovery period

Special Considerations

Keep your fingernails short and filed. Dirt and secretions that
 lodge under fingernails contain microorganisms. Long fingernails can scratch client's skin.

Geriatric
If a client is disoriented and restless, restrain the client during
 procedures that require maintenance of sterile or clean materials.

Pediatric
If a child is restless or too young to understand the importance
 of maintaining a sterile field, restrain the child with linen or
 soft restraints during the medical procedure.

Home Health
Restrict pets from the room in which a medical procedure is
 being performed.
Most procedures are performed with clean, rather than sterile,
 technique.

Implementation

Action	Rationale
Hand Washing—Medical 1. Perform 2- to 4-minute hand washing:	Reduces microorganisms from hands

Action	Rationale
– Remove rings (often may retain wedding band) and chipped nail polish; move watch to position high on wrist.	Removes sources that harbor and promote growth of microorganisms
– Wet hands from wrist to fingertips under flowing water.	Cleans from least to most dirty Aids in removal of micro-organisms
– Keep hands and fore-arms lower than elbows during washing.	Hands are the most contam-inated parts to be washed Water flows from least to most contaminated area
– Place soap, preferably bacteriostatic, on hands and rub vigorously for 15 to 30 seconds, massag-ing all skin areas, joints, fingernails, between fin-gers, and so forth; slide ring up and down while rubbing fingers (if un-able to remove).	Creates friction to remove organisms

Permits cleaning around and under ring |
– Rinse hands from fingers to wrist under flow of water.	Washes dirt and organisms from cleanest to least clean area
– Repeat soaping, rubbing, and rinsing until hands are clean.	
– Dry hands with paper towel moving from fin-gers to wrist to forearm.	Dries hands from clean to least clean area
– Turn off faucet with paper towel.	Prevents recontamination of hand
2. **Management of contami-nated materials:**	
– Don gloves when contact with body fluids or in-fected area is possible.	Prevents contamination of hands Prevents contact with secre-tions
– Don mask if organism can be transmitted by airborne route through contact with mucous membranes.	Prevents exposure to airborne microorganisms or projectile body fluids
– Don gown if contact with body secretions	Avoids contact with poten-tially infectious material

Action	Rationale
or contaminated area is likely, if client has highly contagious condition, or if client is immuno-suppressed.	Avoids spread of infection Protects client from exposure to microorganisms
– Place disposable contam-inated materials in bag before leaving bedside; place in dirty utility. room or send for waste disposal personnel; or place in isolation bag or mark "isolation" on bag; use double-bagging, if agency policy.	Provides added protection against exposure to body fluids or infectious materials Alerts housekeeping to dis-pose of materials properly
– Reusable items should be bagged, labeled "Isolation," and sent to central supply unit for sterilization or to appro-priate department for cleaning; items too large to bag should be sprayed with disinfectant and sent for thorough cleaning.	Decreases spread of micro-organisms on used medical equipment
– Linens should be placed in linen bags before leav-ing bedside and placed in central hamper or linen chute (agency may require double bagging).	
– Clean stethoscope be-tween use with different clients with soap and water and wipe with al-cohol swab (if used in an infected area or with in-fected client, a thorough disassembly and clean-ing may be needed); use a separate stethoscope for an infected client, if possible.	Decreases spread of micro-organisms on stethoscope Limits exposure to infection
– Sphygmomanometers, thermometers, EKG	Decreases exposure to poten-tially infectious medium

Action	Rationale
leads, or similar daily-use items should be sprayed or wiped with a bacteriostatic substance between use with different clients.	These items provide a good medium for organism growth
– Used syringes and needles, scalpels and other sharp disposables should be placed in appropriately marked container.	Prevents accidental stick and contact with client's blood
DO NOT REPLACE CAPS ON NEEDLES.	Prevents accidental sticks during attempts to recap needle
– Discard gown, gloves, and mask before leaving client's room.	Prevents spread of infection

3. **Handling of personal effects of patients with infection:**

Action	Rationale
– Items should be placed in bags and sent home with family; if client is discharged and does not want certain items, dispose of these as in step 2. NEVER SHARE PERSONAL-CARE ITEMS BETWEEN CLIENTS.	Prevents general spread of infection
– If papers, books, or other items become soiled with infectious material, items should be discarded unless sterilization is possible and desired.	

4. **Room assignment:**

Action	Rationale
– A private room is preferable but is required only when a highly virulent or infectious microorganism is present, the microorganism is airborne, or the client is highly susceptible to infection.	Protects other clients or client from cross-contamination
– A semiprivate room may be used when the micro-	

Action	Rationale

organism is limited to one body area; however, good medical asepsis must be maintained by staff, client, family, and visitors to prevent spread of infection.

5. **Room cleaning:**
   - Room should be cleaned with disinfectant daily.

   Reduces microorganisms in the environment

   - If soiled materials spill on floor, clean area with disinfectant or bacteriocidal agent specific to organism, if known.
   - When client with known infection is discharged, is transferred, or dies, room should be cleaned and disinfected thoroughly and allowed to remain vacant 12 to 24 hours (see Procedure 12.3 for postmortem care and Procedure 10.8 for additional information on isolation techniques).

   Promotes thorough removal of microorganisms

Evaluation

Goals met, partially met, or unmet?

Desired Outcomes (sample)

Client shows no signs of infection or of additional infection. Medical procedures are performed with no evidence of exposure to microorganisms.

Documentation

The following should be noted on the client's chart:

- Status of source of infection/potential infection (wound, dressing, breath sounds, secretions)

- Procedure performed
- Protective garments used
- Client teaching completed

Sample Documentation

DATE	TIME	
1/2/94	1200	Abdominal abscess site dressed. Site clean and without redness. Drains intact. Client tolerated procedure without complaint of unusual discomfort. States understands dressing change process and would like to change dressing in morning.

✋ Principles of Surgical Asepsis (Aseptic Technique)

☒ Equipment

- Bacteriocidal or antimicrobial soap
- Sink with side or foot pedal
- Surgical scrub brush
- Sterile gloves
- Sterile gown
- Mask
- Hair covering and booties (optional)
- Sterile materials (dressing, instruments)
- Sterile sheets or towels (occasionally found in dressing tray)
- Waste disposal materials: trash can, bags (isolation bags optional)

Purpose

Avoids the introduction of microorganisms onto a designated field

Assessment

Assessment should focus on the following:

Data from medical history and physical or diagnostic studies indicating susceptibility to infection (decreased leukocyte count, history of immunosuppression, or steroid intake)

Doctor's orders or agency policy regarding dressing changes and isolation procedures

Client or nurse's allergy to soap or bacteriostatic solutions

Client's room assignment (ward, double or single room)

Date of expiration and sterility indicator on sterile supplies and solutions

Client knowledge of principles of asepsis

Client's ability to cooperate and not contaminate sterile field
Agency policy regarding surgical scrub procedure

Nursing Diagnoses

The nursing diagnoses may include the following:

Potential altered biological safety: infection related to central
line insertion and total parenteral nutrition (TPN) therapy
Potential for infection related to immunosuppression from renal
transplant therapy

Planning

Key Goals and Sample Goal Criteria

The client will

Demonstrate no signs of infection throughout TPN therapy and
central line maintenance
Demonstrate no signs of infection during postoperative recovery period

Special Considerations

Variations in sterile technique—e.g., the omission of some
protective coverings (hair cover, booties, mask)—may be used
in performing some procedures. CONTINUE TO USE
ASEPTIC PRINCIPLES TO GOVERN ACTIONS DURING A
PROCEDURE.
IF UNSURE OF STERILITY OF MATERIAL, GLOVE, OR
FIELD, CONSIDER IT CONTAMINATED.

Geriatric
If a client is disoriented and restless, restrain the client during
procedures requiring maintenance of sterile materials. Enlist
assistance for manual restraint of the client or use mechanical
restraints (see Procedure 10.11).

Pediatric
If a child is restless or too young to understand the importance
of maintaining a sterile field, restrain the child with linen or
soft restraints during the procedure. Use a family member to
assist in restraining the child and allaying fears, if possible.
Provide sedation or pain medication before the procedure to
comfort and calm the child.

Home Health
Restrict pets from the room in which a sterile or clean procedure is being performed. Most procedures are performed with clean, rather than sterile, technique. Enlist and instruct a family member to serve as an assistant.

Implementation

Action	Rationale
1. A private room is preferable for performance of a sterile procedure; transfer client to treatment room, if necessary.	Minimizes microorganisms in environment

Hand Washing—Surgical

Action	Rationale
2. Don mask, hair cover, and booties, if required.	Prevents introduction of contaminants from mouth, hair or shoes into environment
3. Perform 5- to 10-minute surgical scrub using counted brush stroke method:	Reduces organisms on hands Counted brush method places emphasis on detail to specific areas and ensures that all skin surfaces are exposed to sufficient friction
– Remove rings (often must remove wedding band), chipped nail polish, and watch.	Removes sources that harbor and promote growth of microorganisms
– Wet hands and arms from elbows to fingertips under flowing water (use sink with side or foot pedal).	Cleans from least to most dirty Aids in removal of microorganisms
– Place soap, preferably antimicrobial/bacteriostatic, on hands and rub vigorously for 15 to 30 seconds; use scrub brush gently—*do not abrade skin.*	Creates friction to remove organisms
– Using circular motion scrub all skin areas, joints, fingernails, between fingers, and so	

Action	Rationale
forth (on all sides and 2 inches above elbows); slide ring, if present, up and down while rubbing fingers.	Permits cleaning around and under ring
– Continue scrub for 5 to 10 minutes or per agency policy.	
– Rinse hands from fingers to elbows under flow of water.	Washes dirt and organisms from cleanest to least clean area
– Repeat soaping, rubbing, and rinsing until hands and arms are clean.	
– Pat hands dry with sterile towel moving from fingers to wrist.	Dries hands from clean to least clean area
– Turn off faucet with side or foot pedal.	Prevents recontamination of hand

Sterile Field
4. To create a sterile field:
   – Arrange sterile supplies on overbed table or surgical stand.
   – Never use opened items or items of questionable sterility.
   – Open packages to reveal supplies, using insides of packages to form sterile field; open package's outer flap away from you, open side flaps next, and then pull inner flap toward you (Fig. 10.7.1); spread edges of package cover over table with fingertips.

	Prevents reaching over exposed materials
	Edges are considered unsterile

5. To add items to sterile field:
   – Drop sterile items onto field, keeping packaging between items and hands (Fig. 10.7.2); *use*

	Prevents contamination of supplies

Action	Rationale

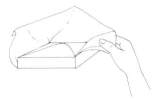

Figure 10.7.1

sterile forceps or tongs to remove items from package, if unable to do so with sterile technique; if unable to remove item from package without contamination, wait until sterile garb is applied, then place items on sterile field.

– Use sterile gloves or *sterile tongs* to remove sterile towel and cover field and supplies if not beginning procedure immediately.

Sterility will be lost if field is exposed to air for extended period of time

DO NOT REACH OVER OPEN STERILE FIELD.

Exposes field to contamination

– Don sterile gown and sterile gloves (see Procedures 10.4 and 10.5).

Prevents exposure of sterile field to hands or clothing

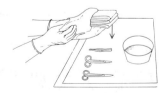

Figure 10.7.2

Action	Rationale
– Begin procedure with hands held above waist.	Area below waist considered nonsterile
6. To maintain a sterile environment:	
– Drape sterile sheets or towels over area surrounding site being treated.	Decreases chance of exposure to nonsterile sites
– *Use tongs or forceps* to clean site thoroughly with bacteriocidal agent.	Maintains sterility of gloves Reduces microorganisms
– Discard *tongs* from sterile field.	Prevents field contamination
– Pour liquids into a sterile basin held by an assistant in sterile garb or by holding bottle over 1-inch outer parameter of field; avoid splashing on field.	Prevents reaching over sterile field
IF FIELD BECOMES WET, CONSIDER IT CONTAMINATED.	Water conducts microorganisms from nonsterile area to sterile field

Maintain Asepsis During Procedure

Action	Rationale
7. As procedure is performed:	
– Remove soiled equipment from area or sterile field; drop trash in bag or receptacle.	
– Avoid touching nonsterile surfaces.	
– When procedure is complete and dressing is intact, label dressing with date, time, and your initials.	Indicates when next dressing change is due
8. Decrease exposure of immunosuppressed clients or burn clients to microorganisms by maintaining sterile environment:	Limits exposure to microorganisms from other clients
– Place client in single room.	
– Use a separate stethoscope, sphygmomano-	

Action	Rationale
meter, and thermometer for client, if possible.	
– Only hospital gowns, linens, and materials should be used; allow no items from home unless approved and sterilized by hospital.	Prevents introduction of possible source of contamination
– When client is severely immunosuppressed, papers, books, and other personal items should be removed from immediate area, unless sterilization is possible.	
– Special food trays, disposable or presterilized, should be used.	

Evaluation

Goals met, partially met, or unmet?

Desired Outcomes (sample)

Client shows no signs of infection or of additional infection.
Procedures are performed with no evidence of exposure to microorganisms.

Documentation

The following should be noted on the client's chart:

- Status of wound, dressing, and incision site with indication of signs of infection, if any
- Procedure performed
- Protective garments used
- Client teaching done regarding maintenance of dressing and sterile protective environment and verbalized understanding by client

Sample Documentation

DATE	TIME	
1/2/94	1200	Temporary pacemaker inserted at bedside by Dr. Hope using sterile technique. Site clean and without redness. Client tolerated procedure without complaint of unusual discomfort. Clients states understands dressing change process and need for sterility.

🖐 Isolation Techniques

☒ Equipment

- Isolation cart or the following supplies:
  - masks
  - gloves (nonsterile or sterile)
  - gowns
  - plastic bags (or cloth linen bags)
  - tape or bag ties or fasteners
- Isolation card, indicating requirements for type of isolation (see Appendix E)
- Soap and source of water
- Paper towels

Purpose

Prevents spread of infection from client to others
Decreases exposure of susceptible client to infection

Assessment

Assessment should focus on the following:

Type of isolation indicated
Site of infection
Kind of restrictions needed in addition to universal precautions
Perceptions of client and family regarding information provided by doctor
Usual duration of infection
Adequate ventilation in room (often door is kept closed)
Associated physical symptoms of client, such as elevated temperature, chills, stiff neck

Nursing Diagnoses

The nursing diagnoses may include the following:

Altered safety related to presence of infection
Potential sepsis related to decreased resistance to infection
Potential for spread of infection related to knowledge deficit
Impaired skin integrity related to burn

Planning

Key Goals and Sample Goal Criteria

The client will

Experience no cross-contamination (*i.e.*, no additional infected
    sites during confinement)
Attain or maintain skin integrity
Verbalize three procedures needed to maintain specified isola-
    tion by end of day

Special Considerations

Hand washing is the single most important measure used to
    prevent the spread of infection. Hands should be washed be-
    fore entering and upon leaving isolation rooms as well as be-
    tween care procedures for different clients.
Most hospital policies require a nurse to obtain a culture from a
    draining body area and to initiate isolation procedures when
    positive cultures are reported. Consult the agency policy
    manual.
A client may become withdrawn, depressed, and harbor feel-
    ings of abandonment due to isolation. Plan frequent visitation
    times with the client and follow through as promised.

Home Health

An isolation card or information sheet, with clear instructions to
    family members, should be provided.

Implementation

Action	Rationale
1. Clearly explain to client and family the isolation type, reason initiated, how	Increases compliance of client, family, and visitors and decreases anxiety.

Action	Rationale
microorganisms are spread, staff and visitor restrictions related to dress and duration of contact (if applicable), and compliance needed; demonstrate procedure for applying sterile mask and gown. THE DOCTOR SHOULD INITIALLY INFORM THE CLIENT OF THE DIAGNOSED INFECTION.	
2. Ensure that isolation cart is complete and that sufficient trash cans and linen bags are in room.	Promotes proper disposal of contaminated materials
3. Keep sufficient linens and towels in room.	Avoids unnecessary trips in and out of room Decreases spread of microorganisms
4. Have housekeeping check room daily for sufficient soap and paper towels.	Promotes hand washing
5. Wash hands and organize equipment.	Reduces microorganism transfer Promotes efficiency
6. Note doctor's orders or refer to isolation guidelines adopted by agency for precautions necessary to establish appropriate type of isolation (see Appendix E).	Provides sufficient protection from microorganisms with minimum stress and restriction on client, visitors, and staff
7. Obtain appropriate isolation card and place on client's door.	Alerts visitors and staff to follow dress and hand-washing restrictions
8. If card must be filled out, include instructions on hand washing; use of masks, gloves and gowns; handling of linen and disposable items; need for private room, if appropriate.	
9. Review disinfectants needed to eliminate specific microorganism.	Prepares nurse for environmental and client management

Action	Rationale
10. Inform family members and visitors of necessary isolation precautions.	Allays fears to prevent withdrawal of friends and family from client Increases compliance
11. Install isolation supplies and cart outside client door.	Facilitates maintenance of isolation
12. Obtain supplies needed for wound care, if required, and keep sufficient supplies in client's room.	Avoids unnecessary trips in and out of room Decreases spread of microorganisms
13. Dispose of supplies taken into room or place them inside appropriate isolation bag for removal.	Prevents spread of infection from objects used on or by client
14. Use plastic bags for garbage and reusable equipment; bag all disposable drainage systems before delivering to agency's disposal unit. Label reusable equipment.	Prevents spread of infection from contaminated materials
15. Place soiled linens in proper linen bags; double bag linens if required by agency.	Allows for washing without removing bag
16. Clean room thoroughly with appropriate antimicrobial agent and leave room unoccupied after client discharge for appropriate time period.	Kills virulent organisms Prevents exposure of other clients to infection
17. Wash hands.	Reduces microorganism transfer

Evaluation

Goals met, partially met, or unmet?

Desired Outcomes (sample)

Infection is cleared, with no spread to other body areas or to other clients, family members, visitors, or staff.

Client demonstrates use of mask, proper disposal of infected tissues, and good hand-washing technique.

Client speaks freely about isolation, with no complaints of a sense of neglect by staff or abandonment.

Documentation

The following should be noted on the client's chart:

- Status of client's infection (identity and extent of areas involved)
- Client, family, and visitors' understanding of and compliance with isolation and required precautions
- Staff compliance with isolation precautions
- Periodic culture reports to establish need for continued isolation

Sample Documentation

DATE	TIME	
2/3/94	1400	Lab report obtained on culture of sputum specimen with results showing pneumococcal pneumonia. Doctor notified. Client and family instructed on isolation procedures; understanding voiced. Respiratory precautions sign placed on door. Masks and gloves placed outside of room. Visitors instructed on use of mask. Understanding verbalized by visitors and compliance noted.

🖐 Preoperative Care

☒ Equipment

- Assessment equipment (*e.g.*, blood pressure cuff, stethoscope, pen light)
- Scale
- Teaching materials (films, booklet, sample equipment)
- Preoperative checklist
- Shave and preparation kit (razor, soap, sponge, tray for water) (optional) Check agency policy.
- Procedure (hospital) gown
- Fingernail polish remover
- Denture cup (optional)
- Envelope for valuables (optional)
- Preoperative medications and administration equipment
- Nonsterile gloves

Purpose

Prepares client physically and emotionally for impending surgery

Assessment

Assessment should focus on the following:

Type of surgery
Preparatory regimen for type of surgery (per doctor's order or agency policy)
Perceptions of previous surgical experiences
Admission history and physical for factors increasing risks of surgery (*e.g.*, age, chronic or acute illness, depression, fluid and electrolyte imbalance)
Learning or comprehension ability
Reading ability
Language barriers

Nursing Diagnoses

The nursing diagnoses may include the following:

Knowledge deficit related to postoperative regimen
Anxiety related to impending surgery

Planning

Key Goals and Sample Goal Criteria

The client will

Verbalize purpose of surgery and the general surgical procedure before day of surgery
Demonstrate understanding of postoperative pulmonary and
circulatory regimen

Special Considerations

Assess the client's readiness to learn and, if preoperative teaching time is limited, gear teaching toward essential items of
concern.
Prior exposure to the postoperative environment, staff, and regimen often decreases the client's anxiety and promotes cooperation postoperatively.

Geriatric

Fear of death may be particularly profound in some elderly
clients, especially if this is a first hospitalization or first
surgery. Supply clear and thorough explanations of all procedures. Encourage the client to participate in preoperative
preparations.

Pediatric

Puppets may be used to explain surgical procedure, preoperative
care, and the postoperative regimen. Answer questions simply,
providing only necessary information and explanations.

Implementation

Action	Rationale
1. Wash hands and organize supplies.	Reduces microorganism transfer Promotes efficiency

Action	Rationale
2. Assess client's knowledge of impending surgery; reinforce information and correct errors in understanding. *Note*, it is the physician's responsibility initially to inform client about surgery, options, and risks.	Determines client's teaching needs Clarifies misinformation
3. Show films and provide booklets regarding surgery and postoperative care; encourage questions; answer questions clearly.	Reduces anxiety Imparts knowledge
4. Verify that operative permit is signed and on chart. *Note*, it is the physician's responsibility to obtain proper informed consent.	Avoids error in sending client to surgery without written consent
5. Verify that ordered lab work and diagnostic studies (x-ray films, EKGs) have been done; check results of diagnostic studies, place copies on chart, and include results on preoperative checklist; alert doctor to abnormal values.	Assesses client preparation and readiness for surgery Determines if treatment of abnormalities is needed or if surgery must be postponed
6. Check to be certain preoperative medications are available.	Avoids delays for client and surgical team on day of surgery
7. Obtain client's height and weight; perform head-to-toe assessment with in-depth assessment of areas related to surgery (see Procedure 3.1).	Provides baseline data
8. Instruct client about procedures or equipment that will be used to provide adequate oxygenation: – Demonstrate use of oxygen mask/cannula, or of endotracheal tube and ventilator	Prepares client for postoperative regimen

Action	Rationale
– Explain related noises and sensations.	Decreases anxiety produced by postoperative regimen
– Arrange introduction to respiratory therapy personnel.	Facilitates cooperation
– Demonstrate turning, coughing, and deep-breathing exercises, demonstrating use of pillow to splint incision site.	
– Explain techniques of chest physiotherapy, if applicable.	
– Stress the importance of pulmonary toilet in prevention of secretion buildup.	
9. Discuss and demonstrate, if applicable, techniques for maintaining adequate circulation and pain control:	
– Demonstrate range-of-motion and leg exercises, and check client's technique.	Maintains circulation while client is bedridden
– If transcutaneous electrical stimulation (TENS) unit is to be used, explain procedure to client.	Prepares client for use of TENS unit postoperatively
– Arrange for physical therapist to visit client.	Facilitates postoperative relationship and cooperation
10. Discuss with client and family the postoperative unit or environment; tour unit and introduce client to staff; inform family of special visitation hours, if applicable; review tentative timetable of surgery and recovery room period; instruct family on agency's methods of	Reduces anxiety about unfamiliar setting and care-givers

Action	Rationale
communicating status updates during and after surgery.	
11. **On the night before surgery:**	
– Don gloves.	
– Shave designated body areas.	Prevents postoperative infection
– Instruct client to shower with povidone solution, if ordered or agency policy.	
– Administer laxative or other medications, if ordered.	Helps flush bowel to prevent contamination of sterile field
– Perform enema and check results.	Evacuates bowel to prevent sterile field contamination
– Withhold foods and fluids after midnight the night before surgery (clear fluids may often be administered up to 3 to 4 hours before surgery, particularly if no IV fluids are infusing); consult agency policy.	Prevents sterile field contamination Prevents bowel and bladder puncture because of distended organs
– Check chart to determine which, if any, medications are to be given (permit sips of water) and at what time.	Delivers drugs client needs to maintain therapeutic levels during surgery while eliminating those that may cause compatibility problems with drugs given in surgery
12. **On day before or morning of surgery, prepare client:**	
– Verify presence of identification band (obtain duplicate band if needed).	Facilitates identification of client
– Remove jewelry (may retain wedding ring—wrap with tape); ask client to send valuables and jewelry home with family or place in valu-	Prevents loss during surgery Secures valuables and belongings

Action	Rationale
ables envelope and store with security department or according to agency policy.	
– Remove nail polish.	Allows for good visualization of nail beds to monitor oxygenation status
– Remove and label glasses, contact lenses, or other prostheses.	Prevents loss
– Remove full or partial dentures and label container (place with family or security department).	Prevents loss
– Assist client into hospital gown.	
13. **Thirty to 60 minutes before surgery** (when operating room signals that client's preoperative medication is to be given):	
– Check client identification band.	Verifies client's identity
– Encourage client to void.	Prevents field contamination and accidental bladder puncture
– Obtain vital signs.	Provides baseline data
– Administer ordered medication.	Induces mild sedation and achieves or maintains therapeutic levels
– Raise side rails and instruct client to stay in bed.	Prevents falls after client has been sedated
– Place call bell within reach and instruct client to call for assistance.	Facilitates communication and safety
– Encourage family to sit with client until stretcher arrives.	Decreases anxiety
14. When operating room personnel arrive to take client to surgery:	Prepares client for transport

Action	Rationale

– Compare client ident-
    ification band with
    surgery call slip; note
    spelling of name and
    identification number.
  – Assist client onto
    stretcher.
  – Write final note in chart.
  – Place chart, stamp plate,
    and ordered medica-
    tions on stretcher with
    client.
15. Assist family to appropri-
    ate postoperative waiting
    room, or remain in client's
    room, if ordered by doctor.
	Confirms correspondence of
	  client identity with impend-
	  ing surgical procedure

Evaluation

Goals met, partially met, or unmet?

Desired Outcomes (sample)

Client verbalizes purpose of postoperative regimen.
Client correctly demonstrates pulmonary and cardiovascular
   exercise regimens.

Documentation

The following should be noted on the client's chart:

* Presence of signed consent form
* Preoperative teaching done and client response
* Preparation procedures performed (*e.g.*, enema, shave)
* Vital signs and other clinical data
* Preoperative medications given
* Disposition of valuables
* Completed preoperative checklist or areas pending comple-
   tion
* Abnormal test results and time doctor was notified of these
* Further teaching or preparation needed

Sample Documentation

DATE	TIME	
1/2/94	1200	Preoperative teaching done with instructions on importance of pulmonary toilet, range-of-motion and calf exercises. Client verbalizes understanding. Preoperative checklist completed, except final vital signs and medication.

🖐 Postoperative Care

☒ Equipment (consult Procedure Manual for detailed lists)

- Assessment equipment (*e.g.,* blood pressure cuff, stethoscope, pen light, scale)
- Respiratory therapy equipment (*e.g.,* oxygen unit, incentive spirometer, nebulizer)
- Physical therapy equipment (*e.g.,* TENS unit, mechanical percussor, vibrator)
- Emesis basin
- IV therapy equipment
- Nasogastric (NG) suction equipment
- Medications and medication administration record
- Teaching materials (films, booklets, sample equipment)
- Sterile gloves

Purpose

Promotes return to state of physical and emotional well-being

Detects complications related to postsurgical status at early stage

Prevents postoperative complications

Facilitates wound healing

Assessment

Assessment should focus on the following:

Type of surgery

Nature of supportive therapy (ventilator, feeding tube, IV therapy)

Medication infusions

Preoperative physiological status

History of chronic or concurrent illnesses which could delay
  recovery
Monitoring equipment (*e.g.*, telemetry unit, central venous pres-
  sure)
Drainage systems (*e.g.*, chest tube, wound, NG, or urine
  drainage systems)
Communication barriers (*e.g.*, language barrier, neurological
  damage, presence of endotracheal tube)
Level of consciousness and orientation
Family support
Emotional state

Nursing Diagnoses

The nursing diagnoses may include the following:

Knowledge deficit related to postoperative regimen
Anxiety related to postoperative situation
Pain related to surgical incision
Potential infection related to disruption in skin integrity

Planning

Key Goals and Sample Goal Criteria

The client will

Attain and maintain clear breath sounds within 24 to 72 hours
  of surgery
Verbalize decreased discomfort within 30 minutes of complaint
  of pain
Perform postoperative pulmonary and circulatory exercises
  every 1 to 2 hours

Special Considerations

Geriatric

Anesthesia may cause temporary disorientation and personality
  change. Reorient the client frequently; allow family members
  to remain with client as much as possible.

Pediatric

Puppets may be used to encourage cooperation with the postoperative regimen. Family members may be effective in persuad-
  ing client to participate.

Home Health

If client has had outpatient surgery, arrange for follow-up by home-health or public-health nurse. Teach client and family information needed for safe and complete healing after surgery.

Implementation

Action	Rationale
1. Wash hands and organize supplies.	Reduces microorganism transfer Provides efficiency
2. When client is admitted to unit:	
– Assist client from stretcher to bed; remove excess linens and cover client with sheet.	Promotes warmth and privacy
– Orient to staff and environment, especially location of call button.	Decreases anxiety Promotes client–staff communication
– Hook up oxygen, connect telemetry, begin drainage systems; position client as ordered or with head of bed elevated 30 to 45 degrees.	Initiates support therapy Facilitates lung expansion
– Assess respiratory, neurological and neurovascular status, vital signs, apical pulse, bowel sounds, and EKG tracing from telemetry as well as other parameters pertaining to specific body systems affected by surgery.	Provides baseline data on postoperative status
– Assess incisional dressings and surgical-wound drainage systems.	
– Note urine output and output from drainage systems as well as diaphoresis, emesis, and diarrhea.	Enables early detection of fluid imbalances or systemic changes

Action	Rationale
3. Allow family members at bedside as soon as possible.	Reassures family Facilitates client comfort and orientation
4. Review postoperative orders:	Updates nurse on postoperative therapy program
– Contact departments to schedule ordered lab work, x-ray films, EKGs, and other diagnostic tests.	Facilitates early detection of complications
– Note medications given post-surgery and in recovery room and arrange medication schedule at appropriate intervals.	Returns client to routine medication regime
– Administer initial medication doses and treatments as soon as appropriate (if oral medication is needed, wait until client is able to tolerate fluids).	Prevents gastrointestinal upset from decreased peristalsis related to anesthesia
– Monitor for nausea or vomiting and return of bowel sounds.	Indicates activity of bowel and possible ileus development
5. Monitor vital signs as indicated by client status or as ordered by routine postoperative protocol (*e.g.,* every ½ hour times 2, every hour times 2, then every 2 to 4 hours if vital signs are stable).	Facilitates early detection of postoperative complications
6. Assess pain level and medicate as ordered; encourage client to request pain medication before onset of severe pain; medicate client 30 minutes before exercises and pulmonary toilet.	Promotes deep breathing and effective coughing Decreases the pain of turning
7. Begin pulmonary toilet immediately (if not contraindicated).	Prevents buildup of secretions

Action	Rationale
– Turn, deep breathe, and cough/suction client every 2 hours.	
– Instruct client in use of incentive spirometry equipment and encourage use every hour.	Facilitates lung expansion Mobilizes secretions
8. Initiate range-of-motion and leg exercises as well as chest physiotherapy, if applicable; if transcutaneous electrical nerve stimulation (TENS) unit is to be used, apply and turn on (see Procedure 8.9).	Maintains circulation while client is bedridden Facilitates removal of accumulated secretions Promotes comfort by blocking pain reception of nerves
9. Monitor surgical dressing and change or reinforce as needed and permitted. MANY DOCTORS PREFER TO REMOVE INITIAL DRESSING.	Promotes sense of well-being Increases self-esteem and sense of self-control
10. Help client to resume a normal state of personal grooming and hygiene:	
– Obtain glasses, contact lenses, dentures, or other prostheses and apply, if appropriate and client desires.	
– Obtain valuables from security when client is fully awake and requests them.	
– Assist client in personal hygiene and grooming, when desired and not prohibited.	Increases self-esteem

Evaluation

Goals met, partially met, or unmet?

Desired Outcomes (sample)

Client verbalizes purpose of postoperative regimen.
Client correctly demonstrates pulmonary and cardiovascular
  exercise regimen.

Documentation

The following should be noted on the client's chart:

- Time of admission of client to room and area admitted from
- Complete assessment with emphasis on abnormal findings
- Status of operative dressings, tubes, drains, and incisions
- Support equipment initiated
- Procedures performed
- Client tolerance to therapy
- Abnormal test results noted and time doctor is notified
- Medications administered
- Client and family concerns
- Teaching needs noted

Sample Documentation

DATE	TIME	
1/2/94	1200	Client admitted from recovery room post right thoracotomy. Alert and oriented. Vital signs obtained every ½ hour with stable results. Skin warm and dry. Respirations deep regular at rate of 16. Denies pain. Mediastinal tube to 20 cm H_2O suction. Serosanguineous drainage (50 ml) noted in pleurevac. Chest dressing clean, dry, and intact.

Use of Limb and Body Restraints

☒ Equipment

- Restraint appropriate for limb or body area (*i.e.*, wrist, ankle, vest or waist restraint)
- Wash cloths for each limb restraint
- Lotion and powder (optional)
- Kerlix gauze (3- or 4-inch roll)
- 2-inch tape

Purpose

Prevents injury to client from falls, wound contamination, and tube dislodgment

Prevents injury to others from disoriented or hostile client when other methods of control have been ineffective

Assessment

Assessment should focus on the following:

Doctor's order (obtain if not on chart)
Agency policy regarding use of restraints
Client's orientation and level of consciousness
Skin status in areas requiring restraint
Effectiveness of other safety controls and precautions
Availability of staff or family members to sit with client

Nursing Diagnoses

The nursing diagnoses may include the following:

Potential for injury related to confusion and disorientation

Planning

Key Goal and Sample Goal Criterion

The client will

Experience no physical injury related to falls during hospitalization.

Special Considerations

A doctor's order should be obtained before applying restraints.

Learn standing orders or agency policy regarding use of restraints.

Some agencies require that restraints be used in certain situations (such as presence of endotracheal tube).

Geriatric

The skin of elderly clients is often very sensitive, and the blood vessels are easily collapsed. Restrain such clients loosely with linen or soft restraints and check the circulation frequently. Remove restraints frequently to check the skin beneath them.

Pediatric

Mittens may be preferable to wrist restraints because they are less restrictive than restraints and permit growth and developmental activities.

Home Health

Sheets may be used to tie client securely to a bed or chair to prevent falls. Socks or other soft pieces of cloth may be fashioned into wrist restraints and mittens may be used to prevent pulling of tubes.

Implementation

Action	Rationale
1. Wash hands and organize equipment.	Prevents microorganism transfer
	Promotes efficiency
2. Explain procedure to client and state why restraints are needed.	Promotes cooperation
	Reduces anxiety
3. Place client in a comfortable position with good body alignment.	

Action	**Rationale**
4. Wash and dry area to which restraint will be applied; massage area and apply lotion if skin is dry; apply powder, if desired.	Facilitates circulation to skin
	Decreases friction on skin from dirt and dead skin cells
5. To apply wrist or ankle restraints:	
– Use 10-inch strip of Kerlix gauze folded to 2-inch width; wrap strip in a figure eight (Fig. 10.11) and fold the circles of the figure over one another; slip wrist or ankle through loop	
– To use commercial restraints, wrap padded portion of restraint around wrist or ankle, thread tie through slit in restraint, and fasten to second tie with secure knot	Holds restraint intact around wrist/ankle
– Secure ends of ties to bed frame. DO NOT SECURE TO BED RAILS	Prevents accidental pull on limb with movement of bed rail

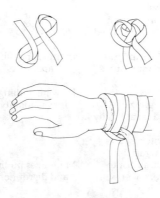

Figure 10.11

Action	Rationale
(with some two-part restraints, the wrist section snaps into a separate section that is secured to bed frame)	Allows removal of restraint for skin care without removal of portion secured to bed
6. Vest restraint: – Place vest on client with opening in front.	Prevents client from getting out of bed without restricting arm and hand mobility
– Pull tie on end of vest flap across chest and slip through slit in opposite side of vest.	
– Wrap other end of flap across client and around chair or upper portion of bed.	Secures vest to client
– Fasten ends of ties together behind chair or to sides of bed frame.	
– Check respiratory status for distress related to restriction from vest.	
– Reposition client for minimal pressure on chest.	
7. Waist restraint: – Wrap restraint around waist.	Prevents client from getting out of bed without binding chest
– Slip end of one tie through slit in restraint.	
– Secure ends of ties to bed frame.	
– Monitor for complaints of nausea or abdominal distress.	Indicates possible restriction on abdomen
8. Hand mittens: – Wrap Kerlix gauze around hand until totally covered.	Prevents pulling of tubes Allows mobility of limb
– Fold hand into fist and continue to wrap fist.	
– Put tape around fist to secure gauze; cover with sock or stocking.	Minimizes pulling of gauze and disruption of mitt

Action	Rationale
9. When a client is in re-straints:	
– Remove restraint every 4 to 8 hours as well as when staff or family are at bedside to prevent injury.	Decreases continuous pressure on skin
– Massage skin beneath restraint and apply lotion or powder; wrap folded washcloth around limb and place restraint on top of cloth.	Increases circulation to skin Decreases friction and skin irritation
– Monitor the extremity distal to the restraint every 1 to 2 hours for color, temperature, and capillary refill.	Determines adequacy of circulation below restraint Identifies need for removal
– Monitor for skin irritation.	
– Check every hour for added pull on restraints and limb, tangled ties, or pressure points from knots; remove and adjust restraint to eliminate problem.	Prevents loss of skin integrity due to excessive pressure
10. Continually assess client's orientation and continued need for restraints and remove as soon as safe to do so.	Decreases risk of disruption of skin integrity Restores sense of self-control

Evaluation

Goals met, partially met, or unmet?

Desired Outcomes (sample)

Client experiences no falls or injury while under nurse's care.
Skin remains intact at site of restraint.

Documentation

The following should be noted on the client's chart:

- Reason for restraint application
- Time doctor's order obtained
- Type of restraint applied
- Client's response to restraints
- Periodic removal of restraints
- Skin care performed

Sample Documentation

DATE	TIME	
1/2/94	1200	Admission history reveals frequent falls and pulling of tubes during recent stay at nursing home. Client diagnosed with senile dementia, anorexia, and severe dehydration. IV and feeding tube inserted. Bilateral wrist restraints applied loosely with waist restraint secured to bed. No family available at this time.

🖐 Decubitus Care

✖ Equipment

- Dressing change materials (see Procedure 10.2); use multi-pack gauze in plastic container
- Nonsterile gloves and sterile gloves
- Towel or linen saver pad
- Sterile irrigation saline
- Povidone-iodine (Betadine) solution or peroxide, as ordered
- Povidone-iodine (Betadine) swabs
- Topical-care agents (may vary from agency to agency, case to case):
  - Karaya Gum patches (Duraderm)
  - gelatin sponge
  - Silvadene cream (Duraprep)
  - zinc oxide
  - granulated sugar
  - topical antibiotics (when infection has been confirmed)
  - antacid (*e.g.*, Maalox, Riopan)
- Moist wound barrier/transparent wound dressing (Duoderm)
- Overbed table or bedside stand
- Paper bag, trash bag
- Pressure relief pad:
  - sheepskin mattress
  - egg crate mattress
  - water mattress
  - gel flotation pads

Purpose

Removes accumulated secretions and dead tissue from wound or incision

Decreases microorganism growth on wounds or incision site

Promotes wound healing

Assessment

Assessment should focus on the following:

Doctor's order regarding type of dressing change, procedure, and frequency of change

Type and location of decubitus

Client factors contributing to development of decubitus (*e.g.,* prolonged immobility, poor circulation, nutritional status, incontinence, seepage of wound drainage onto skin)

Time of last pain medication

Allergies to iodine (*i.e.,* shellfish or seafood) or tape

Protective bed cover (sheepskin, egg crate, flotation mattress)

Client's activity regimen (frequency of turning, getting out of bed)

Client knowledge regarding factors contributing to development of decubitus

Risk assessment for development of decubitus

Nursing Diagnoses

The nursing diagnoses may include the following:

Impaired tissue integrity related to pressure sore
Potential infection related to decreased skin integrity

Planning

Key Goals and Sample Goal Criteria

The client will

Regain skin integrity within 3 weeks
Demonstrate no signs of infection or further infection during confinement

Special Considerations

Decubitus care is often painful. Assess the client's pain needs and provide medication 30 minutes before beginning the procedure.

A clean, instead of sterile, dressing change is often permitted.

Decubitus care tends to vary among agencies; consult the agency manual for guidelines.

Geriatric

Debilitation and decreased activity often accompany advanced age. Family members should be informed of the importance of preventing pressure to certain skin areas for extended periods of time.

Home Health

Newspaper should be used to cover the table surface during a dressing change and animals in the home should be restricted from the area during the procedure.

Implementation

Action	Rationale
1. Wash hands and organize equipment.	Reduces microorganism transfer Promotes efficiency
2. Explain procedure and assistance needed from client.	Promotes cooperation
3. Assess pain level; deliver medication, if needed, and wait for medication to take effect before beginning.	Decreases discomfort of dressing change
4. Place bedside table close to area being dressed and prepare supplies:	Facilitates management of sterile field and supplies
– Place supplies on bed-side table.	
– Tape paper bag or trash bag to side of table.	Facilitates easy disposal of contaminated waste
– Open sterile gloves and use inside of glove package as sterile field.	Promotes use of supplies without contamination and prepares work field
– Open gauze-pad packages and drop several onto sterile field (leave remaining gauze pads in plastic container).	
– Open dressing tray.	
– Open liquids and pour saline on two gauze pads and Betadine on four gauze pads (or more if	

Action	Rationale
wet-to-dry dressing change).	
– Open Betadine swabs, if used, to expose end of plastic stick.	
– Place several sterile cotton-tip swabs and cotton balls on sterile field.	
5. Don nonsterile gloves.	Prevents exposure to damage
6. Place towel or pad under wound area.	
7. Loosen tape by pulling toward the decubitus and remove soiled dressing;	Exposes site for cleaning
note appearance of dressing and wound. SOAK DRESSING WITH SALINE IF IT ADHERES TO WOUND AND THEN GENTLY PULL FREE.	Permits assessment of site
8. Place soiled dressing in paper bag.	Prevents spread of organisms
9. Discard gloves and wash hands.	
10. Don sterile gloves.	
11. Pick up saline-soaked dressing pad with forceps and form a large swab.	
12. Cleanse away debris and drainage from decubitus, moving from center outward; use a new pad for each area cleaned, discarding the old pads.	Prevents contamination of wound from organisms on skin surface Maintains sterility of supplies
13. Wipe decubitus with povidone-soaked pads moving from center of wound outward using a circular motion; use a dry pad to dry the wound and surrounding skin and a skin prep or tincture of benzoin on the surrounding skin; discard forceps.	Decreases microorganisms Facilitates adherence of dressings/pads

Action	Rationale
DO NOT ALLOW TINCTURE OF BENZOIN TO TOUCH BROKEN SKIN AREAS.	Sometimes causes painful tissue erosion
14. Place ordered topical agent onto or into decubitus; may place povidone pads in decubitus and allow to remain until dry.	Provides antiinfective agent
15. Dress decubitus by covering with a single 4 × 4-inch gauze pad or a transparent wound dressing; secure dressing with tape.	Allows air to reach wound but removes drainage
16. Write date and time of dressing change on a strip of tape and place tape across top of dressing.	Indicates last dressing change and need for next change within 24 to 48 hours
17. Dispose of gloves and materials and store supplies appropriately.	Decreases spread of microorganisms
18. Position client for comfort with call bell within reach.	Promotes comfort and communication
19. Wash hands.	Decreases spread of microorganisms

Evaluation

Goals met, partially met, or unmet?

Desired Outcomes (sample)

Client regains skin integrity within 3 weeks.
Client demonstrates no signs of infection or of further infection during confinement.

Documentation

The following should be noted in the client's chart:

- Materials and procedure used for decubitus care
- Location, size, and type of wound or incision

- Status of the decubitus site and stage of healing
- Status of previous dressing
- Solution and medications applied to wound
- Frequency of turning and repositioning client
- Client teaching done and additional learning needs
- Client tolerance to procedure

Sample Documentation

DATE	TIME	
1/2/94	0600	Decubitis site cleaned with saline and povidone swabs. Sacral decubitus approximately 5 cm in diameter, pink, with slightly granulated edges; no drainage or foul odor noted. Povidone pads placed into and over wound. Wound covered with 4 × 4-inch pad. Client turned to side with pillow at back. Tolerated decubitus care with minimal discomfort.

🖐 Wound Irrigation

✖ Equipment

- Irrigation solution
- Sterile irrigation set, including sterile syringe with sterile tubing (or catheter) attached
- Sterile basin
- Gauze pads
- Materials for dressing change, if applicable (see Procedure 10.2)
- Linen saver
- Large towel
- Waste receptacle
- Sterile gloves

Purpose

Facilitates removal of secretions and microorganisms from wound

Assessment

Assessment should focus on the following:

Doctor's order for irrigation orders
Type and location of wound
Irrigant (type of medication added, if applicable)
Pain status and time of last pain medication

Nursing Diagnoses

The nursing diagnoses may include the following:

Potential for infection related to open abdominal incision line

Planning

Key Goals and Sample Goal Criteria

The client will

Regain skin integrity within 1 month
Demonstrate no signs of infection during confinement

Special Considerations

Wound irrigation can be painful; medicate client 30 minutes before beginning the procedure.

Pediatric

Children might contaminate the sterile field, gown, or gloves accidentally. Restrain them with linen or soft restraints during the procedure. Encourage a parent to sit with the child during the procedure, if possible, to provide reassurance and to help calm the child.

Home Health

Newspaper should be used to cover the table surface during wound irrigation and animals in the home should be restricted from the area during the procedure.

Implementation

Action	Rationale
1. Assess pain level; deliver medication, if needed, and wait for medication to take effect.	Decreases discomfort during procedure
2. Wash hands and organize supplies.	Reduces microorganism transfer
	Promotes efficiency
3. Explain procedure and assistance needed from client; provide privacy.	Facilitates cooperation
	Decreases anxiety
4. Place bedside table near wound area and open supplies (arrange for dressing change in addition to wound irrigation).	Permits replacement of dressing after wound irrigation
5. Don nonsterile gloves and remove dressing.	

Action	Rationale
6. Place linen saver and towel under wound.	Catches overflow of irrigant
7. Discard nonsterile gloves, wash hands, and don sterile gloves.	Maintains sterility of process
8. Place basin beside wound and tilt client to side toward basin.	Facilitates drainage of irrigation into basin
9. Irrigate wound: – Insert irrigation tubing into upper portion of wound (or above cleanest portion of wound so that fluid flows from cleanest to dirtiest portion of wound; Fig. 10.13). – Attach syringe to tubing or catheter and pour in irrigant; continue to pour irrigant until wound debris and drainage are washed into basin. – Move catheter to different part of wound and repeat irrigation until total wound area has been irrigated and all irrigant has been used.	Flushes debris and contaminants from wound

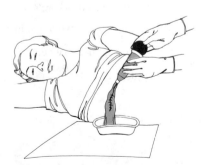

Figure 10.13

Action	Rationale
10. Use sterile pads, if needed, to remove additional debris; pack wound with gauze pads, if ordered; apply sterile dressing.	
11. Write the date and time of dressing change on a strip of tape and place tape across dressing.	Indicates last dressing change and need for next change within 24 to 48 hours
12. Dispose of gloves and materials and store supplies appropriately.	Decreases spread of microorganisms
13. Position client for comfort with call bell within reach.	Promotes comfort and communication
14. Wash hands.	Decreases spread of microorganisms

Evaluation

Goals met, partially met, or unmet?

Desired Outcomes (sample)

Client regains skin integrity within 1 month.
Client demonstrates no signs of infection during confinement.

Documentation

The following should be noted on the client's chart:

- Location, appearance, and type of wound or incision
- Status of previous dressing
- Solution and medications applied to wound
- Client teaching done
- Client tolerance to procedure

Sample Documentation

DATE	TIME	
1/12/94	0600	Gaping abdominal incisional wound irrigated with sterile saline. Incision about 8 inches in length and gapes open at 2 cm crosswise along entire length of incision. No purulent drainage from wound. Open area pink with whitish yellow edges. Wound packed with moist saline gauze. Client turned to side with pillow at back. Tolerated procedure with minimal discomfort.

✋ Wound Drain Management

☒ Equipment

- Graduated container
- Sterile dressing tray (forceps, scissors, gauze pads [optional])
- Sterile gauze dressing pads (2 × 2-inch, 4 × 4-inch, or surgical [ABD] pads, depending on drainage and size of area to be covered), or transparent dressing
- Sterile bowl
- 2-inch tape or Montgomery straps (paper tape, if allergic to others)
- Sterile gloves
- Nonsterile gloves
- Towel or linen-saver pad
- Cotton balls and cotton-tip swabs (optional)
- Sterile irrigation saline or sterile water
- Povidone-iodine (Betadine) solution or peroxide, as ordered
- Povidone-iodine (Betadine) swabs
- Bacteriostatic ointment
- Overbed table or bedside stand
- Paper bag, trash bag
- Additional gauze pads

Purpose

Removes accumulated secretions and dead tissue from wound or incision

Decreases microorganism growth on wounds or incision site

Promotes wound healing

Assessment

Assessment should focus on the following:

Type of drain

Doctor's order or agency policy regarding frequency of drainage measurement

Type, appearance, and location of wound or incision
Time of last pain medication
Client allergies to iodine (shellfish or seafood) or tape

Nursing Diagnoses

The nursing diagnoses may include the following:

Impaired tissue integrity related to draining abscess
Potential infection related to decreased skin integrity

Planning

Key Goals and Sample Goal Criteria

The client will

Regain skin integrity within 3 weeks
Demonstrate no signs of infection in the wound, such as redness, pain, purulent drainage, or foul odor

Special Considerations

Dressing changes and drain manipulation are often painful. Assess client's pain needs and medicate, if needed, 30 minutes before beginning procedure.

Pediatric

It may be necessary to have a parent assist while the procedure is being performed.
Using dolls may be helpful in explaining to the child what drain management entails.

Home Health

Newspaper should be used to cover the table surface before arranging a sterile field. Animals in the home should be restricted from the area during the procedure.

Implementation

Action	Rationale
1. Wash hands and organize equipment.	Reduces microorganism transfer

Action	Rationale
2. Explain procedure and assistance needed from client; provide privacy.	Promotes efficiency Promotes cooperation Avoids embarrassment
3. Assess pain level and administer pain medication, if needed; wait for medication to take effect before beginning.	Decreases discomfort of dressing change
4. Place bedside table close to area being dressed.	Facilitates management of sterile field and supplies
5. Place towel or pad under wound area.	Eliminates drainage onto surrounding skin
6. Perform dressing change (see Procedure 10.2); during wound cleaning, note condition of drain-insertion site (intactness of sutures, presence of redness or purulent drainage).	
7. Clean wound with Betadine-soaked pads or swabs, moving from drain outward in a circular motion; place gauze dressing around drain-insertion site (Fig. 10.14.1).	Prevents contamination of wound with microorganisms Decreases skin irritation from drainage
8. Check that tubings are not kinked, twisted, or dislodged.	
9. Continue procedure by performing steps appropri-	

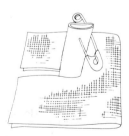

Figure 10.14.1

Action	Rationale

ate for type of drain used;
then proceed to steps 18
through 20 for completion
of procedure.

Penrose Drains

10. Place extra 4 × 4-inch
    pads over drain.

    Facilitates absorption of
    drainage

11. Cover with one or two
    surgical pads and tape
    securely.

Hemovac

12. Apply and secure dress-
    ing; note drainage color
    and amount; empty if half-
    full or more by opening
    pouring spout, holding it
    inverted over graduated
    container, and squeezing
    hemovac gently.

    Assesses drainage
    Empties drain to prevent
    overfilling and applying
    tension on suture areas

    Facilitates flow of clots and
    drainage

13. Compress evacuator after
    emptying:
    - Place palm of hand on
      top of evacuator and
      press flat with top of
      spout open.
    - Replace stopper to spout
      while holding evacuator
      flat (Fig. 10.14.2.).
    - Remove hand from
      evacuator and check
      that it remains flat.

    Activates suction needed to
    maintain drainage evacu-
    ation

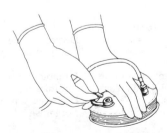

Figure 10.14.2

Action	Rationale
14. When assessing wound, drainage, and drain, check to be sure evacuator is still compressed; if not, empty drain and recompress.	Maintains suction pressure
Jackson-Pratt (Bulb Drain)	
15. Apply and secure dressing; note drainage color and amount; empty if half-full or more by opening pouring spout, inverting over graduated container, and squeezing bulb.	Assesses drainage Prevents overfilling and tension pull on suture line Releases contents from the bulb drain
16. After emptying, recompress bulb by squeezing bulb in palm of hand with top of spout open, then closing spout and releasing bulb.	Initiates suction needed for drainage evacuation
17. When assessing wound, drainage, and drain, check to be sure evacuator is still compressed; if not, empty drain and recompress.	Maintains suction pressure
T-tube	
18. Apply and secure dressing; hang bag off trunk of body.	Facilitates use of gravity for drainage
19. To empty, open pouring spout, tilt to side with spout positioned over graduated container, pour, and recap spout.	Prevents overfill of tube and tension on suture line
20. Dispose of gloves and materials and store supplies appropriately.	Decreases spread of micro-organisms
21. Position client for comfort with call bell within reach.	Promotes comfort and communication
22. Wash hands.	Decreases spread of micro-organisms

Evaluation

Goals met, partially met, or unmet?

Desired Outcomes (sample)

Client regains skin integrity within 3 weeks.
Client demonstrates no signs of infection in wound.

Documentation

The following should be noted in the client's chart:

- Location and type of wound or incision
- Status of previous dressing
- Status of the wound or incision site and drain
- Type and amount of drainage
- Solution and medications applied to wound
- Client teaching done
- Client's tolerance to procedure

Sample Documentation

DATE	TIME	
1/12/94	0600	Abdominal-wound dressing saturated with serous drainage. Dressing removed, Penrose drain intact with moderate drainage. Area surrounding drain intact without redness. Site cleaned and wiped with Betadine swabs. Dressing change performed. Client tolerated dressing change with minimal discomfort.

CHAPTER 11

Medication Administration

OVERVIEW

- Medication administration is one of the most frequently performed procedures executed by the nurse.
- Precision is essential in the performance of these skills; otherwise, fatalities may occur.
- To administer drugs safely, the nurse must make decisions regarding alterations in technique based on the age, developmental stage, weight, physiologic status, mental

Jean Smith-Temple and Joyce Young Johnson:
Nurses' Guide to Clinical Procedures, Second Edition.© 1994
J. B. Lippincott Company

status, educational level, and past physical history of the client.

- Legal liability remains a major concern in medication administration; however, using a few basic guidelines can significantly decrease the nurse's risk of involvement in a lawsuit:
  - Know the medication being administered.
  - Know the correct technique for administration.
  - Know the client in relation to factors that might affect administration methodology (see above).
  - Know the agency policy on administering drugs by any technique.
  - Know the client's rights in relation to medication administration.
  - REMEMBER THE FIVE "RIGHTS" OF MEDICATION ADMINISTRATION *EACH TIME* DRUGS ARE ADMINISTERED: THE RIGHT *CLIENT, DRUG, ROUTE, TIME, AND AMOUNT*.
  - Document administration immediately after giving medication.
  - If you are unsure about any aspect of drug therapy or administration, ASK!
- Generally, medications given by parenteral techniques act faster and have more reliable results than drugs given by other routes. Because errors in parenteral medication can quickly become debilitating or lethal, USE SPECIAL CAUTION!
- Medications given orally are least expensive, but the oral route is the least dependable route of administration.
- Although exposure to blood is often minimal during parenteral medication administration, gloves are recommended.
- Administration of parenteral medications often requires manipulation of needles, placing the nurse at risk for a needle-stick injury. When available, the nurse should use a needleless methodology and equipment for medication administration.
- Before administering ordered medication, be sure that no folk medications or over-the-counter medications have been ingested that may result in a drug interaction.

☙ Principles of Medication Administration

☒ Equipment

- Physician's order
- Medication-administration record
- Medication cards, if used at agency
- Ink pen
- Disposable gloves
- Medication to be administered
- Drug reference book
- Medicine tray

Optional, depending on route of administration
- Syringes with appropriate-size needles
- Alcohol swabs
- Medication cups
- Cup of water
- Drinking straw
- Medication labels
- Calculator
- Lubricant
- Medicine dropper
- Needleless system equipment (access pins, caps, etc.)

Purpose

Uses basic safety factors of drug administration in preparing and administering medications

Avoids client injury due to drug errors

Assessment

Assessment should focus on the following:

Clarity and legibility of physician's order
Age and weight of client
Lighting in medication preparation area

Planning

Key Goal and Sample Goal Criterion

The client will

Receive correct drug and dosage at the correct time without injury.

Special Considerations

Consult a drug reference manual or pharmacist for information on drugs with which you are unfamiliar.

Pediatric

Infants and children often require very small dosages of medications.

Use a syringe instead of a medication cup for the most accurate measurement of liquid medications.

Home Health and Geriatric

Administer medications only to the client admitted to the home-health service (*i.e.,* not to a spouse or relative).

Administer only drugs prescribed by the tending physician.

For elderly clients at home who have problems with memory, use devices that remind client when drugs must be taken (*e.g.,* calendars, daily pill dispensers).

Implementation

Action	Rationale
1. Wash hands.	Reduces microorganism transfer
2. Gather equipment and unlock medication cart or cabinet.	Promotes efficiency

Action	Rationale

3. Compare medication-administration record to physician's order, adhering to principles of the five rights of drug administration; use these principles throughout preparation and administration. Check for the *right:*

- *Client*—includes checking name, identification number, room number, prescribing doctor's name on the order, medication-administration record, medication cards, and client-identification band
- *Drug*—includes ascertaining that generic names are compatible with brand names (if both are used) and that client has no allergies to ingredients of ordered medications; includes checking drug labels with medication-administration records or cards
- *Dosage*—includes determining that dosage ordered is within usual dosage range for route of administration, weight and age of client; checking dosages on drug labels for compatibility with dosages written on medication-administration record or cards; and performing accurate dose calculations
- *Time*—includes checking that medication-administration frequency (*e.g.,*

Promotes safety
Avoids client injury related to wrong dose, drug, route, time, or client

Action	Rationale

"every 12 hours" [q 12 hours] or "three times a day" [t.i.d.]) is compatible with times (*i.e.*, 6 A.M. and 6 P.M., or 10 A.M., 2 P.M., and 6 P.M.) listed on medication-administration record or medication cards

- *Route*—includes checking drug label to ascertain if medication can be administered by ordered route and checking that route recorded on medication-administration record and cards corresponds to the doctor's order

4. If client has allergy to any ordered medication, notify physician.

Prevents unnecessary allergic reactions and injury

5. Focusing on one medication at a time, begin label checks by comparing the actual drug labels to the order, as transcribed on the medication-administration record or cards; if using a medication-administration record, begin at the top and systematically move down the page; if using cards, group the cards according to route of administration (*e.g.*, oral medications, IM medications) and focus on one card at a time.

Prevents error in preparation
Promotes systematic preparation

6. Comparing drug labels with the orders on the medication-administration record or cards, determine if dosage calculations are necessary.

Action	Rationale

7. Perform calculations using
   one of the following formulas:

$$\frac{\text{DESIRED DOSAGE}}{\text{AVAILABLE DOSAGE}} \times \frac{\text{VEHICLE}}{\text{(ML, TABLET)}} = \frac{\text{CORRECT DOSAGE}}{\text{(ML, TABLETS, MINIMS)}}$$

Example: Doctor's order: 15 mEq potassium per liter of D_5W
        Available dose: 40 mEq potassium per 20-ml vial
                                     (2 mEq per ml)

$$\frac{15\ \text{mEq potassium}}{40\ \text{mEq potassium}} \times 20\ \text{ml} = 7.5\ \text{ml}$$
                                     (inject into liter D_5W)

OR

DESIRED DOSAGE: AVAILABLE DOSAGE

=

DESIRED VOLUME: AVAILABLE VOLUME

Example: D is desired volume (amount to be administered)
15 mEq potassium: 40 mEq potassium = D:20 ml
  Multiply the means by the extremes

$$300 = 40\,D$$

$$\frac{300}{40} = D$$

$$D = 7.5\ \text{ml}$$

Desired dosage is the dosage ordered
Available dosage equals the dosage on hand (*e.g.,* the number of
  milligrams or the number of milliequivalents)
Vehicle is the drug form (number of tablets or amount of solution containing the available dosage)
Desired volume is the volume of the drug to be administered (*e.g.,*
  number of milliliters, minims, tablets)
Available volume is the amount of solution or number of tablets
  containing the drug (*e.g.,* ml minims, tablets) on hand

IF YOU ARE UNCERTAIN OF THE ACCURACY OF YOUR CALCULATIONS, CHECK WITH ANOTHER NURSE.	Provides safety check

Action	Rationale

8. Check label on each medication:
   - Before removing drug from drawer or storage area
   - Before pouring or drawing up medication (or once medication is in hand, if unit dose)
   - Before replacing multiple-dose containers on shelf (or before removing your hands from the drug once it is on the medicine tray, if unit dose)

9. Recheck medication-administration record for appropriate client-identification record.

   Ensures nurse is focusing on right client record

10. Using aseptic technique, pour or draw up each medication after second label check (Fig. 11.1); use guidelines in Table 11.1 in preparing drugs for various routes of administration.

    Prepares drug using aseptic technique

    Ensures accurate measurement of drug amount

11. Place each drug on medication tray after checking label a third time and before proceeding to prepare the next drug.

    Provides third label check

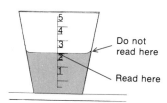

Do not read here

Read here

Figure 11.1

Action	Rationale
12. Recheck medication record or cards with each drug on tray; if using medication cards, make certain medicines are	Provides safety check and identifying information on drug once on medication tray

TABLE 11.1   Guidelines for Preparing Various Forms of Medication

Guideline	Rationale
1. Most agencies require that certain medications (such as heparin, insulin, intravenous digoxin) be checked by a second nurse *during* preparation. Check agency policy and procedure manuals for the full listing of these drugs.	Prevents error in preparation of drugs with potentially lethal effects
2. Do not open unit-dose packages in advance if dosages are exact (*i.e.*, pills, oral liquids, and suppositories). Open just before administering.	Provides identifying drug information Prevents waste
3. When preparing topical, nasal, ophthalmic, and other boxed medications, remove medication from box and check labels of actual containers.	Prevents administration of wrong drug
4. If pouring pills from multiple-dose containers, pour pill into cap and then into medicine cup.	Maintains asepsis
Pour liquids away from label. Read amount of medication poured in medicine cups at bottom of meniscus (see Fig. 11.1).	Prevents destruction of label Measures liquid drug correctly
5. Separate drugs requiring preassessment data, such as vital signs.	Prevents administration prior to vital sign assessment
6. When preparing any drug, check for expiration date.	Eliminates administering drugs that no longer have full therapeutic effect

See Procedures 11.2 through 11.18 for additional information on the preparation and administration of drugs for various routes.

Action	Rationale
placed in front of appropriate cards.	
13. Place all administration equipment on tray.	Ensures that proper equipment for administration is present
14. Lock medication cart or cabinet.	Adheres to accreditation guidelines

Evaluation

Goals met, partially met, or unmet?

Desired Outcome (sample)

Client received correct drug and dosage at the correct time without injury.

✋ Eye (Ophthalmic) Instillation

✖ Equipment

- Two to six cotton balls, one to three cotton balls per eye (some agencies recommend use of sterile cotton balls)
- Disposable gloves
- Medication record or card
- Pen
- Medication to be administered

Purpose

Instills medications in mucous membranes of eye for various therapeutic effects, such as decreasing inflammatory and infectious processes and preventing drying of cornea, conjunctiva, and other delicate eye structures

Assessment

Assessment should focus on the following:

Presence in structures of eye (sclera, cornea, conjunctival sacs, eyelids) of lesions, redness, or drainage
Status of vision prior to drug administration
Complaints of pain or eye discomfort

Nursing Diagnoses

The nursing diagnoses may include the following:

Altered comfort: pain related to infectious process

Planning

Key Goal and Sample Goal Criterion

The client will

Show signs of resolved inflammatory process of eye, as indicated by the absence of redness, drainage, edema, swelling, and pain

Special Considerations

Geriatric and Home Health

For elderly clients at home who have difficulty remembering, use a calendar to remind them when to administer eye medication.

 Transcultural

In some cultures (such as Vietnamese) touching the head may be viewed as taking away the spirit. The nurse should consult the client, or parents if a child is involved, regarding what is culturally appropriate.

A family member may be instructed to assist in positioning the client, if necessary or desired.

Implementation

Action	Rationale
1. Wash hands.	Decreases microorganism transfer
2. Prepare drug to be administered according to the five rights of drug administration (see Procedure 11.1, Principles of Medication Administration).	Promotes safe drug administration
3. Identify client by identification bracelet and by addressing client by name.	Verifies identity of client
4. Explain procedure and purpose of medication to client.	Reduces anxiety Promotes cooperation
5. Don gloves.	Prevents exposure to secretions from eye

Action	Rationale
6. Position client in supine or sitting position with forehead tilted back slightly.	Facilitates proper placement of medication
7. If drainage or excess tearing is noted around lower lashes and eyelids, wipe eye with a cotton ball from the inner to outer aspect (if both eyes need to be wiped, use a separate cotton ball for each eye).	Removes excess secretions and debris to facilitate absorption of medication through mucous membranes Prevents cross-contamination
8. If using bottle with a dropper, squeeze top of medication dropper to aspirate solution into dropper tube.	Creates suction to draw up medication in dropper
9. Holding dropper or ointment to be administered in dominant hand, place heel of dominant hand on client's forehead (Fig. 11.2).	Provides strategic placement of nurse's hand to prevent accidental eye injury to client
10. Using cotton ball, gently pull lower eyelid downward.	Exposes lower conjunctival sac for placement of medication
11. Instruct client to look up towards forehead.	Eliminates corneal-reflex stimulation

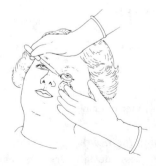

Figure 11.2

Action	Rationale
12. Administer ordered number of drops (or quantity of ointment) into conjunctival sac of appropriate eye without letting dropper touch client; apply ointments from inner to outer canthus, ending ointment administration smoothly with a twisting motion.	Places medication in conjunctival sac for absorption without contaminating dropper
13. Remove hands and instruct client to close and roll eyes around, unless prohibited or client is unable to do so.	Spreads medication evenly over eye
14. Remove excess medication and secretions from around eye with cotton balls.	Prevents local irritation and discomfort
15. Discard gloves.	Reduces microorganism transfer
16. If ointments or drops temporarily affect vision, instruct client not to move about until vision is clearer.	Prevents accidental injury
17. Lift side rails.	Prevents falling accidents
18. Place call light within reach.	Facilitates communication with nurse
19. Discard or restore equipment properly.	Facilitates clean and orderly environment
20. Document administration on medication record.	Provides legal record of medication administration and prevents accidental remediation

Evaluation

Goals met, partially met, or unmet?

Desired Outcome (sample)

Client shows no redness, edema, or drainage from eye.

Documentation

The following should be noted on the client's chart:

- Condition of eye structures (appearance of skin, presence of drainage, redness, lesions)
- Status of vision
- Reports of pain or tenderness
- Eye in which drug was instilled
- Name of drug, amount, and date and time administered
- Adverse reactions to medication
- Effects of drug
- Teaching regarding drug and self-administration of medications

Sample Documentation

DATE	TIME	
7/7/94	1115	One drop of gentamycin solution (3 mg/ml) administered in each eye as initial dose of medication. Client states left eye is slightly painful but no blurred vision. Slight redness in right eye and small amount of creamy, mucous-colored secretions from right eye.

🖐 Ear (Otic) Instillation

☒ Equipment

- Two or three cotton balls or tissue
- Disposable gloves
- Small basin of warm water
- Soap
- Washcloth
- Small dry towel
- Medication record or card
- Pen
- Medication to be administered

Purpose

Instills liquid medication into external auditory canal for such therapeutic effects as decreasing inflammation and infection and softening ear wax for easy removal

Assessment

Assessment should focus on the following:

Condition of external ear (excess wax production, cleanliness, drainage, and odor)
Hearing ability of client
Client balance and coordination
Ability of client to follow instructions

Nursing Diagnoses

The nursing diagnoses may include the following:

Altered comfort related to inner ear inflammation
Impaired hearing ability related to excessive wax buildup

Planning

Key Goals and Sample Goal Criteria

The client will

Verbalize relief of ear discomfort

Show signs of resolved infection and inflammation, as indicated by the absence of redness, swelling, drainage, and pain in ear, prior to hospital discharge

Show no signs of excess wax buildup in ear

Special Considerations

Geriatric

For elderly clients who have difficulty remembering, use a calendar to remind them when to administer ear medication.

Pediatric

It may be necessary to have a parent assist by holding the child in position in order to avoid ear damage when administering ear medications.

 Transcultural

In some cultures (such as the Vietnamese), touching the head may be viewed as taking away the spirit. The nurse should consult the client, or parent if a child is involved, regarding what is culturally appropriate.

Ask a family member to assist in positioning the client's head if necessary or desired.

Implementation

Action	Rationale
1. Wash hands.	Reduces spread of microorganisms
2. Prepare medication, adhering to the five rights of drug administration (see Procedure 11.1, Principles of Medication Administration).	Decreases chance of drug error
3. Identify client by reading identification bracelet and by addressing client by name.	Confirms identity of client

Action	**Rationale**
4. Explain procedure and purpose of drug.	Decreases anxiety
5. Verify client's allergies.	Prevents unnecessary allergic reactions and injury
6. Don gloves.	Decreases nurse's exposure to ear secretions
7. Wash ear if excess wax is noted.	Helps clear path for channeling of drug into ear canal
8. Assist client into side-lying, sitting, or semi-Fowler's position, with ear to receive medication either facing directly upward (in side-lying position) or forehead tilted upward and turned toward opposite side (in sitting or semi-Fowler's position).	Positions client for channeling of drug into ear canal
9. Using nondominant hand, gently pull auricle of the ear up and back (for adults and children older than three years [Fig. 11.3]) or down and back (for children younger than 3 years).	Straightens ear canal for correct channeling of drug into ear
10. While resting heel of dominant hand on side of client's face near temporal	Prevents accidental injury of tympanic membrane

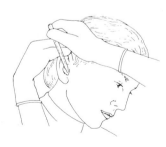

Figure 11.3

Action	Rationale
area, drop ordered number of ear drops into ear canal without touching ear with medicine dropper.	Delivers medication Decreases contamination of solution remaining in bottle
11. Release ear and remove excess medication from around outside of ear with cotton ball or tissue.	Reduces skin irritation and promotes comfort
12. Replace cap on medicine container.	Maintains medication sterility
13. Instruct client to remain in position for 3 to 5 minutes.	Allows time for medication to be absorbed
14. Remove gloves and discard with soiled materials.	Reduces transfer of microorganisms
15. Raise side rails and place call light within reach.	Prevents falls due to disequilibrium and facilitates communication with nurse
16. Wash hands.	Reduces spread of microorganisms
17. Document administration on medication record.	Provides legal record of medication administration and prevents accidental remedication

Evaluation

Goals met, partially met, or unmet?

Desired Outcomes (sample)

Client states that pain is relieved.
There is no evidence of redness, edema, or discharge from the affected ear.
Ear canal is clear with no excess wax buildup.

Documentation

The following should be noted on the client's chart:

- Condition of ear (appearance of skin, presence of drainage, redness, edema, excess wax buildup)
- Status of hearing
- Reports of pain or tenderness

- Ear in which drug was instilled
- Name and amount of drug
- Adverse reactions to medication
- Effects of drug
- Teaching regarding drug information and techniques for self-administration of medications

---

Sample Documentation

DATE	TIME	
4/7/94	1100	Client received first dose of neomycin (0.01%) ear drops. Given 2 drops in right ear without report of pain. Slight redness and a small amount of yellowish discharge from ear. No excess wax buildup noted. Client able to repeat statements without visual cues, indicating unimpaired hearing.

🖐 Nasal Instillation

✖ Equipment

- Nasal drops to be given
- Medication record or card
- Pen
- Disposable gloves
- Tissue
- Pillow roll (or large towel made into pillow roll)
- Wet washcloth

Purpose

Delivers medication for local or systemic absorption through nasal membranes for such therapeutic effects as resolving infections, treating inflammation, and relieving congestion

Assessment

Assessment should focus on the following:

Condition of nasal mucosa
Patency of nasal airway
Presence of nosebleed or discharge
Respiratory character
Contraindications, if any, to client blowing nose

Nursing Diagnoses

The nursing diagnoses may include the following:

Ineffective breathing pattern related to bronchial congestion and nasal inflammation

Planning

Key Goals and Sample Goal Criterion

The client will

Show signs of breathing, as evidenced by smooth, nonlabored respirations, a breathing rate of 12 to 16 breaths per minute, and no cyanosis.

Special Considerations

Geriatric

For elderly clients who have difficulty remembering, use a calendar to remind them when to use nose drops.

Pediatric

It may be necessary to obtain the assistance of a parent to hold the child in position for nasal instillations.

Home Health

Instruct client on administration of nasal medications and provide information about the drugs involved. Caution client against overuse of nasal medications.

 Transcultural

In some cultures (such as the Vietnamese), touching the head may be viewed as taking away the spirit. The nurse should consult the client, or parent if a child is involved, regarding what is culturally appropriate.

Ask a family member to assist in positioning the client's head if necessary or desired.

Implementation

Action	Rationale
1. Wash hands.	Reduces microorganism transfer
2. Prepare medication adhering to the five rights of drug administration (see Procedure 11.1, Principles of Medication Administration).	Decreases chance of drug error
3. Identify client by reading identification bracelet and	Confirms identity of client

Action	Rationale
by addressing client by name.	
4. Explain procedure and purpose of drug.	Decreases anxiety
5. Verify client's allergies listed on medication record or card.	Prevents unnecessary allergic reactions and injury
6. Don gloves.	Decreases nurse's exposure to nasal secretions
7. If excess mucus is noted in nares, instruct client to blow nose gently (unless contraindicated).	Clears nares for proper medication absorption
8. Wipe excess secretions with tissue.	Removes secretions and cleans skin
9. Position client in sitting position with head tilted slightly backwards, or supine with head tilted back in a slightly hyperextended position (it may be necessary to place a pillow roll or rolled towel under client's neck).	Facilitates proper channeling of drug through nasal passage for optimal absorption
10. Squeeze top of medication dropper with dominant hand.	Suctions solution into dropper
11. Stabilize client's forehead with palm of nondominant hand while gently lifting nose open (Fig. 11.4).	Prevents accidental damage to nasal mucosa if client suddenly tries to move head when dropper is in place

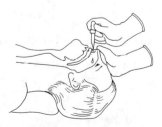

Figure 11.4

Action	Rationale
12. Without touching client's nose or skin with dropper, hold dropper about ¼ to ½ inch above naris and tilt tip of dropper towards nasal septum (center of nose).	Maintains asepsis of remaining drug
	Directs dropper to center of nose for proper placement of drug
13. Squeeze top of dropper and deliver the appropriate number of drops.	Delivers correct dose of medication
14. Instruct client to take one short deep breath and to remain in position for 3 to 5 minutes.	Facilitates full absorption of drug
15. Replace dropper in bottle.	Maintains medication sterility
16. Remove nasal secretions or solution from client's skin (use warm wet washcloth, if necessary).	Prevents local skin irritation and client discomfort
17. Lift side rails and place call light within reach.	Facilitates client–nurse communication
18. Discard gloves and restore other equipment properly.	Promotes cleanliness
19. Wash hands.	Prevents spread of infection
20. Document administration on medication-administration record.	Serves as legal record of medication administration and prevents accidental remedication

Evaluation

Goals met, partially met, or unmet?

Desired Outcomes (sample)

Client's respirations are even and smooth at rate of 16 breaths per minute.
Nasal passage is clear; septum is pink.

Documentation

The following should be noted on the client's chart:

- Name, dosage, and route of medication
- Assessment data relevant to purpose of medication
- Effects of medication
- Teaching of information about drug used and techniques of self-administration of medication

---

Sample Documentation

DATE	TIME	
9/6/94	2100	Client received final dose of Neosynephrine nasally, 2 drops in right naris. Client states pain in nose relieved. No redness or swelling of nasal mucosa. No drainage from nares. Respirations smooth and even.

🖐 Administration of Oral Medication

⊠ Equipment

- Medication record or cards
- Pen
- Disposable gloves, if possibility of exposure to oral secretions
- Medication to be administered
- Medication cup
- Water, juice, or beverage
- Drinking straw

Purpose

Delivers medication for absorption through alimentary tract

Assessment

Assessment should focus on the following:

Complete medication order
Condition of client's mouth (presence of lesions, tears, bleeding, tenderness)
Ability of client to swallow without difficulty
Client nausea or inability to retain oral medications

Nursing Diagnoses

The nursing diagnoses may include the following:

Altered comfort: pain related to surgical incision
Altered sleep pattern related to unfamiliarity with hospital environment

Planning

Key Goals and Sample Goal Criteria

The client will

Verbalize relief of pain within 1 hour of onset
Fall asleep within 1 hour of sleep-medication administration

Special Considerations

When preparing and administering oral drugs, many factors must be taken into account to ensure adequate drug absorption and proper action.

Consult a drug reference manual or pharmacist about drugs with which you are unfamiliar. Some general factors to take into consideration are the following:

- Many solid forms of medication (*e.g.*, capsules, enteric-coated tablets) should not be crushed or chewed.
- Many oral medications require administration with milk or food in order to avoid gastric irritation.
- Frequently, several oral medications are given at the same time. When this occurs, the effects of one or more drugs may be potentiated or decreased.
- When a client receives a medication for the first time, monitor the client closely for an adverse reaction or sensitivity.
- Schedule first doses of new medications on different hours from other medications to obtain a clear picture of the client's response to the new drug.

Geriatric

For elderly clients who have difficulty remembering, use devices that remind client to take medications, such as daily pill dispensers and calendars.

Pediatric

Holding and cuddling an infant may elicit a positive response when administering oral medications. If drugs are being mixed with food or liquid, use as small an amount of these as possible so that the child will take all of the drug.

Medicine can also be given through nipples or droppers.

Toddlers tend to cooperate more when they are given a choice of method of drug delivery—spoon, dropper, syringe—and are allowed to help with drug administration. Most prefer to hold and take pills without assistance.

Home Health
Be alert for self-prescribed medications, usually obtained from
previous doctors, friends, or family members. These medications may have adverse reactions when combined with current medications. Ask to see *all* drugs taken within the past
24 to 72 hours.

 Transcultural
If client prefers a substance that is hot or cold for treatment of
the condition, and the medication can be warmed or cooled
without contraindications, the nurse should acknowledge
and accommodate cultural beliefs.
The nurse should inquire if folk medications have been or are
currently being ingested before administering ordered medications to prevent potential drug interactions. Consult pharmacy and the physician as indicated.

Implementation

Action	Rationale
1. Wash hands.	Reduces microorganism transfer
2. Prepare medication, adhering to the five rights of drug administration (see Procedure 11.1).	Prepares drug Decreases chance of drug error
3. Identify client by reading identification bracelet and by addressing client by name.	Confirms identity of client
4. Explain procedure and purpose of drug.	Decreases anxiety Promotes cooperation
5. Verify client's allergies listed on medication record or card.	Alerts nurse to potential allergic reaction
6. Separate drugs to be withheld, based on assessment data.	Prevents accidental administration of drugs
7. Obtain preassessment data if needed prior to administration.	Determines if medication should be held or given
8. Assist client into semi-Fowler's or sitting position.	Prevents aspiration

Action	Rationale
9. Don gloves if there is a possibility of nurse's exposure to oral secretions.	Avoids exposure to client secretions
10. Open unit-dose packages and place one drug in client's hand *or* pour in medication cup and give to client; provide assistance if needed.	Maintains asepsis while administering
11. Instruct client to place tablets or capsules into mouth and to follow with enough liquid to ensure that drug is swallowed.	Ensures drug is swallowed and that tablets are not lodged in throat or esophagus
12. Administer liquid medications after pills, instructing client to drink all of the solution; provide assistance, if needed.	Facilitates proper absorption of certain liquids that are not to be followed by a beverage
13. Remain with client until all medications are taken; check client's mouth if there is any question whether drug has actually been swallowed.	Ensures that drug is taken
14. Reposition client and place call bell within reach.	Facilitates comfort and communication
15. Lift side rails.	Prevents accidental falls
16. Discard or restore equipment properly:	Promotes clean environment
– If client refuses drug or drug has not been given for any reason, DO NOT leave drug at the bedside.	Eliminates question as to what happened to drug at later time
– Remove drug from room and restore in medication drawer or cabinet only if in unopened unit-dose package.	Allows nurse to administer drug at later date
– If unit-dose package has been opened, discard in sink with witness present, if necessary.	Witness needed when destroying controlled drugs for compliance with federal regulations

Action	Rationale
17. Wash hands.	Prevents spread of infection
18. Document administration on medication record.	Serves as legal record of medication administration and prevents accidental remediation
19. Check client 30 to 60 minutes later for effects of medication.	Detects beneficial or toxic effects of drug

Evaluation

Goals met, partially met, or unmet?

Desired Outcomes (sample)

Client states that pain is relieved within an hour of administration of pain-killing drug.
Client falls asleep within 1 hour of administration of sleep enhancer.

Documentation

The following should be noted on the client's chart:

- Name, amount, and route of drug given
- Purpose of administration if drug is given on a when-needed (p.r.n.) basis
- Assessment data relevant to purpose of medication
- Effects of medication on client
- Teaching of information about drug used or about self-administration technique

Sample Documentation

DATE	TIME	
7/8/94	2200	Dalmane (15 mg PO) given for complaint of inability to sleep at 2100. Client asleep with even, nonlabored respirations; rate 16.

🖐 Administration of Buccal and Sublingual Medication

☒ Equipment

- Medication record or card
- Pen
- Disposable gloves
- Medication to be administered

Purpose

Delivers medication for absorption through oral mucous membranes

Assessment

Assessment should include the following:

Complete medication order
Condition of mouth (presence of lesions, tears, bleeding, tenderness)

Nursing Diagnoses

The nursing diagnoses may include the following:

Altered comfort: chest pain related to oxygen deficit to cardiac muscle
Anxiety related to learning results of diagnostic tests

Planning

Key Goals and Sample Goal Criteria

The client will

Verbalize relief of pain within 10 minutes of onset
Show signs of relaxation (respiratory rate of 20 breaths per minute, calm facial expression) within 15 minutes of medication administration

Special Considerations

Geriatric and Home Health

For elderly clients at home who have difficulty remembering, use devices that remind the client when to take medications, such as calendars and daily pill dispensers).

Implementation

Action	Rationale
1. Wash hands.	Reduces microorganism transfer
2. Prepare medication, adhering to the five rights of drug administration (see Procedure 11.1, Principles of Medication Administration).	Prepares drug Decreases chance of drug error
3. Identify client by reading identification bracelet and addressing client by name.	Confirms identity of client
4. Explain procedure and purpose of drug.	Decreases anxiety Promotes cooperation
5. Verify allergies listed on medication record or card.	
6. Don gloves.	Decreases nurse's exposure to client's body secretions
7. Place tablet: – Under tongue for sublingual medication	Facilitates dissolving and absorption through oral mucous membranes
– Between cheek and gum on either side of mouth for buccal administration (avoid broken or irritated areas)	Reduces additional irritation

Action	Rationale
Note: If client's mucous membranes are dry, offer a sip of water before giving medication.	
8. Instruct client not to swallow drug but to let drug dissolve.	Facilitates absorption by proper route
9. Discard gloves and wash hands.	Reduces transfer of microorganisms
10. Document administration on medication record.	Serves as legal record of medication administration and prevents accidental remedication

Evaluation

Goals met, partially met, or unmet?

Desired Outcomes (sample)

Client states pain is relieved within 5 minutes of administration of one sublingual nitroglycerin

Client demonstrates signs of decreased anxiety (relaxed facial expression and respiratory rate of 20 breaths per minute).

Documentation

The following should be noted on the client's chart:

- Name, amount, and route of drug given
- Purpose of administration if drug is given on a when-needed (p.r.n.) basis
- Assessment data relevant to purpose of medication
- Effects of medication on client
- Teaching of information about drug used or about self-administration of medication

---

Sample Documentation

DATE	TIME	
1/9/94	1100	Nitroglycerin gr. 1/150 SL for c/o sharp, nonradiating, midsternal chest pain with relief in 2 minutes. No dysrhythmias noted. Blood pressure 110/70 after 1 tablet.

Medication Preparation
From a Vial

☒ Equipment

- Medication administration record or medication card
- Vial with prescribed medication
- Appropriate-sized syringe and needle for type of injection and viscosity of solution
- Extra needle
- Alcohol swabs
- Medication label or small piece of tape
- Medication tray
- Access pin and sterile cap (for needleless procedure) and multidose vials

Purpose

Obtains medication from vial, using aseptic technique, for administration by a parenteral route

Assessment

Assessment should focus on the following:

Appearance of solution (clarity, absence of sediment, color indicated on instruction label)
Vial label for expiration date of drug

Planning

Special Considerations

If medication requires reconstitution, follow the guidelines on the vial.

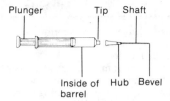

Figure 11.7.1

Sterility of the syringe, needle, and medication must be maintained while preparing the drug. Figure 11.7.1 identifies
those parts of a syringe and needle assembly that must be
kept sterile.

In a needleless system, the needle will be replaced by an access
pin with a sterile cap to allow frequent withdrawal of medication. Although exposure to a contaminated needle by the
nurse is unlikely at this point in the medication administration
procedure, use of a needleless system minimizes risk to the
nurse for broken skin integrity.

Geriatric
For elderly clients who have difficulty remembering, use devices that remind the client when to take medications, such as
calendars and daily medication dispensers.

For elderly clients with special visual deficits, carefully note if
client is able to withdraw an accurate amount of solution from
the vial.

Home Health
Assess area in which client or family member will be preparing
drug for adequacy of lighting.

Implementation

Action	Rationale
1. Wash hands.	Reduces microorganism transfer
2. Organize equipment.	Promotes efficiency
3. Check label of medication vial with medication record or card, using principles of the five rights of drug administration.	Avoids client injury from wrong drug or dosage

Action	Rationale
4. Perform dosage calculations if vial contains more medication than client requires.	Determines correct amount of solution to be prepared
5. Remove thin seal cap from top of vial without touching rubber stopper.	Exposes rubber top for insertion of needle while maintaining asepsis
6. Firmly wipe rubber stopper on top of vial with alcohol swab. If **needleless system** is used, insert the spike of the access pin into the vial until the "wing" of the pin touches the vial's rubber stopper. Remove the sterile cap without touching the top of the access pin (Fig 11.7.2).	Ensures asepsis Permits access to the fluid in the vial using a syringe only
7. Pull end of plunger back to fill syringe with a volume of air equal to the amount of solution to be drawn up (Fig. 11.7.3); do not touch inside of plunger.	Draws air into syringe to create positive pressure in vial Maintains plunger sterility

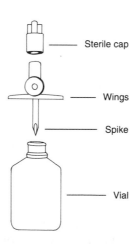

Sterile cap

Wings

Spike

Vial

Figure 11.7.2

Action   **Rationale**

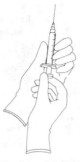

Figure 11.7.3

8. Remove needle cap. (For **needleless system** use syringe only. Remove cap and needle if necessary. Screw syringe onto access pin and skip steps 9 and 10.)	Prepares for insertion
9. Using a slightly slanted angle, firmly insert needle into center of rubber top of vial with the sharpest point of the needle (tip of bevel) entering first.	Prevents solution contamination with sediment from rubber top
10. Continue insertion until needle is securely in vial.	Prevents accidental slip of needle from vial
11. Press end of plunger down.	Infuses air to create positive pressure in vial
12. Hold vial with nondominant hand and turn it upward, keeping needle/spike inserted; control syringe with dominant hand and keep plunger down with thumb.	Moves solution to area of vial closest to rubber stopper for easy removal
13. Pull needle/spike back to point at which bevel is beneath fluid level; keep needle/spike beneath	Places needle in position in which fluid can be obtained (below level of fluid)

Action	Rationale
fluid level as long as fluid is being withdrawn.	
14. Slowly pull end of plunger back until appropriate amount of solution is aspirated into syringe.	Ensures delivery of prescribed amount of medication
15. If air bubbles enter syringe, gently flick syringe barrel with fingers of dominant hand while keeping a finger on end of plunger; continue holding vial with nondominant hand.	Congregates bubbles in one area for removal Prevents plunger from popping out of barrel
16. Push plunger in until air is out of syringe.	Displaces bubble of air into vial
17. Withdraw additional solution, if needed.	Replaces solution lost when clearing bubbles
18. Pull needle out of bottle while keeping a finger on end of plunger. (For **needleless system,** screw syringe off and detach from access pin; cover pin with a sterile cap. Apply sterile needle to syringe if IM/SQ injection will be given.)	Prevents plunger from popping out of barrel
19. If bubbles remain in syringe: – Hold syringe vertically, (with needle pointing up, if attached). – Pull back slightly on plunger and flick syringe with fingers. – Slowly push plunger up to release air but not to the point of expelling the solution.	Removes remaining air bubbles from syringe using principle that air rises
20. Recheck amount of solution in syringe, comparing with drug volume required.	Ensures that correct amount of drug has been prepared

Action	Rationale
21. Compare drug label with medication record or card.	Provides additional identification check of drug
22. Change needle if drug is known to be irritating to tissue; replace cap.	Prevents tissue irritation from drug clinging to outer surfaces of needle when solution is injected into skin; cap replacement is unnecessary if the needleless system is used
23. Label syringe with drug label; include name and amount of drug.	Provides identification information once at client bedside
24. Place syringe, medication cards, and additional alcohol swabs on medication tray.	Organizes equipment for administration of drug
25. Discard or restore all equipment appropriately.	Promotes clean and organized environment
26. Wash hands.	Prevents spread of microorganisms

Evaluation

Goals met, partially met, or unmet?

Desired Outcome (sample)

Correct amount and type of drug is drawn into syringe using aseptic technique.

Medication Preparation From an Ampule

☒ Equipment

- Medication administration record or medication card
- Ampule with prescribed medication
- Appropriate-sized syringe and needle for type of injection and viscosity of solution
- Medication label or small piece of tape
- Extra needle
- Medication tray
- Alcohol swabs
- Paper towel

Purpose

Obtains medication from ampule, using aseptic technique, for administration by a parenteral route

Assessment

Assessment should focus on the following:

Appearance of solution (clarity, absence of sediment, color indicated on instruction label)

Ampule label for expiration date of drug

Planning

Special Considerations

The sterility of syringe, needle, and medication must be maintained while preparing the drug by using principles of asepsis (see Fig. 11.7.1 for identification of the parts of a syringe and needle assembly that must be kept sterile).

Home Health
In the home, instruct client to discard ampules by wrapping in paper towel and dropping into large-size coffee can with hole cut in lid. Store can in safe place (away from children) until it becomes full, then transfer to garbage. Evidence of "injectable" goods is not readily detected.

Implementation

Action	**Rationale**
1. Wash hands.	Reduces microorganism transfer
2. Organize equipment.	Promotes efficiency
3. Check label of medication vial with medication record or card, using principles of the five rights of drug administration.	Avoids client injury from wrong drug or dosage
4. Perform dosage calculation if dosage in ampule differs from amount required.	Determines correct amount of solution to be withdrawn
5. Holding ampule, gently tap neck (top of ampule) with fingers (Fig. 11.8.1) *or* make a complete circle with the ampule by rotating wrist.	Displaces solution from top of ampule to bottom
	Prevents waste of drug
6. Place alcohol swab or gauze pad around neck of ampule with fingers of dominant	Promotes easy opening of ampule

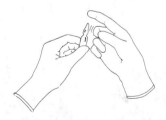

Figure 11.8.1

Action	Rationale
hand; firmly place fingers of nondominant hand around lower part of ampule with thumb placed firmly against junction.	Provides protection against finger cuts
7. With a quick jolting motion of the wrists, break top of ampule by snapping away from you and others who may be near you (Fig. 11.8.2).	Opens ampule Prevents injury from glass pieces
8. Place top of ampule on paper towel or immediately discard.	Prevents injury from picking up edges of jagged glass
9. Remove needle cap.	
10. Press plunger of syringe all the way down; *do not* aspirate air into syringe.	Prevents accidental displacement and waste of solution
11. Place needle into ampule without letting needle or hub touch cut edges of the ampule (Fig. 11.8.3).	Maintains needle sterility
12. Withdraw appropriate amount of solution into syringe and remove needle from ampule.	
13. Place ampule on paper towel or discard immediately.	Prevents injury from picking up edges of jagged glass
14. If bubbles are in syringe: – Hold syringe vertically, with needle pointing up.	Removes remaining air bubbles from syringe using principle that air rises

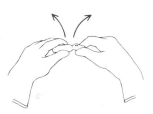

Figure 11.8.2

Action	Rationale

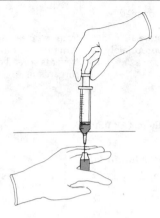

Figure 11.8.3

- Pull back slightly on plunger and flick syringe with fingers.
- Slowly push plunger up to release air but not to the point of expelling the solution.

15. Recheck amount of solution in syringe, comparing with drug volume required.

Ensures that correct amount of drug has been prepared

16. Compare drug label with medication record or card.

Provides additional identification check of drug

17. Change needle if drug is known to cause tissue irritation; replace cap.

Prevents tissue irritation from drug clinging to outer surfaces of needle when solution is injected into skin

18. Label syringe with drug label (or tape, if more than one parenteral drug is being given); label should include name and amount of drug.

Provides identification information once at client bedside

19. Place syringe, medication cards, and additional

Organizes equipment for administration of drug

Action	Rationale
alcohol swabs on medication tray.	
20. Discard or restore all equipment appropriately.	Promotes clean and organized environment
21. Wash hands.	Prevents spread of microorganisms

Evaluation

Goals met, partially met, or unmet?

Desired Outcome (sample)

Correct amount and type of drug drawn into syringe using aseptic technique.

Medication Preparation With a Cartridge System

❌ Equipment

- Medication administration record or medication card
- Prefilled medication cartridge with appropriate medication
- Plastic or metal cartridge holder
- Medication tray

Purpose

Secures prefilled medication cartridge in holder
Prepares cartridge medication for administration

Assessment

Assessment should focus on the following:

Sterility of needle on medication cartridge, as indicated by intact needle cover
Adequacy of medication cartridge, as indicated by absence of cracks
Color and clarity of medication solution
Expiration date of medication
Cleanliness of cartridge holder

Planning

Key Goal and Sample Goal Criterion

The client will

Show no signs of tissue damage or infection from injections received during period of confinement.

Special Considerations

Do not use cartridge if there is any indication of previous opening, inappropriate color, or sediment or if expiration date has
passed.

Clean reusable cartridge holders with an appropriate disinfectant solution between uses with different clients.

Implementation

Action	Rationale
1. Wash hands.	Reduces microorganism transfer
2. Organize equipment.	Promotes efficiency
3. Check label of prefilled medication cartridge with medication record or card, using principles of the five rights of drug administra-tion.	Avoids client injury from wrong drug or dosage
4. Open cartridge holder, slide cartridge (leave nee-dle covered) into barrel, and secure as follows:	Prevents cartridge movement in holder during usage Maintains needle sterility

Metal Holders
- Pull plunger straight back (all the way out) and then down at about a 90-degree angle (Fig. 11.9.1*A*).
- Insert cartridge, needle end first, into barrel (Fig. 11.9.1*B*).
- Pull plunger back up di-rectly in line with barrel of syringe (Fig. 11.9.1*C*).

Plastic Holders
- Pull plunger straight back.
- Insert cartridge through large opening of barrel and guide covered needle through hub of holder (Fig. 11.9.2).

Action	Rationale

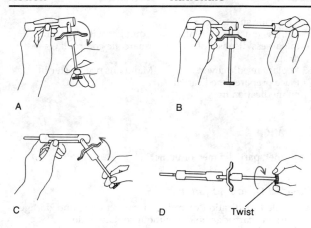

Figure 11.9.1

Metal and Plastic Holders
- Hold cartridge and barrel stable close to end that has needle.
- Gently twist plunger in a clockwise direction until plunger locks onto cartridge (Fig. 11.9.1*D*).
5. Remove needle cover and eject air and excess medication (if discarding

Obtains accurate dosage

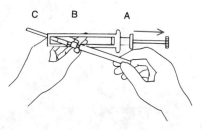

Figure 11.9.2

Action	Rationale
a narcotic substance, a witness must be present to witness disposal of drug).	Complies with federal narcotic-control laws
6. Replace needle cover.	Maintains needle sterility
7. Place prepared medication on medication tray.	

Evaluation

Goals met, partially met, or unmet?

Desired Outcome (sample)

A prefilled medication cartridge of correct drug and dosage is secured in cartridge holder without contamination.

Mixing Medications

☒ Equipment

- Medication administration record or medication cards
- Prescribed medication
- Appropriate-sized syringe and three needles for type of injection and viscosity of solutions
- Medication label or small piece of tape
- Alcohol swabs
- Medication tray

Purpose

Mixes medications (including insulin) from multiple containers into one syringe for parenteral administration

Assessment

Assessment should focus on the following:

Appearance of solutions (clarity, absence of sediment, color indicated on instruction labels)
Drug labels for expiration dates of drugs
Parenteral-drug compatibility charts for drug compatibility

Planning

Key Goal and Sample Goal Criterion
The client will

Receive appropriately mixed and sterile medications

Special Considerations

If a medication requires reconstitution, follow the guidelines on the vial.

If you are uncomfortable with the mixing process provided in this procedure, draw up medications using two syringes (one with removable needle cap), remove cap from one syringe, and aspirate medication into the other.

Implementation

Action	Rationale
1. Wash hands.	Reduces microorganism transfer
2. Organize equipment.	Promotes efficiency
3. Check label of medications to be mixed with medication record or cards, using principles of the five rights of drug administration (see Procedure 11.1).	Avoids client injury from wrong drug or dosage
4. Perform dosage calculations, if needed.	Determines correct amount of solution to be prepared
5. Remove thin seal caps from tops of both vials without touching rubber stoppers.	Exposes rubber tops Maintains asepsis
6. Firmly wipe rubber stoppers on top of both vials with alcohol swabs.	Maintains asepsis
7. Pull end of plunger of syringe back to fill syringe with air equal to amount of solution to be drawn from first vial (vial A).	Draws air into syringe needed for creating positive pressure in vial
(*Note:* If one solution is colored and the other is clear, the colored solution should be vial B and the clear solution should be vial A. INSULIN IS OFTEN THE EXCEPTION [CHECK AGENCY POLICY]: WITH NPH AND REGULAR INSULIN, REGULAR INSULIN SHOULD BE	Allows nurse to determine if clear solution has been contaminated with other solution PREVENTS CONTAMINATION OF SHORT-ACTING REGULAR INSULIN,

Action	Rationale
VIAL B AND NPH INSULIN SHOULD BE VIAL A.)	WHICH IS OFTEN USED IN ACUTE SITUATIONS, WITH NPH INSULIN
– If one vial is multiple dose and one single dose, the single-dose vial will be vial A and the multiple-dose dose vial will be vial B (Fig. 11.10*A*).	Prevents contamination of solution in multiple-dose container with other solution
8. Insert air into vial A equal to the volume of solution to be withdrawn (Fig. 11.10*B*).	Creates positive pressure in vial
	Prevents excess pressure on plunger that could cause plunger to pop out of barrel when withdrawing solution

A Two multiple-dose vials

B A: Single-dose vial
   B: Multiple-dose vial

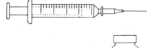

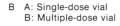

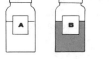

C

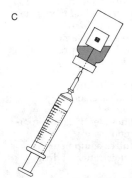

D

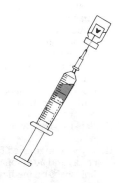

Figure 11.10

Action	Rationale
9. Remove needle from vial A and complete additional steps using *same* syringe.	
10. Pull end of plunger back to fill syringe with air equal to amount of solution to be drawn up from vial B.	Draws air into syringe sufficient to create positive pressure in vial
11. Insert air into vial B in same manner as first vial; do not, however, remove needle from vial B when air insertion is completed (Fig. 11.10C).	Creates positive pressure in vial
12. Invert vial and withdraw exact amount of solution needed from vial B.	Aspirates solution into syringe
13. Attach new needle to syringe.	Prevents dull needle from pushing pieces of rubber top into vial and contaminating solution
14. Insert needle into vial A, gently holding finger on end of plunger.	Stabilizes plunger so that drug in syringe does not accidentally spill into vial
15. Invert vial and withdraw exact amount of solution needed from vial A (Fig. 11.10D).	Withdraws solution from vial A
16. Leaving needle cap on, attach new needle to same syringe.	Prevents tissue irritation from dull needle and medication on needle
17. Recheck amount of solution in syringe.	Ensures correct amount of drug has been prepared
18. Pull plunger back another 0.1 ml.	Makes air lock
19. Compare drug labels with medication record or card.	Provides additional identification check of drug
20. Label syringe with drug labels.	Provides identification information
21. Place syringe, medication cards, and additional alcohol swabs on medication tray.	Organizes equipment for administration of drug

Action	Rationale
22. Discard or restore all equipment appropriately.	Promotes clean and organized environment
23. Wash hands.	Prevents spread of micro-organisms

Evaluation

Goals met, partially met, or unmet?

Desired Outcome (sample)

Correct amounts of correct drugs mixed in syringe without incompatibility or contamination.

Documentation

See specific administration procedure.

✋ Intradermal Injection

☒ Equipment

- Medication record or card
- Pen (ink or felt)
- Two alcohol swabs
- Nonsterile gloves
- Medication to be administered
- 1-ml syringe with 26- to 28-gauge needle
- Medication tray

Purpose

Permits exposure of client to small amount of toxin or medication deposited under the skin for absorption

Serves as method of diagnostic testing for allergens or for exposure to specific diseases

Assessment

Assessment should focus on the following:

Complete medication order

Agency protocol regarding specific sites of skin tests

Condition of client's skin (*e.g.*, presence of redness, hematomas, scarring, swelling, tears, abrasions, lesions, excoriation, and excessive hair)

Nursing Diagnoses

The nursing diagnoses may include the following:

Potential for biological injury related to allergen sensitivity

Planning

Key Goal and Sample Goal Criterion

The client will

Experience no undetected signs of local or systemic reaction to drug or allergen.

Special Considerations

Allergens used in testing could cause a sensitivity or anaphylactic reaction. Be certain that appropriate antidotal drugs (usually epinephrine hydrochloride, a bronchodilator, and an antihistamine) are available on the unit *before* beginning. REACTIONS MAY BE FATAL.

Home Health

In the client's home, administer intradermal medication only by order of the attending physician (or with the attending physician's permission, if ordered by another physician).

Implementation

Action	Rationale
1. Wash hands.	Reduces microorganism transfer
2. Prepare medication, adhering to the five rights of drug administration (see Procedures 11.1 and 11.7 through 11.9).	Decreases chance of drug error Prepares drug appropriately from form in which it is supplied
3. Identify client by reading identification bracelet and addressing client by name.	Confirms identity of client
4. Explain procedure and purpose of drug.	Decreases anxiety Promotes cooperation
5. Verify allergies listed on medication record or card.	Alerts nurse to possibility of allergic reaction
6. Don gloves.	Prevents direct contact with body contaminants
7. Select injection site on forearm if no other site is required by agency policy or doctor's orders; use	Forearm is standard beginning point for intradermal injections and the area at which subcutaneous fat is least

Action	Rationale
alternative sites designated in Figure 11.11.1 if forearm cannot be used.	likely to interfere with administration and absorption
8. Position client with forearm facing upward.	Accesses injection area
9. Cleanse site with alcohol.	Decreases microorganisms
10. Remove needle cap.	
11. Place nondominant thumb about one inch below insertion site and pull skin downward (toward hand).	Pulls skin taut for injection
12. With bevel up and using dominant hand, insert needle just below the skin at a 10- to 15-degree angle (Fig. 11.11.2).	Places needle just below epidermis
13. Once entry into skin surface is made, advance needle another 1/8 inch.	Prevents back leakage of medication
14. Inject drug slowly and smoothly while observing for bleb (a raised welt) to form. The bleb *should* be present.	Delivers medication slowly and allows chance to stop administration if systemic reaction begins. Provides visual feedback of proper drug administration
15. Remove needle at same angle inserted.	Prevents tearing of skin
16. Gently remove blood, if any, by dabbing with second alcohol swab.	Cleans area while avoiding pushing medication out

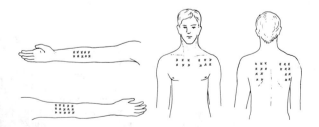

Figure 11.11.1

Action	**Rationale**

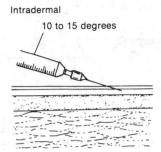

Intradermal
10 to 15 degrees

Figure 11.11.2

Action	**Rationale**
17. Observe skin for redness or swelling; if this is an allergy test, observe for systemic reaction (*e.g.,* respiratory difficulty, sweating, faintness, decreased blood pressure, nausea, vomiting, cyanosis).	Provides visual assessment of local or systemic reaction
18. Reassess client and injection site after 5 minutes, 15 minutes, then periodically thereafter during shift.	Detects occurrence of subsequent reaction
19. Place uncapped needle on tray.	Prevents needle sticks
20. Place a 1-inch circle around bleb and instruct client not to rub the area.	Serves as guide in locating and reassessing area later
21. Reposition client.	Promotes comfort
22. Discard equipment appropriately.	Promotes clean and organized environment
23. Wash hands.	Decreases transfer of microorganisms
24. Document administration on medication record.	Serves as legal record of administration and prevents accidental remediation

Evaluation

Goals met, partially met, or unmet?

Desired Outcome (sample)
Client shows no signs of local or systemic reaction.

Documentation

The following should be noted on the client's chart:

- Name of allergen or toxin, dosage, injection site, and route of administration
- Indicators of local or systemic reaction, if any
- Abnormal findings in local skin area
- Results of test 24 to 48 hours after administration
- Teaching of information about drug or injection technique

Sample Documentation		
DATE	**TIME**	
2/13/94	1440	Tuberculin skin test (0.1 ml) given intradermally in right lower forearm and circled. Noted a 0.5-cm reddened area surrounding injection site after injection, but no other reactions noted.

Intramuscular Injection

☒ Equipment

- Medication record or card
- Pen
- Two alcohol swabs
- Disposable gloves
- Medication tray
- Medication to be administered
- 3-ml syringe with 1-, 1.5-, or 2-inch needle (21, 22, or 23 gauge)

Purpose

Delivers ordered medication into muscle tissue

Assessment

Assessment should focus on the following:

- Medication order
- Site of last injection, allergies, and client response to previous injections, as noted in client's chart
- Intended injection site (presence of bruises, tenderness, skin breaks, nodules, or edema)
- Factors that determine appropriate size and gauge of needle (client size and age, site of injection, viscosity and residual effects of medication)

Nursing Diagnoses

The nursing diagnoses may include the following:

Altered comfort: abdominal pain related to incision
Anxiety related to pain from injections

Planning

Key Goals and Sample Goal Criteria

The client will

State the major purpose of the injection before receiving it
Verbalize minimum discomfort related to injection

Special Considerations

If nausea or pain medication has been ordered in multiple forms (oral, parenteral, or rectal), determine client preference before preparing the medication.

Geriatric and Pediatric

If client is confused or combative, obtain assistance to stabilize the injection site and avoid tissue damage from the needle.

Implementation

Action	Rationale
1. Wash hands.	Reduces microorganism transfer
2. Prepare medication, adhering to the five rights of drug administration (see Procedures 11.1 and 11.7 through 11.10).	Decreases chance of drug error Prepares drug properly from form in which it is supplied
3. Identify client by reading identification bracelet and addressing client by name.	Confirms identity of client
4. Explain procedure and purpose of drug.	Decreases anxiety Promotes cooperation
5. Verify allergies listed on medication record or card.	Alerts nurse to possibility of allergic reaction
6. Don gloves.	Prevents contact with body fluids
7. Select injection site appropriate for client's size and age (see Fig. 11.12.1 for injection sites located by anatomical landmarks).	
8. Assist client into position for comfort and easy visibility of injection site.	

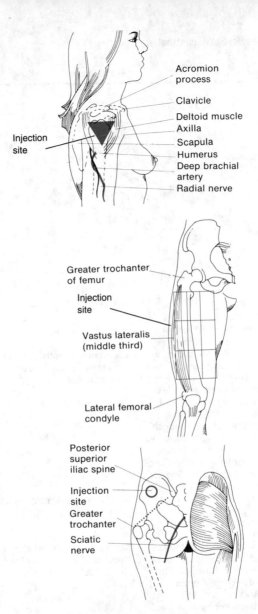

Figure 11.12.1
(continues next page)

Action	Rationale

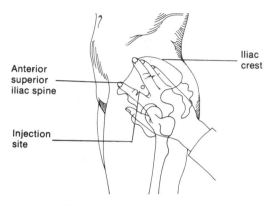

Anterior superior iliac spine

Injection site

Iliac crest

Figure 11.12.1 (cont.)

Action	Rationale
9. Clean site with alcohol.	Maintains asepsis
10. Remove needle cap.	
11. Pull skin taut at insertion area by using the following sequence: – Place thumb and index finger of nondominant hand over injection site (taking care not to touch cleaned area) to form a **V.** – Pull thumb and index finger in opposing directions, spreading fingers about 3 inches apart.	Facilitates smooth and complete insertion of needle into muscle
12. Quickly insert needle at a 90-degree angle with dominant hand (as if throwing a dart).	Minimizes pain from needle insertion
13. Move thumb and first finger of nondominant hand from skin to support barrel of syringe; fingers should be placed on barrel so that when you aspirate, you can see the barrel clearly (Fig. 11.12.2).	Maintains steady position of needle and prevents tearing of tissue

Action	**Rationale**

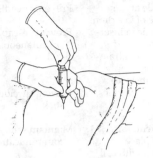

Figure 11.12.2

14. Pull back on plunger and observe for possible blood return in syringe (Fig. 11.12.3).

Determines if needle is in a blood vessel rather than in muscle

15. If blood does return when aspirating, pull the needle out, apply pressure to the insertion site, and repeat steps 7 to 14.

Prevents inadvertent intra-venous injection

16. If no blood returns, push plunger down slowly and smoothly; encourage client to talk.

Delivers medication
Decreases client anxiety

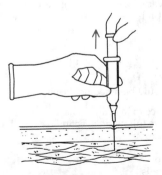

Figure 11.12.3

Action	Rationale
17. Remove needle at same angle as angle of insertion.	Prevents needless tearing of tissue
18. Massage and clean insertion area with second alcohol wipe (if contraindicated for drug, apply firm pressure instead).	Prevents escape of drug into subcutaneous tissue
19. Place needle on tray; do not recap.	Prevents accidental needle stick
20. Remove gloves.	
21. Reposition client; raise side rails and place bed in lowest position with call button within reach.	Maintain safety, comfort, and communication
22. Dispose of equipment properly.	Prevents injury and spread of infection
23. Wash hands.	Reduces microorganism transfer
24. Document administration on medication record.	Serves as legal record of administration and prevents accidental remediation

Evaluation

Goals met, partially met, or unmet?

Desired Outcomes (sample)

There is no redness, edema, or pain at injection site.
Client correctly verbalizes purpose of injection.
Client states that minimum pain was experienced during injection.

Documentation

The following should be noted on the client's chart:

- Client's tolerance to injection
- Condition of site following injection (*i.e.,* local reactions)
- Effect of medication
- Injection site
- Time of injection
- Status of side rails

Sample Documentation

DATE	TIME	
7/8/94	1200	50 mg Demerol given intramuscularly in right deltoid for complaint of nagging pain in left hip. No local redness or swelling after injection. Side rails up and bed in low position.

🖐 Z-Track Injection

☒ Equipment

- Medication record or card
- Pen
- Two alcohol swabs
- Disposable gloves
- Medication tray
- Medication to be administered
- 3-ml syringe with 2- to 3-inch needle (20 to 22 gauge)

Purpose

Delivers irritating or caustic medications deep into muscle tissue to prevent seepage

Assessment

Assessment should focus on the following:

Complete medication order

Intended injection site (presence of bruising, tenderness, skin breaks, nodules, or edema)

Site of last injection, allergies, and client response to previous injections

Factors that determine size and gauge of needle (client size and age, site of injection, viscosity and residual effects of medication)

Nursing Diagnoses

The nursing diagnoses may include the following:

Altered nutrition: less iron intake than required to support bodily functions

Planning

Key Goals and Sample Goal Criteria

The client will

Verbalize no extreme discomfort after injection
Experience no tissue damage from medication leakage into subcutaneous tissue

Special Considerations

Skin staining can occur if incorrect technique is used in giving
iron injections. Drugs given by this method are generally so irritating to the skin and subcutaneous tissue as to cause
sloughing.

Implementation

Action	Rationale
1. Wash hands.	Reduces microorganism transfer
2. Prepare syringe with medication, adhering to the five rights of drug administration (see Procedures 11.1 and 11.7 through 11.10).	Prepares drug properly Decreases chance of drug error Prepares drug properly from form in which it is supplied
3. Change needle after drug has been fully drawn up.	Prevents staining and irritation of skin and subcutaneous tissue when needle is inserted into skin
4. Pull plunger back another 0.3 ml.	Makes air lock in syringe
5. Identify client by reading identification bracelet and addressing client by name.	Confirms identity of client
6. Explain procedure and purpose of drug.	Decreases anxiety Promotes cooperation
7. Verify allergies listed on medication record or card.	Alerts nurse to possibility of allergic reaction
8. Provide privacy.	Decreases embarrassment
9. Don gloves.	Prevents direct contact with body secretions
10. Assist client into prone position with toes pointed inward.	Promotes comfort by relaxing gluteal muscles

Action	Rationale
11. Outline dorsogluteal site by identifying appropriate landmarks (may also use ventrogluteal and vastus lateralis areas); see Procedure 11.12 and Fig. 11.12.1 for information on locating injection sites using anatomical landmarks.	Prevents sciatic nerve damage
12. Clean site with alcohol.	Maintains asepsis
13. Remove needle cap.	
14. Hold syringe with needle pointed downward and observe for air bubble to rise to top (away from needle).	Ensures that air clears needle after drug so drug can be "sealed" into muscle tissue
15. Using fingers of nondominant hand, pull skin laterally (away from midline) about 1 inch and downward (Fig. 11.13.1).	Retracts skin and subcutaneous tissue from muscle
16. While maintaining skin retraction, rest heel of nondominant hand on skin below fingers (Fig. 11.13.2).	Allows nurse to maintain retraction and stability of needle while aspirating or if client suddenly moves
17. Talk to client, pausing to warn of impending needle stick.	Provides distraction Prevents jerking response

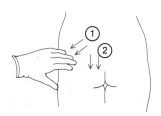

Figure 11.13.1

Action	Rationale

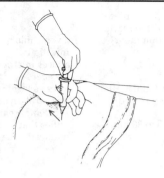

Figure 11.13.3

Action	Rationale
18. With dominant hand, quickly insert needle at a 90-degree angle (as if throwing a dart).	Minimizes pain from insertion Ensures needle enters muscle mass
19. Pull plunger back and aspirate for blood return.	Determines if accidental insertion into blood vessel has occurred
20. If blood returns, remove needle, clean site with antiseptic swab, assess site, apply adhesive bandage, and begin at step 1.	
21. If no blood returns, inject drug slowly and hold needle in place for 10 seconds.	Prevents leakage into subcutaneous tissue Gives adequate absorption time
22. Remove needle at same angle as angle of insertion while releasing skin at the same time.	Prevents needless tearing of tissue Avoids direct track between muscle and surface of skin
23. Place alcohol swab over insertion area, but DO NOT MASSAGE.	Avoids displacing drug into tissues and causing irritation and pain
24. Place needle on tray; do not recap.	Prevents accidental needle stick
25. Reposition client, raise side rails, and lower bed	Maintains safety, comfort, and communication

Action	Rationale
to lowest position; place call button within reach.	
26. Dispose of equipment properly.	Prevents injury and spread of infection
27. Wash hands.	Reduces microorganism transfer
28. Document administration on medication record.	Serves as legal record of administration and prevents accidental remedication
29. Check site 15 to 30 minutes later.	Verifies that no seepage of medication has occurred

Evaluation

Goals met, partially met, or unmet?

Desired Outcomes (sample)

Client offers no complaint of extreme pain after medication is administered by Z-track method.
Skin remains intact without bruise or hematoma formation.

Documentation

The following should be noted on the client's chart:

Name of medication, dosage, route, and site of injection
Assessment and laboratory data relevant to purpose of medication
Effects of medication
Condition of site following injection
Teaching of information about drug or injection technique

Sample Documentation

DATE	TIME	
7/8/94	1600	Client received first dose of Imferon 150 mg by Z-track injection in left dorsogluteal area. No local redness, swelling, or skin stain. No complaint of nausea or headache.

✋ Intermittent Intravenous Medication

✖ Equipment

- Medication record or card
- Pen
- Disposable gloves
- Four or five alcohol swabs
- Medication to be administered mixed in 50 to 100 ml of appropriate intravenous fluid (usually 0.9% saline or 5% dextrose) and attached to 22- or 23-gauge needle
- Small roll of 1/2- to 1-inch width tape

If administering medication by piggyback method, include:
- 1 ml of sterile saline

If administering medication through heparin lock, include:
- Two syringes of sterile saline (1.5 to 2 ml)
- One syringe with 1 to 2 ml of heparin flush solution

Purpose

Intermittently delivers medication through intravenous route for various therapeutic effects, most frequently treatment of infections

Assessment

Assessment should focus on the following:

Complete medication order
Condition of intravenous site (patency, discoloration, edema, and pain)
Appearance of intravenous fluid with added medication (discoloration, sediment)

Expiration dates on medication that has been mixed
Condition of tubing presently hanging, if any

Nursing Diagnoses

The nursing diagnoses may include the following:

Potential for infection related to open abdominal skin wound
Altered comfort: pain related to increased gastric secretion of
hydrochloric acid

Planning

Key Goals and Sample Goal Criteria
The client will

Show no undetected signs of infection
Show a decrease in the symptom precipitating use of the intermittent drug infusion within three days of beginning the medication

Special Considerations

Pediatric
When infusing intermittent medications to pediatric clients, always regulate by an electronic infusion regulator (IV pump or
controller) and a volume-controlled chamber (such as a
Buretrol or Volutrol) in order to prevent infusion errors related to increased rates or volumes (see Procedure 5.6). Check
the agency procedure manual.

Implementation

Action	Rationale
1. Wash hands.	Reduces microorganism transfer
2. Prepare medication, adhering to the five rights of drug administration (see Procedure 11.1).	Prepares drug Decreases chance of drug error

Action	Rationale
3. Calculate infusion flow rate (see Procedure 5.5).	Determines accurate infusion rate
4. Identify client by reading identification bracelet and addressing client by name.	Confirms identity of client
5. Explain procedure and purpose of drug.	Decreases anxiety Promotes cooperation
6. Verify allergies listed on medication record or card.	Alerts nurse to possibility of allergic reaction
7. Hang medication with attached tubing and needle on IV pole.	
8. Don gloves at any point during procedure where there is a risk of exposure to blood or body secretions (such as when untaping site for in-depth assessment).	Decreases nurse's exposure to body secretions
9. Assess patency of catheter or heparin lock:	Confirms that established intravenous line is open
Heparin Lock	
– Cleanse rubber port of lock with alcohol.	Reduces microorganisms
– Stabilize lock with thumb and first finger of nondominant hand.	Prevents pulling out of catheter
– Insert needle of sterile saline syringe into lock.	
– Pull back on end of plunger and observe for blood return.	Aspirates blood Ensures catheter is functional
– If no blood returns, reposition extremity in which catheter is placed and reassess site for redness, edema, or pain.	Checks for problems related to positioning, local infiltration, or phlebitis
– Discontinue heparin lock and restart if unable to get blood return (see Procedures 5.2 and 5.4).	Discontinues nonfunctional catheter Establishes functional line
– *If blood returns,* insert saline and proceed to next step.	Flushes catheter

Action	Rationale

Primary Line

   – Insert needle of syringe containing sterile saline into center of port nearest insertion site. | Provides access to port near catheter site for easy observation when aspirating

   – Pinch intravenous tubing just above the port (Fig. 11.14.1). | Allows for one-way flow during aspiration

   – Pull back on plunger and observe for blood return in the tubing; or lower fluid and tubing below level of extremity for 1 to 2 minutes. | Aspirates for blood return

    | Verifies catheter placement

   – If no blood returns, reposition extremity in which catheter is placed and reassess site for redness, edema, or pain. | Checks for problems related to positioning, phlebitis, or infiltration

   – Discontinue primary IV and restart if unable to get blood return (see Procedures 5.2 through 5.4). | Establishes patent IV line

   – If blood returns, instill saline and proceed to next step. | Flushes blood from catheter

10. Cleanse rubber port to be used (see step 11) with alcohol. | Reduces microorganisms

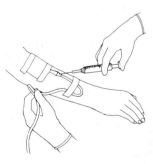

Figure 11.14.1

Action	Rationale
11. Insert needle attached to tubing of mixed medication into heparin lock port; for piggyback method, insert needle into port closest to top of primary tubing.	Connects to main infusion line
12. Secure needle with tape.	Prevents needle dislodgment
13. For piggyback method, lower primary bag to about 6 inches below secondary bag (mixed-medication bag; Fig. 11.14.2).	Provides more gravitational pull for secondary bag than for primary infusion
14. Slowly open tubing roller clamp and adjust drip rate (see Procedure 5.6).	Prevents adverse reactions from too rapid an infusion rate
15. Periodically assess client during infusion.	Monitors for adverse reactions and good infusion
16. When infusion is complete, leave medication and tubing on pole if tubing is not expired; for	

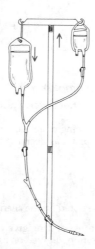

Figure 11.14.2

Action	Rationale
heparin lock (and when administering several different piggyback medications), carefully remove needle from primary tubing and recap; for piggyback method, leave connected to port.	Provides greater mobility for client while maintaining cleanliness of IV tubing for future use
	Decreases destruction of primary tubing port
17. If tubing has expired, disconnect and discard.	Reduces contamination of system
18. Insert needle of second syringe of sterile saline and inject into heparin lock; then insert heparin flush *or* readjust drip rate for primary infusion.	Clears catheter and tubing
19. Discard or restore all equipment appropriately.	Promotes clean environment
20. Wash hands.	Reduces microorganism transfer
21. Document administration on medication record.	Serves as legal record of administration and prevents accidental remediation

Evaluation

Goals met, partially met, or unmet?

Desired Outcomes (sample)

IV antibiotics and medications were infused without signs of contamination.

Within two days of beginning cimetidine infusions, client states that upper abdominal pain has decreased.

Documentation

The following should be noted on the client's chart:

- Name, amount, and route of drug given
- Purpose of administration, if given on a when-needed (p.r.n.) basis or one-time order

- Assessment data relevant to purpose of medication
- Effects of medication on client
- Teaching of information about drug

Sample Documentation

DATE	TIME	
7/8/94	1100	Client received initial dose of IV tobramycin, 80 mg. No redness or drainage from abdominal wound. Client denies having abdominal pain. Temperature, 99.8°F. Other vital signs within normal limits.

✋ Administration of Subcutaneous Medication

❌ Equipment

- Pen
- Medication record or card
- Two alcohol swabs
- Nonsterile gloves
- Adhesive bandage
- Medication to be administered
- 2- to 3-ml syringe with $^1/_2$- to $^7/_8$-inch needle (25, 26, or 27 gauge) or insulin syringe
- Medication tray

Purpose

Delivers medication into subcutaneous tissues for absorption

Assessment

Assessment should focus on the following:

Medication order
Condition of skin at intended injection site (presence of tears, abrasions, lesions, and scars)
Chart or medication administration record for site of last injection

Nursing Diagnoses

The nursing diagnoses may include the following:
Potential altered skin integrity related to repeated insulin injections
Knowledge deficit regarding technique for self-administration of insulin related to newly diagnosed diabetic status

Planning

Key Goals and Sample Goal Criteria

The client will

Show no signs of tissue damage from insulin injections
Demonstrate correct technique for insulin injection with 100%
   accuracy within 1 week

Special Considerations

Some agencies recommend that aspiration after needle insertion
   not be performed with heparin administration. Check agency
   procedure manual BEFORE heparin administration.
Many agencies require that heparin and insulin be checked with
   another nurse when preparing. Check agency policy manual
   before beginning.

Geriatric

Elderly clients often experience a loss of subcutaneous fat tissue.
Choose needle length carefully to avoid painful injections and
   trauma to the underlying bone.

Pediatric

For clients less than 1 year old, SUBCUTANEOUS INJECTION
   IN THE DORSAL GLUTEAL AREA CAN BE HAZARDOUS
   because of possible damage to sciatic nerve.
Enlist assistant to restrain child during procedure to avoid tissue damage from needle during sudden movement.

Home Health

Arrange supplies (*e.g.,* insulin, alcohol, needles) in line on a
   table to assist the client and family in learning the sequence of
   steps in the procedure.

Implementation

Action	Rationale
1. Wash hands.	Reduces microorganism transfer
2. Prepare medication, adhering to the five rights of drug administration (see Procedures 11.1 and 11.7 through 11.10).	Prepares drug Decreases chance of drug error Prepares drug properly from form in which it is supplied

Action	Rationale
3. Identify client by reading identification bracelet and addressing client by name.	Confirms identity of client
4. Explain procedure and purpose of drug.	Decreases anxiety Promotes cooperation
5. Verify allergies listed on medication record or card.	Alerts nurse to possible allergic reaction
6. Provide privacy.	Decreases embarrassment
7. Don gloves.	Prevents direct contact with body fluids
8. Perform or instruct client to perform the remaining steps.	Helps client learn procedures
9. Select injection site on upper arm or abdomen. (*Note:* Heparin should be injected in abdomen.) Use one of the following alternative sites if these two areas are not available because of tissue irritation, scarring, tubes, or dressings: thighs, upper chest, scapular areas (Fig. 11.15.1); the sites should be rotated.	Prevents repeated and permanent tissue damage

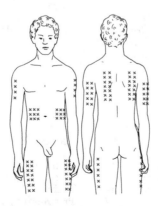

Figure 11.15.1

Action	**Rationale**
10. Position client for site selected.	Accesses injection area Promotes comfort
11. Cleanse site with alcohol.	Reduces microorganism transfer
12. Remove needle cap.	
13. Grasp about 1 inch of skin and fatty tissue between thumb and fingers. (*Note:* For heparin injection, hold skin gently; do not pinch.)	Prevents trauma to tissue
14. With dominant hand, insert needle at a 45-degree angle quickly and smoothly; for a larger person, insert at a 90-degree angle (Fig. 11.15.2).	Facilitates injection into subcutaneous tissue (a large person has a thicker layer of subcutaneous tissue)
15. Quickly release skin fold with nondominant hand.	Facilitates spread of medication
16. Aspirate with plunger and observe barrel of syringe for blood return.	Determines if needle is in a blood vessel
17. If blood does not return, inject drug slowly and smoothly.	Delivers the medication
18. *If blood returns:* – Withdraw needle from skin. – Apply pressure to site for about 2 minutes.	Prevents injection into blood vessels

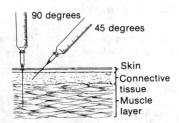

90 degrees

45 degrees

Skin
Connective tissue
Muscle layer

Figure 11.15.2

Action	Rationale
– Observe for hematoma or bruising.	
– Apply adhesive bandage, if needed.	
– Prepare new medication, beginning with step 1, and select new site.	
19. Remove needle at same angle at which it was inserted.	Prevents tissue damage
20. Cleanse injection site with second alcohol swab and lightly massage. DO NOT massage after heparin injection.	Promotes comfort Prevents bruising and tissue damage
21. Apply adhesive bandage, if needed.	Contains residual bleeding
22. Place uncapped needle on tray.	Prevents needle stick
23. Discard all equipment appropriately.	Promotes cleanliness
24. Wash hands.	Decreases microorganism transfer
25. Document administration on medication record.	Serves as legal record of administration and prevents accidental remedication

Evaluation

Goals met, partially met, or unmet?

Desired Outcomes (sample)

No scars, craters, or lumps are noted on skin.
Client performs insulin self-injection with 100% accuracy within 1 week of receiving instructions.

Documentation

The following should be noted on the client's chart:

• Name, dosage, and route of medication; site of injection

- Assessment and laboratory data relevant to purpose of medication
- Effects of medication
- Teaching of information about drug or injection technique

Sample Documentation

DATE	TIME	
7/8/94	1400	Client received first dose of regular insulin, 15 units subcutaneously in right upper arm. No scars, abrasions, or lumps noted on skin.

Administration of Rectal Medication

Equipment

- Medication record card
- Pen
- Disposable gloves
- Suppository to be administered
- Packet of water-soluble lubricant

Purpose

Delivers medication for absorption through mucous membranes of rectum

Assessment

Assessment should focus on the following:

Complete medication order
Condition of anus and skin surrounding buttocks (presence of ulcerations, tears, hemorrhoids, excoriation, abnormal discharge, and foul odor)
Abdominal girth, if distension is present
Client knowledge regarding use of suppositories

Nursing Diagnoses

The nursing diagnoses may include the following:

Altered elimination: constipation related to decreased peristalsis
Altered comfort: pain related to abdominal distension

Planning

Key Goals and Sample Goal Criteria

The client will

Have bowel movement within 24 hours
Show a decrease in abdominal distension, as indicated by an abdominal girth of less than 40 inches and a soft abdomen
Verbalize relief of pain

Implementation

Action	Rationale
1. Wash hands.	Reduces microorganism transfer
2. Prepare medication, adhering to the five rights of drug administration (see Procedure 11.1).	Prepares drug Decreases chance of drug error
3. Identify client by reading identification bracelet and addressing client by name.	Confirms identity of client
4. Explain procedure and purpose of drug.	Decreases anxiety Promotes cooperation
5. Verify allergies listed on medication record or card.	Alerts nurse to possible allergic reaction
6. Don gloves.	Decreases nurse's exposure to client body secretions
7. Position client in prone or side-lying position.	Places client for good exposure of anal opening
8. Place towel or linen saver under buttocks.	Protects sheets
9. Remove suppository from wrapper and inspect tip.	Detects sharp tip
10. If pointed end of suppository is sharp, gently rub sharp tip until slightly rounded.	Decreases chance of tearing rectal membranes
11. Lubricate rounded tip with lubricating jelly.	Decreases chance of tearing membranes
12. Gently spread buttocks with nondominant hand.	Exposes anal opening

Action	Rationale
13. Instruct client to take slow, deep breaths through mouth.	Relaxes sphincter muscles, facilitating insertion
14. Insert suppository into rectum until closure of anal ring is felt (Fig. 11.16).	
15. Remove finger, wipe excess lubricant away from skin, and release buttocks.	Promotes client comfort
16. Instruct client to squeeze buttocks together for 3 to 4 minutes and to remain in position for 15 to 20 minutes. (*Note:* Suppositories given to expel gas may be released at any time.)	Decreases urge to release suppository
17. Discard gloves and paper wrapper.	Promotes clean environment
18. Raise side rails.	Promotes safety
19. Place call light and bedpan within reach.	Facilitates communication Anticipates premature expulsion of suppository or feces
20. Wash hands.	Reduces microorganism transfer
21. Document administration on medication record.	Serves as legal record of administration and prevents accidental remediation

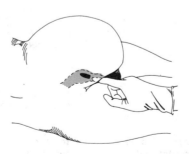

Figure 11.16

Evaluation

Goals met, partially met, or unmet?

Desired Outcomes (sample)

Client has normal bowel movement within 24 hours.
Abdominal girth decreases to 36 inches in 24 hours.
Client verbalizes absence of abdominal pain.

Documentation

The following should be noted on the client's chart:

- Name, dosage, and route of drug
- Condition of anus and surrounding area, if abnormal
- Assessment date relevant to purpose and effects of medication
- Teaching of knowledge about drug and self-administration of medication

---

Sample Documentation

DATE	TIME	
7/8/94	1400	Acetaminophen, gr. XX suppository given for rectal temperature of 103.4°F. Slight protrusion of hemorrhoids noted. Client denies discomfort in anal area.

📋 Topical Application

✖ Equipment

- Medication to be applied (creams, ointments, gels, medicated disks, sprays)
- Medication record or card
- Pen

For creams, gels, ointments, lotions:
- Two pairs of disposable gloves
- Tongue blade
- Mild soap
- Small towel
- Basin of warm water

For sterile application to open wound or incision:
- Two pairs of sterile gloves
- Sterile gauze
- Sterile towel
- Sterile water
- Sterile cleansing solution
- Sterile tongue blade

Purpose

Delivers medication to skin for local or systemic effects, such as skin lubrication and reduction of inflammation

Assessment

Assessment should focus on the following:

Complete medication order
Condition of last treatment area and intended site of this application

Nursing Diagnoses

The nursing diagnoses may include the following:

Altered skin integrity related to local inflammation

Planning

Key Goal and Sample Goal Criterion

The client will

Show no signs of inflammation in lower left leg, such as redness, heat, swelling, pain, and skin tears

Special Considerations

Geriatric

For elderly clients who have problems with memory, use devices that remind them that medication is to be taken (*e.g.,* calendars, daily pill dispenser).

Pediatric

Client cooperation may be improved if the child is allowed to apply the medication under your supervision.

Home Health

Instruct client and family to monitor for side-effects and possible reactions to medications.

Implementation

Action	Rationale
1. Wash hands.	Reduces microorganism transfer
2. Prepare medication, adhering to the five rights of drug administration (see Procedure 11.1, Principles of Medication Administration).	Prepares drug Decreases chance of drug error
3. Identify client by reading identification bracelet and addressing client by name.	Confirms identity of client

Action	Rationale
4. Explain procedure and purpose of drug.	Decreases anxiety Promotes cooperation
5. Verify allergies listed on medication record or card.	Alerts nurse to possibility of an allergic reaction
6. Don disposable gloves if applying gel, cream, ointment, or lotion; apply sterile gloves if applying to open wound or incision and use sterile technique throughout procedure.	Decreases nurse's exposure to client body secretions Protects nurse from receiving effects from the drug
7. Wash intended application site with warm, soapy water, rinse, and pat dry (unless contraindicated); if applying drug to open skin area, use sterile cleaning solution and gauze to clean area.	Removes surface skin debris Facilitates absorption
8. Wash hands and change gloves.	Maintains asepsis
9. Apply drug to treatment area, using appropriate application method:	Delivers medication with appropriate technique

Ointments, Creams, Lotions, Gels

– Pour or squeeze ordered amount onto palmar surface of fingers; or use tongue blade to obtain if removing from multiple-dose container or jar.	Removes drug from container
– Lightly spread with fingers of other hand.	Thins texture of the substance Warms cold gels and creams
– Gently apply to treatment area, lightly massaging until absorbed or as per package directions.	Spreads drug for intended effect

Nitroglycerin Ointment
(Special preparation and application)

– Remove previous ointment pad and wash area.	Prevents adverse reactions from dose greater than ordered dose

Action	Rationale
– Squeeze ordered number of inches of drug onto paper measuring rule that comes with ointment.	Obtains ordered amount of drug
– Place on skin surface that is less hairy than other areas (such as upper chest, upper arm); DO NOT apply to areas where there is a heavy skinfold (abdomen) or heavy muscle mass (gluteal muscles) or to the axilla or groin.	Facilitates optimal absorption for dilation of coronary vessels
– Secure with adhesive application pad (comes with ointment) or plastic wrap or tape.	Prevents premature removal of pad

Medication Disks
(such as nitroglycerin or clonidine [Catapres])

– Remove outer package.	
– Carefully remove protective back (usually a plastic shield).	Obtains disk containing premeasured drug
– Place patch on skin surface that is less hairy than other areas (such as upper chest, upper arm); DO NOT apply to areas where there is a heavy skinfold (abdomen) or heavy muscle mass (gluteal muscles) or to the axilla or groin.	Facilitates optimal absorption
– Gently press around edges with fingers.	Provides for stability during long-term use

Sprays

– Instruct client to close eyes or turn head if spray is being applied to upper chest and above.	Protects against inhaling aerosol particles
– Apply a light coat of spray onto treatment	

Action	Rationale
area (usually 2 to 10 seconds, depending upon size of treatment area)	
10. Discard or restore all equipment properly.	Promotes cleanliness
11. Wash hands.	Prevents spread of infection
12. Document administration on medication-administration record.	Serves as legal record of administration and prevents accidental remediation

Evaluation

Goals met, partially met, or unmet?

Desired Outcome (sample)

Client displays no redness, swelling, drainage, pain, or open skin areas on lower left leg.

Documentation

The following should be noted on the client's chart:

• Name, dosage, and route of medication
• Assessment data relevant to purpose of medication
• Condition of treatment area
• Effects of medication
• Teaching of information about medication and techniques of self-administration

---

Sample Documentation

DATE	TIME	
7/8/94	2100	Tolnaftate 1% cream applied to abdomen for treatment of tinea. Client still has dry, flaky circles (2 cm in diameter) scattered on left lower quadrant of abdomen. States no itching. No other skin abnormalities noted.

Administration of Vaginal Medication

☒ Equipment

- Medication record or card
- Pen
- Basin of warm water
- Disposable gloves
- Washcloth
- Soap
- Towel
- Sanitary pad
- Vaginal applicator
- Vaginal suppository or cream to be administered

Purpose

Delivers medication for absorption through vaginal membranes for such therapeutic effects as resolving infections and treating inflammation

Assessment

Assessment should focus on the following:

Complete medication order
Condition of vaginal area (presence of lesions, tears, bleeding, tenderness, discharge, or odor)

Nursing Diagnoses

The nursing diagnoses may include the following:

Altered vaginal mucous membranes related to inflammatory process

Planning

Key Goals and Sample Goal Criterion

The client will

Demonstrate no signs of inflammation, such as redness, itching, edema, abnormal drainage and pain, within 1 week of medication initiation.

Implementation

Action	Rationale
1. Wash hands.	Reduces microorganism transfer
2. Prepare medication, adhering to the five rights of drug administration (see Procedure 11.1, Principles of Medication Administration).	Prepares drug Decreases chance of drug error
3. Identify client by reading identification bracelet and addressing client by name.	Confirms identity of client
4. Explain procedure and purpose of drug.	Decreases anxiety Promotes cooperation
5. Verify allergies listed on medication record or card.	Alerts nurse to possibility of allergic reaction
6. Provide privacy.	Decreases embarrassment
7. Don gloves.	Decreases nurse's exposure to client body secretions
8. Assist client into dorsal recumbent or Sims' position.	Places client in appropriate position for drug placement
9. Wash and dry perineum, if discharge or odor noted.	Promotes cleanliness Facilitates drug absorption Removes excess secretions
10. Insert medication into vaginal applicator:	Assists nurse with insertion of drug into vagina at length necessary to facilitate absorption
– Cream—place applicator over top of open medication tube, invert applicator–tube combination, and squeeze tube	Forces medication into applicator

Action	Rationale
– Suppository—insert suppository into applicator (or insert suppository without applicator, if desired).	
11. Spread labia if vagina is not easily visible.	Exposes vaginal opening
12. Insert applicator into vagina about 2.5 to 3.0 inches and press applicator top down (Fig. 11.18); if using finger to insert suppository, also insert 2.5 to 3.0 inches.	
13. Remove applicator or finger.	Completes process
14. Instruct client to remain in bed in a flat position for 15 to 20 minutes.	Allows time for medication to be absorbed
15. Apply sanitary pad.	Contains discharge secretions
16. Discard gloves.	Decreases transfer of microorganisms
17. Raise side rails.	Facilitates client safety
18. Place call light within reach.	Provides client with means to communicate needs
19. Discard or restore equipment properly (applicators may be washed with soap and water and	Promotes cleanliness

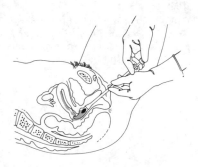

Figure 11.18

Action	Rationale
stored in plastic wrapping, box, or washcloth).	
20. Wash hands.	Reduces microorganism transfer
21. Document administration on medication record.	Provides legal record of administration and prevents accidental remedication

Evaluation

Goals met, partially met, or unmet?

Desired Outcomes (sample)

No redness, heat, swelling, abnormal drainage, or pain is present in vaginal area.

Documentation

The following should be noted on the client's chart:

- Name, dosage, and route of medication
- Assessment data relevant to purpose of medication
- Effects of medication
- Teaching of information about medication and techniques of self-administration

Sample Documentation

DATE	TIME	
7/8/94	2100	Client received final dose of Monistat vaginally. States pain and itching relieved. No redness, edema, or drainage in vaginal area.

CHAPTER 12

Special Procedures

12.1 Central Venous Pressure Line Management
12.2 Hyperthermia/Hypothermia Unit Management
12.3 Postmortem Care

OVERVIEW

- Central venous pressure (CVP) can provide important information about the maintenance of fluid balance. However, CVP lines can predispose the client to complications during insertion and throughout residence of the catheter. Complications include arrhythmias, pulmonary embolism, sepsis, phlebitis, pneumothorax, and hemothorax.

- Aggressive temperature-control therapy is crucial to regain the delicate balance necessary for vital organ function. If not closely monitored, temperature-control techniques can cause problems greater than those originally being treated. Potential complications of hypothermia/hyperthermia include cardiac, vascular, pulmonary, or metabolic compromise.

- A thorough assessment is imperative before beginning any intervention. Improperly performed postmortem techniques could result in serious legal, ethnic/cultural, or ethical/moral dilemmas.

- When there is a threatened or actual death, the care of significant others also becomes a nursing concern.

- Any exposure to body fluids presents a threat to the safety of the care-giver. Self-protective precautions, such as the use of gloves and gown in postmortem care, should be taken.

Jean Smith-Temple and Joyce Young Johnson:
Nurses' Guide to Clinical Procedures, Second Edition.© 1994
J. B. Lippincott Company

✋ Central Venous Pressure Line Management

✖ Equipment

- Manometer setup
- IV infusion tubing
- Yardstick or carpenter's level
- IV pole
- Masks (for client and nurse)
- Appropriate fluid
- 4 × 4-inch gauze
- Tape
- Sterile gloves

Purpose

Assess client's blood volume status and pressure in right atrium

Prevents, or assists in treatment of, fluid overload and dehydration

Assessment

Assessment should focus on the following:

Ordered rate of infusion and frequency of manometer readings

Circumstances necessitating central venous pressure (CVP) readings

Client knowledge of procedure

Status of central line and date inserted

Condition of central line insertion site (*e.g.,* presence of redness, edema, or pain)

Other clinical indicators of fluid status (*e.g.,* neck vein distension, edema, pulmonary congestion)

Nursing Diagnoses

The nursing diagnoses may include the following:

Altered fluid balance: deficit, related to decreased fluid intake
Possible fluid overload related to IV infusion
Altered circulation: decreased capillary refill, related to fluid
overload and congestive heart failure

Planning

Key Goals and Sample Goal Criteria
The client will

Demonstrate no undetected increase or decrease in fluid volume
for duration of CVP line maintenance
Verbalize no extreme anxiety regarding the CVP insertion, monitoring, and maintenance
Maintain infection-free status of CVP catheter site with no pain,
redness, or swelling

Special Considerations

Check patency of central line if CVP manometer is applied after
initial catheter insertion. Readings will not be accurate if CVP
line is obstructed.
Abnormal CVP readings should be reported to the physician.
Normal CVP is 5 to 10 cm H_2O. However, "normal" CVP may
vary for each client, so consult physician for guidelines.

Implementation

Action	Rationale
Assisting with Initial CVP Line Insertion	
1. Explain procedure to client.	Decreases anxiety
2. Wash hands and organize equipment.	Reduces microorganism transfer
	Promotes efficiency
3. Prepare IV fluids and tubing for infusion (see Procedure 5.3).	Manometer readings are inter-mittent, and fluid is infused at other times
4. Attach one end of mano-meter tubing (near stop-cock) to IV fluid tubing;	Flushes air from manometer tubing

Action	Rationale
position stopcock off to manometer and open to cup tubing and IV fluid and infuse slowly (Fig. 12.1.1).	
5. Turn stopcock off to CVP tubing and on to IV fluids and CVP manometer tube (Fig. 12.1.2); fill tube to ¾ full.	Allows for measurement of elevated readings, if present
6. Turn stopcock off to manometer and open to IV fluid and CVP tubing; maintain sterility.	Bypasses manometer, leaving tubing status equivalent to infusion tubing
7. Don gloves and mask and apply mask to client.	Prevents exposure to blood Prevents site contamination with respiratory tract microorganisms
8. Once central line catheter is inserted by physician, connect tubing to catheter; flush catheter with fluid; proceed to step 16.	Prevents clotting of line and reveals positional blockages to flow that might affect CVP readings

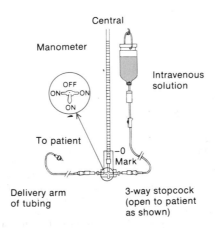

Figure 12.1.1

Action	Rationale

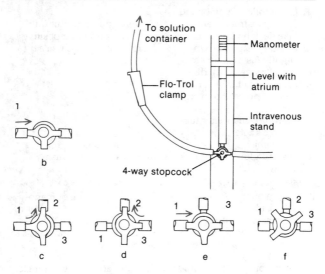

Figure 12.1.2

Addition of Manometer to Established Line

9. Complete steps 1 and 2 and then obtain new tubing, unless recently changed; slow flow rate of old tubing; disconnect tubing from bag/bottle and tape tubing to IV pole.

Minimizes contaminants

Maintains fluid flow through catheter, preventing clotting

10. Prepare new IV tubing; then fill CVP tubing and manometer as described in steps 4 to 6.

11. Using sterile dressing change technique, remove dressing; see Procedure 5.9 for central line dressing change technique.

Allows observation of site

12. Place 4 × 4-inch gauze under catheter hub.

Protects hub from skin contaminants

Action	Rationale

13. Close roller clamp on old tubing; instruct client to take deep breath and hold it while bearing down slightly (as if having a bowel movement); disconnect old tubing and quickly proceed to next step. — Prevents pulling of air into vein by providing positive pressure via Valsalva's maneuver

14. Connect manometer tubing to catheter.
15. Flush line. — Maintains patency
16. Discard gloves and masks and wash hands. — Reduces microorganism transfer

Obtaining Readings

17. Tape manometer to pole at bedside; use yardstick or level to line up zero point of manometer with client's right atrium (Fig. 12.1.3). — Stabilizes position of manometer

Ensures accuracy and consistency of readings

18. Turn stopcock off to fluids (open to client's IV catheter and manometer). — Provides access of manometer to pressures in right atrium

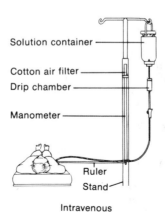

Solution container

Cotton air filter

Drip chamber

Manometer

Ruler

Stand

Intravenous

Figure 12.1.3

Action	Rationale
19. Watch fluid fluctuations and read value when fluctuations have stabilized; read at end of exhalation phase of respirations.	Eliminates interferences and results in more accurate CVP readings
20. Refill manometer as in step 5 and repeat reading process, steps 18 and 19.	Ensures accuracy by revealing large fluctuations in readings caused by factors other than client's blood levels
21. Turn stopcock off to manometer.	Re-establishes flow to IV catheter from IV fluids
22. Position client for comfort with side rails up and call bell within reach.	Facilitates comfort, safety, and communication
23. Discard or restore supplies.	Maintains clean and orderly environment

Evaluation

Goals met, partially met, or unmet?

Desired Outcomes (sample)

Fluid volume is within acceptable limits, due to accurate reading and recording of CVP values and prompt reporting of abnormalities.

Insertion site is clean and dry with no pain, redness, swelling, or drainage.

Client is calm with slow, unlabored respirations.

Client verbalizes understanding of purpose of CVP monitoring.

Documentation

The following should be noted on the client's chart:

- Readings obtained, with changes in trend of values noted
- Consistency of clinical signs and symptoms with readings obtained
- Status of central line
- Client's tolerance of line insertion
- Client's tolerance of dressing change and attachment of manometer to established line
- Client's understanding of teaching regarding CVP line and readings

Sample Documentation

Date	Time	
12/3/94	1400	CVP reading of 7. Skin warm and dry. No pedal or sacral edema noted. Central line dressing dry and intact, fluid infusing well per Dial-A-Flo at 50 ml/hr.

🖐 Hyperthermia/Hypothermia Unit Management

☒ Equipment

- Hyperthermia/hypothermia unit
- Hyperthermia/hypothermia blanket
- Disposable gloves
- Rectal probe
- Linen blanket (optional)
- Two sheets
- Linen savers (optional)

Purpose

To attain and maintain client's body temperature within acceptable to normal range

Assessment

Assessment should focus on the following:

Baseline data (*i.e.,* vital signs, temperature, neurostatus, skin condition, circulation, and EKG)

Signs of shivering

Hyperthermia/hypothermia unit and blanket (properly functioning)

Condition of electrical plugs (properly grounded) and wires (not frayed or exposed)

Nursing Diagnoses

The nursing diagnoses may include the following:

Altered temperature: elevation, related to sepsis

Altered temperature: decreased, related to prolonged exposure to cold

Potential skin impairment related to excess exposure to heating/cooling unit

Planning

Key Goals and Sample Goal Criteria

The client will

Demonstrate acceptable to normal temperature
Maintain adequate tissue perfusion with capillary refill time of less than 10 seconds
Demonstrate no skin breakdown
Demonstrate minimal or no shivering

Special Considerations

There is a potential for skin damage with any electrical temperature-control device; therefore, treatment and temperature must be monitored closely.

Geriatric and Pediatric
The temperature-control mechanisms of chronically ill elderly and very young pediatric clients are often very sensitive to changes in heat and cold.
Use blanket device to decrease or increase temperature gradually.

Implementation

Action	Rationale
1. Wash hands and organize equipment.	Reduces microorganism transfer Promotes efficiency
2. Connect the blanket pad (may cover with clear plastic cover) to the operating unit:	Protects blanket from secretions
– Insert male tubing connector of blanket into inlet opening on unit (Fig. 12.2).	Secures blanket tubing–unit connection and prevents solution leakage
– Repeat same for outlet opening.	
– Connect second pad, if used, in same manner.	

Action   **Rationale**

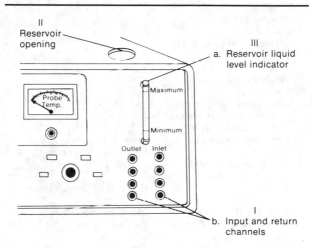

II
Reservoir opening

III
a. Reservoir liquid level indicator

Probe Temp.

Maximum

Minimum

Outlet   Inlet

I
b. Input and return channels

Figure 12.2

Action	Rationale
3. Check blanket solution-level gauge and add more recommended solution (usually alcohol-distilled water mixture; see user's manual) into reservoir cap; add solution until it reaches the "fill line."	Facilitates proper functioning Solution is circulated through coils in blanket and warmed/cooled to maintain blanket at the desired temperature
4. Turn the unit on by moving the temperature control knob to desired temperature (blanket coils will fill with solution automatically).	Activates unit
5. Monitor blanket for adequate filling, watching gauge and adding solution to reservoir as needed to maintain fluid level.	Prevents inadequate filling of blanket and improper functioning of system
6. Turn unit off.	Allows safe transport of unit
7. Set master temperature control knob to either manual or automatic operation.	Adjusts unit to be controlled by temperature probe (automatic) or by nurse (manual)

Action	Rationale
If using automatic control: – Insert thermistor-probe plug into thermistor-probe jack on unit. When using manual control: – Set master temperature-control knob to desired temperature.	
8. Explain procedure to client.	Reduces anxiety Promotes cooperation
9. Transport equipment into client's room.	
10. Don gloves.	Prevents microorganism transfer
11. Bathe client and apply cream, lotion, or oil to skin.	Increases circulation Provides opportunity for skin assessment
12. Place blanket on bed, place a sheet over the blanket, and apply linen saver, if needed.	Protects skin from direct contact with blanket, and decreases soiling of blanket
13. Place client on blanket (may use side-to-side rolling, bed scales, or lifting apparatus).	
14. Remove gloves.	
15. Obtain baseline assessment data.	Allows detection of changes in status
16. Initiate therapy: don gloves, lubricate rectal probe, and insert probe into rectum.	Allows machine to warm or cool to desired temperature with constant automatic monitoring to ensure safe regulation of temperature to desired range
17. Automatic control: – Check temperature control for accuracy of setting. – Check that automatic mode light is on. – Check pad temperature range for safe limits.	Ensures machine is functioning properly

Action	Rationale
Manual control: – Check that manual mode light is on. – Check that temperature setting and safety limits are accurate. – Monitor client's temperature. – Adjust blanket temperature to maintain body temperature.	Allows nurse to monitor client's temperature continually and to adjust blanket temperature, as needed, to achieve desired body temperature
18. Monitor client status: – Temperature—every 15 minutes until desired temperature is reached	Assures that no excess change in body temperature occurs
– Vital signs—every 15 to 30 minutes, or as ordered initially, and every 1 to 2 hours until treatment is discontinued	Initial treatment might cause adverse changes—*e.g.,* arrhythmias, hyperventilation
– Onset of shivering—verbalized sensations, muscle twitching, EKG artifact; if present, obtain order for medication to prevent	Shivering increases body metabolism and energy needs Medication (tranquilizer) will decrease shivering
19. Every 4 hours, remove rectal probe and clean; use glass thermometer to check temperature.	Allows monitoring for rectal irritation and maintains probe accuracy
20. Maintain client in supine position with every 2 hour range of motion, massage to bony prominences, and support stockings as ordered.	Provides for maximum body surface area exposure Decreases venous stasis
21. Turn, cough, and deep-breathe client every hour.	Increases ventilation of airways and secretion removal
22. Observe for edema.	Detects edema related to increased cell permeability

Action	Rationale
23. Adjust master temperature control gradually until 37°C is reached over a period of 6 hours.	Rapid changes in temperature could result in severe vital sign changes and/or arrhythmia

Evaluation

Goals met, partially met, or unmet?

Desired Outcomes (sample)

Client's temperature is within acceptable or normal limits.
No skin breakdown or shivering is noted.
Nail beds and mucous membranes are pink; capillary refill time is brisk.

Documentation

The following should be noted on the client's chart:

- Time treatment was initiated and initial temperature settings
- Initial and subsequent client response to treatment
- Baseline vital signs and client status

Sample Documentation

DATE	TIME	
12/3/94	1400	Client placed on hypothermia blanket with master temperature set at 36°C and patient temperature probe indicating 39°C. Vital signs stable. No shivering noted. Skin intact with capillary refill less than 5 seconds.

☝ Postmortem Care

☒ Equipment

- Disposable gloves
- Clean linens
- Clean gown
- Wash basin
- Death certificate
- Isolation bags (optional)
- Cloth or disposable gown
- Two washcloths and towels
- 4 × 4-inch gauze or other dressing (optional)
- Moist cotton balls (optional)
- Identification bracelets or body tags
- Shroud (optional, unless agency policy)
- Dilute bleach mixture (optional)

Purpose

Provides proper preparation of body of deceased client for viewing by family members and for transport to funeral home or morgue with minimum exposure of staff to body fluids and excrement

Assessment

Assessment should focus on the following:

Hospital policy regarding postmortem care and notification process

Need for autopsy (if death occurs within 24 hours of hospitalization or is the result of suicide, homicide, or unknown causes; or if the family requests an autopsy)

Nursing Diagnoses

The nursing diagnoses may include the following:

Potential ineffective coping by family with the death of loved one

Potential spread of infection related to contact with contaminated body fluids

Planning

Key Goals and Sample Goal Criteria

The family will experience no excessive anxiety related to the viewing of the deceased client's body

The body will appear clean and as natural as possible

The environment will appear clean and pleasant

Special Considerations

The bodies of deceased clients with known infections requiring blood and body fluid precautions or isolation (*e.g.*, tuberculosis, AIDS) should be tagged accordingly, and there should be appropriate disposal of soiled items and cleaning of nondisposable items.

Home Health

The client must be "pronounced dead" prior to removal of the body from the home (unless being taken to hospital or health facility). Follow home-health agency policy for recording the pronouncement on the client's chart.

 Transcultural

Many religious rites and cultural practices may be employed by a variety of cultures. It is important that the nurse demonstrate respect for the deceased, as well as allow the family privacy.

Communicate with the family to determine what is important before preparing the body. It may be important to summon a priest, minister, rabbi, or other religious leader after the client is deceased.

Implementation

Action	Rationale
1. Record time of death (cessation of heart function)	Required for death certificate and all official records

Action	Rationale
and time pronounced dead by physician.	
2. Notify family members that client's status has changed for the worse and assist them to a private room until physician is available.	Provides privacy for family during initial grief and allows time for physician to notify family of client's death
3. Close door to client's room.	Prevents exposure of body to other patients and visitors and prevents accidental viewing of body by family before body is prepared
4. Don gloves and isolation gown.	Protects nurse from body secretions
5. Hold eyelids closed until they remain closed or place moist 4 × 4-inch gauze or cotton balls on lids.	Fixes eyelids in a natural, closed position before rigor mortis onset
6. Remove tubes, such as IV, nasogastric (NG) catheter, or urinary catheter, if allowed and no autopsy is to be done.	Provides a more natural appearance for viewing by family members
7. If unable to remove tubes: – Clamp IVs and tubes. – Coil NG and urinary tubes and tape them down. – Cut IV tubings as close to clamp as possible, cover with 4 × 4-inch gauze, tape securely.	Retains secretions and provides as clean and natural an appearance for family viewing as possible
8. Remove extra equipment from room to utility room.	Allows free mobility around bed and improves appearance of environment
9. Wash secretions from face and body.	Improves appearance of body and decreases room odor
10. Replace soiled linens and gown with clean articles.	Provides clean appearance and decreases odor
11. Place linen savers under body and extremities, if needed.	Catches secretions and excrement escaping from open sphincters or oozing wounds

Action	Rationale
12. Put soiled linens and pads in bag (isolation bag, if appropriate) and remove from room.	Decreases exposure to body fluids Removes odor and improves appearance of environment
13. Position body supine with arms at side, palms down.	Provides a natural appearance
14. Place dentures (if present) in mouth, put a pillow under head, close mouth, and place rolled towel under chin.	Gives face a natural appearance and sets mouth closed before onset of rigor mortis
15. Remove all jewelry (except wedding band, unless band is requested by family members) and give to family with other personal belongings; record the name(s) of receiver(s).	Prevents loss of property during transfer of body and ensures proper disposal of belongings
16. Place clean top covering over body leaving face exposed.	Allows family to view client, and covers remaining tubes and dressings
17. Place chair at bedside.	Provides for family member unable to stand or if momentary weakness occurs
18. Dim lighting.	Makes atmosphere more soothing and minimizes abnormal appearance of body
19. After body has been viewed by family, tag with appropriate identification (some agencies require that body be placed in a covering or shroud and that an outer covering identification tag be applied).	Ensures proper identification of body before transfer to funeral home or morgue
20. Send completed death certificate with body to funeral home or complete paperwork as required by hospital and send body to morgue.	Fulfills legal requirements for documentation of death

Action	Rationale
21. Close rooms of clients on hall through which body is transported, if hospital policy.	Prevents distress of other clients and visitors
22. Restore or dispose of equipment, supplies, and linens properly; remove gown and gloves and wash hands.	Reduces microorganism transfer Maintains clean and orderly environment
23. Have room cleaned: use special cleaning supplies if client had infection (*e.g.*, 1:10 chloride dilution for AIDS clients, special germicides for isolation situations).	Prevents transfer of micro-organisms

Evaluation

Goals met, partially met, or unmet?

Desired Outcomes (sample)

Body and environment are clean with a natural appearance.
Family views body with no signs of extreme distress at its physical appearance.
There is no spread of disease.

Documentation

The following should be noted on the client's chart:

- Time of death and code information, if performed
- Notification of physician and family members
- Response of family members
- Disposal of valuables and belongings
- Time body was removed from room

Sample Documentation

Date	Time	
12/3/94	1200	Client pronounced dead by Dr. Brown; family members notified by doctor. Body viewed by family with no unusual reactions. Gold-colored wedding band taped to finger on body; gold-colored watch, clothing, and shoes given to Mr. Dale Smith (son). Body removed to James Funeral Home, accompanied by completed death certificate.

STRESS MANAGEMENT TECHNIQUES*

The following techniques can be taught to provide an individual with an opportunity to control his or her response to stressors and, in turn, to increase his or her ability to manage stress constructively. Suggested readings are listed at the end to provide more specific information.

Progressive Relaxation Technique

Progressive relaxation is a self-taught or instructed exercise that involves learning to constrict and relax muscle groups in a systematic way, beginning with the face and finishing with the feet. This exercise may be combined with breathing exercises that focus on inner body processes. It usually takes 15 to 30 minutes and may be accompanied by a taped instruction that directs the person concerning the sequence of muscles to be relaxed.

1. Wear loose clothing; remove glasses and shoes.
2. Sit or recline in a comfortable position with neck and knees supported; avoid lying completely flat.
3. Begin with slow, rhythmic breathing.
   a. Close your eyes or stare at a spot and take in a slow deep breath.
   b. Exhale slowly.
4. Continue rhythmic breathing at a slow steady pace and feel the tension leaving your body with each breath.
5. Begin progressive relaxation of muscle groups.
   a. Breathe in and tense (tighten) your muscles and then relax the muscles as you breathe out.

*Carpenito LJ: Nursing Diagnosis: Application to Clinical Practice, 4th ed, pp 1089–1091. Philadelphia, JB Lippincott, 1992

b. Suggested order for tension–relaxation cycle (with tension technique in parentheses):

Face, jaw, mouth (squint eyes, wrinkle brow)
Neck (pull chin to neck)
Right hand (make a fist)
Right arm (bend elbow in tightly)
Left hand (make a fist)
Left arm (bend elbow in tightly)
Back, shoulders, chest (shrug shoulders up tightly)
Abdomen (pull stomach in and bear down on chair)
Right upper leg (push leg down)
Right lower leg and foot (point toes toward body)
Left upper leg (push leg down)
Left lower leg and foot (point toes toward body)

6. Practice technique slowly.
7. End relaxation session when you are ready by counting to three, inhaling deeply, and saying, "I am relaxed."

Self-coaching

Self-coaching is a procedure to decrease anxiety by understanding one's own signs of anxiety (such as increased heart rate or sweaty palms) and then coaching oneself to relax.

For example, "I am upset about this situation but I can control how anxious I get. I will take things one step at a time, and I won't focus on my fear. I'll think about what I must do to finish this task. The situation will not be forever. I can manage until it is over. I'll focus on taking deep breaths."

Thought Stopping

Thought stopping is a self-directed behavioral procedure learned to gain control of self-defeating thoughts. Through repeated systematic practice, a person does the following:

1. Says "stop" when a self-defeating thought crosses the mind (*e.g.*, "I'm not smart enough" or "I'm not a good nurse")
2. Allows a brief period—15 to 30 seconds—of conscious relaxation (because of an increased focus on negative thoughts, it may seem at first that self-defeating thoughts increase; however, eventually the self-defeating thoughts will decrease)

Assertive Behavior

Assertive behavior is the open, honest, empathic sharing of your opinions, desires, and feelings. Assertiveness is not a magical acquisition but a learned behavioral skill. Assertive persons do not allow others to take advantage of them and thus are not victims. Assertive behavior is not domineering but remains controlled and nonaggressive. An assertive person

Does not hurt others
Does not wait for things to get better
Does not invite victimization
Listens attentively to the desires and feelings of others
Takes the initiative to make relationships better
Remains in control or uses silences as an alternative
Examines all the risks involved before asserting
Examines personal responsibilities in each situation before asserting

Refer to suggested readings for specific techniques or participate in an assertiveness training course led by a competent instructor. Assertive behavior is best learned slowly in several sessions rather than in one lengthy session or workshop.

Guided Imagery

This technique is the purposeful use of one's imagination in a specific way to achieve relaxation and control. The person concentrates on the image and pictures himself involved in the scene. The following is an example of the technique.

1. Discuss with person an image he or she has experienced that is pleasurable and relaxing, such as

   Lying on a warm beach
   Feeling a cool wave of water
   Floating on a raft
   Watching the sun set

2. Choose a scene that will involve at least two senses.
3. Begin with rhythmic breathing and progressive relaxation.
4. Have person travel mentally to the scene.
5. Have the person slowly experience the scene; how does it look? sound? smell? feel? taste?
6. Practice the imagery.

    a. Suggest tape recording the imagined experience to assist with the technique.

    b. Practice the technique alone to reduce feelings of embarrassment.

7. End the imagery technique by counting to three and saying, "I am relaxed" (if the person does not use a specific ending, he or she may become drowsy and fall asleep, which defeats the purpose of the technique).

Suggested Readings

Alberti, R.E. and Emmons, L. (1974). *Your Perfect Right: A Guide to Assertive Behavior* (2nd ed.). San Luis Obispo, CA: Impact.

Benson, H. (1976). *The Relaxation Response.* New York: Avon Books.

Bloom, L., Coburn, K., and Pearlman, J. (1976). *The New Assertive Woman.* New York: Dell.

Chenevert, M. (1978). *Special Techniques in Assertiveness Training for Women in the Health Professions.* St. Louis: C.V. Mosby.

Gridano, D and Everly, G. (1979). *Controlling Stress and Tension.* Englewood Cliffs, NJ: Prentice-Hall.

Herman, S. (1978). *Becoming Assertive: A Guide for Nurses.* New York: D. Van Nostrand.

Hill, L. and Smith, N. (1985). *Self-Care Nursing.* Englewood Cliffs, NJ: Prentice-Hall. (Especially Part II, Self Care Primarily Associated with the Mind).

McCaffery, M. (1979). *Nursing Management of the Patient with Pain* (2nd ed.). Philadelphia: J.B. Lippincott. (Especially Chap. 10, Imagery, and Chap. 9, Relaxation).

NURSING DIAGNOSES, NORTH AMERICAN NURSING DIAGNOSIS ASSOCIATION, APRIL 1992

Activity Intolerance
Activity Intolerance, High Risk for
Adjustment, Impaired
Airway Clearance, Ineffective
Anxiety
Aspiration, High Risk for
Body Image Disturbance
Body Temperature, High Risk for Altered
Breastfeeding, Effective
Breastfeeding, Ineffective
Breastfeeding, Interrupted*
Breathing Pattern, Ineffective
Cardiac Output, Decreased
Caregiver Role Strain*
Caregiver Role Strain, High Risk for*
Communication, Impaired Verbal
Constipation
Constipation, Colonic
Constipation, Perceived
Coping, Defensive
Coping, Ineffective Individual
Decisional Conflict (Specify)
Denial, Ineffective
Diarrhea
Disuse Syndrome, High Risk for
Diversional Activity Deficit
Dysreflexia
Family Coping: Compromised, Ineffective

Family Coping: Disabling, Ineffective
Family Coping: Potential for Growth
Family Processes, Altered
Fatigue
Fear
Fluid Volume Deficit
Fluid Volume Deficit, High Risk for
Fluid Volume Excess
Gas Exchange, Impaired
Grieving, Anticipatory
Grieving, Dysfunctional
Growth and Development, Altered
Health Maintenance, Altered
Health-Seeking Behaviors (Specify)
Home Maintenance Management, Impaired
Hopelessness
Hyperthermia
Hypothermia
Incontinence, Bowel
Incontinence, Functional
Incontinence, Reflex
Incontinence, Stress
Incontinence, Total
Incontinence, Urge
Infant Feeding Pattern, Ineffective*
Infection, High Risk for
Injury, High Risk for
Knowledge Deficit (Specify)
Noncompliance (Specify)
Nutrition, Altered: Less than Body Requirements
Nutrition, Altered: More than Body Requirements
Nutrition, Altered: Potential for More than Body Requirements
Oral Mucous Membrane, Altered
Pain
Pain, Chronic
Parental Role Conflict
Parenting, Altered
Parenting, High Risk for Altered
Peripheral Neurovascular Dysfunction, High Risk for*
Personal Identity Disturbance
Physical Mobility, Impaired
Poisoning, High Risk for
Post-Trauma Response

Powerlessness
Protection, Altered
Rape Trauma Syndrome
Rape Trauma Syndrome: Compound Reaction
Rape Trauma Syndrome: Silent Reaction
Relocation Stress Syndrome*
Role Performance, Altered
Self-Care Deficit
  Bathing/Hygiene
  Feeding
  Dressing/Grooming
  Toileting
Self-Esteem, Chronic Low
Self-Esteem, Situational Low
Self-Esteem Disturbance
Self-Mutilation, High Risk for*
Sensory-Perceptual Alterations (Specify) (visual, auditory,
  kinesthetic, gustatory, tactile, olfactory)
Sexual Dysfunction
Sexuality Patterns, Altered
Skin Integrity, High Risk for Impaired
Skin Integrity, Impaired
Sleep Pattern Disturbance
Social Interaction, Impaired
Social Isolation
Spiritual Distress
Suffocation, High Risk for
Swallowing, Impaired
Therapeutic Regimen, Ineffective Management of*
Thermoregulation, Ineffective
Thought Processes, Altered
Tissue Integrity, Impaired
Tissue Perfusion, Altered (Specify Type) (renal, cerebral, cardio-
  pulmonary, gastrointestinal, peripheral)
Trauma, High Risk for
Unilateral Neglect
Urinary Elimination, Altered
Urinary Retention
Ventilation, Inability to Sustain Spontaneous*
Ventilatory Weaning Response, Dysfunctional*
Violence, High Risk for: Self-Directed or Directed at Others

*New diagnoses from 1992 conference.

COMMON CLINICAL ABBREVIATIONS

*When multiple meanings are possible, consider context.

abd	abdomen	diab	diabetic
ac	before meals	diag, DX	diagnosis
ADLs	activities of daily living	DOA	dead on arrival
		dr	dram
ad. lib.	as desired	EENT	eye, ear, nose, throat
adm	admission	et	and
AKA	above the knee amputation	EKG	electrocardiogram
		exam	examination
alb	albumin	F	fahrenheit
amb	ambulate	FBS	fasting/fingerstick blood sugar
ant	anterior		
AP	anterior-posterior	FHT	fetal heart tones
ax	axillary	fl, fld	fluid
approx	approximately	ft	feet
b.i.d.	twice a day	fx	fracture/fractional
BKA	below the knee amputation	g/gm	gram
		gr	grain
BM	bowel movement	grav	gravida
BP	blood pressure	gt, gtt	drops
BRP	bathroom privileges	h, hr	hour
C	centigrade, celsius	hg	mercury
c̄	with	hct	hematocrit
Ca	calcium	hgb	hemoglobin
CA	cancer	HOB	head of bed
CC	chief complaint	hs	hour of sleep
cc	cubic centimeter	hx	history
C & S	culture and sensitivity	I & D	incision and drainage
c/o	complains of	I & O	intake and output
CVP	central venous pressure	ID	intradermal
		IM	intramuscular
cysto	cystoscopy	irriga	irrigation
DC	discontinue	IV	intravenous

K	potassium	RLQ	right lower quadrant
kg	kilogram	RO or r/o	rule out
L	liter	ROM	range of motion
L, lt	left	Rx	prescription
lat	lateral	$\bar{s}$	without
lb	pound	SC/sub q	subcutaneous
lymph	lymphatic	sm	small
MAE	moves all extremities	SL	sublingual
m	minims	SOB	short of breath
mcg	microgram		or
mEq	milliequivalent		side of bed
mg, mgm	milligrams	sol	solution
MI	myocardial infarction	sp. gr.	specific gravity
ml	milliliter	S & S	signs/symptoms
neg	negative	stat	immediately
NKA	no known allergies	supp	suppository
noct	nocturnal	T, temp	temperature
NPO	nothing by mouth	T & A	tonsillectomy and
N & V	nausea and vomiting		adenoidectomy
OOB	out of bed	tab	tablet
oz	ounce	tbsp	tablespoon
OD	right eye	t.i.d.	three times a day
OS	left eye	tinc	tincture
OU	each eye	TKO	to keep open
p.c.	after meals	trach	tracheostomy
PO	by mouth, orally	tsp	teaspoon
pr	per rectum	TUR	transurethral
PRN	when needed		resection
q	every	tx	treatment
qAM	every morning	UA	urinalysis
qd	every day	UGI	upper gastro-
q.i.d.	four times a day		intestinal
q.o.d.	every other day	vag	vaginal
qs	quantity sufficient	vol	volume
R	rectal	VS	vital signs
RBC	red blood cell	WBC	white blood cell
rt, R	right	WNL	within normal limits
resp	respirations	wt	weight

Selected Abbreviations Used for Specific Descriptions

ASCVD	arteriosclerotic cardiovascular disease	CNS	central nervous system
			or
ASHD	arteriosclerotic heart disease		Clinical Nurse Specialist
BE	barium enema	DJD	degenerative joint disease
CMS	circulation movement sensation	DOE	dyspnea on exertion

DT's	delerium tremens
D_5W	5% dextrose in water
FUO	fever of unknown origin
GB	gall bladder
GI	gastrointestinal
GYN	gynecology
H_2O_2	hydrogen peroxide
HA	hyperalimentation or headache
HCVD	hypertensive cardiovascular disease
HEENT	head, ear, eye, nose, throat
HVD	hypertensive vascular disease
ICU	intensive care unit
LLE	left lower extremity
LLQ	left lower quadrant
LOC	level of consciousness; laxatives of choice
LMP	last menstrual period
LUE	left upper extremity
LUQ	left upper quadrant
Neuro	neurology; neurosurgery
NS	normal saline
NWB	non-weight bearing
OPD	outpatient department
ORIF	open reduction internal fixation
Ortho	orthopedics
OT	occupational therapy
PAR	post-anesthesia room
PE	physical examination
PERRLA	pupils equal, round, & react to light and accommodation
PID	pelvic inflammatory disease
PI	present illness
PM & R	physical medicine & rehabilitation
Psych	psychology; psychiatric
PT	physical therapy
RL (or LR)	Ringer's lactate; lactated Ringer's
RLE	right lower extremity
RR	recovery room
RUE	right upper extremity
RUQ	right upper quadrant
Rx	prescription
STSG	split-thickness skin graft
Surg	surgery, surgical
THR; TJR	total hip replacement; total joint replacement
URI	upper respiratory infection
UTI	urinary tract infection
VD	venereal disease
WNWD	well-nourished, well-developed

DIAGNOSTIC LABORATORY TESTS: NORMAL VALUES

Test	Normal Values
Serum/Plasma Chemistries	
Arterial blood gases:	
pH	7.35–7.45
pCO₂	35–45 mm Hg
HCO₃	22–26 mEq/L
pO₂	80–100 mm Hg
O₂ saturation	95%–100%
AST (Aspartate aminotransferase), formerly SGOT	5–40 U/ml
Bilirubin:	
Direct (conjugated)	0.1–0.3 mg/dl
Indirect (unconjugated)	0.2–0.8 mg/dl
Total	0.1–1 mg/dl
Newborns	1–12 mg/dl
Blood urea nitrogen (BUN)	5–20 mg/dl
Calcium (total)	8–10 mg/dl
Chloride	90–110 mEq/L
Cholesterol	150–250 mg/dl
Creatinine	0.7–1.5 mg/dl
Creatinine phosphokinase (CPK)	5–75 mU/ml
	MM (skeletal) band present,
CPK isoenzymes	MB band (cardiac) <5%
Glucose	80–120 mg/dl
Erythrocyte sedimentation rate (ESR)	Up to 20 mm/hr
Erythrocyte Indices :	
Mean corpuscular volume (MCV)	80–94 cu micron/micrometer
Mean corpuscular hemoglobin (MCH)	27–32 micromicrograms/cell

Test	Normal Values
Mean corpuscular hemo-globin concentration (MCHC)	33%–38%
Reticulocytes	0.5%–1.5% of red cells
Hematocrit:	
Newborns	44%–64%
Infants	30%–40%
Children	31%–43%
Men	42%–52%
Women	37%–47%
Hemoglobin concentration:	
Newborns	14–24 g/dl
Infants	10–15 g/dl
Children	11–16 g/dl
Men	14–18 g/dl
Women	12–16 g/dl
Lactic dehydrogenase (LDH)	90–200 ImU/ml
Platelet count	150,000–400,000/cu mm
Potassium	3.5–5 mEq/L
Partial thromboplastin time (PTT); (activated—APTT)	20–45 seconds
Prothrombin time	9.5–12 seconds
Red blood cells (RBCs):	
Newborns	4.8–7.1 million/cu mm
Infants/children	3.8–5.5 million/cu mm
Men	4.7–6.1 million/cu mm
Women	4.2–5.4 million/cu mm
Serum glutamic oxaloacetic transaminase (SGOT)	5–40 U/ml
Sodium	138 mEq/L
White blood cells (Leukocyte count)	5000–10,000 cu mm
Neutrophils	60%–70%
Eosinophils	1%–4%
Basophils	0%–0.5%
Lymphocytes	20%–30%
Monocytes	2%–6%
Urine Chemistry	
Calcium	<150 mg/24 h
Creatine	0–200 mg/24 h
Creatinine	0.8–2 g/24 h
Creatinine clearance	100–150 ml of blood cleared of creatinine per minute

Test	Normal Values
Osmolality	Males: 390–1090 mM/kg
	Females: 300–1090 mM/kg
Potassium	40–65 mEq/24 h
Protein	Up to 100 mg/24 h
Sodium	130–200 mmol/24 h
Urea nitrogen	9–16 g/24 h
Uric acid	250–750 mg/24 h

TYPES OF ISOLATION

The four major categories of isolation involve the use of universal precautions in addition to either disease-specific or category-specific isolation precautions, *or* the use of body substance isolation. HAND WASHING IS REQUIRED WITH ALL CLIENT CONTACT AND WITH ALL FORMS OF ISOLATION.

Universal precautions (blood and body fluid) involve the use of protective coverings whenever contact with blood and certain other body fluids is a possibility. These precautions are intended to prevent contact of the skin and mucous membranes of health care workers with blood and body fluids of the client.

Universal precautions are applied to blood; semen or vaginal secretions; and cerebrospinal, pleural, peritoneal, synovial, and amniotic fluid. When used properly, these precautions eliminate the need for the category "Blood and Body Fluid Precautions" used in the category-specific isolation system. Universal precautions do not apply to feces, urine, nasal secretions, sputum, sweat, and tears unless these body fluids contain visible blood. If a client is known to have an infection involving these body fluids, the appropriate disease-specific or category-specific isolation system is initiated (see Table for protective barriers required).

Body substance isolation (BSI) involves the use of protective barrier coverings whenever contact with any body fluid is expected. BSI is based on the principle that not all clients infected with blood-borne pathogens can be reliably identified prior to the possible exposure of health-care team members. Health-team members are instructed to use precautions with all clients, thus eliminating the need for additional disease or category-specific isolation.

BSI precautions are posted in all client rooms. Gloves are used when handling any body secretion or secretion-soiled item. A gown is added when soiling of clothing is likely. A mask and goggles are worn whenever secretions are projectile or when an infection with a microorganism that is transmitted through air (droplet transmission) is suspected (an additional mask-precautions notice may be posted). All linens are handled with care to prevent contamination of the nurse's clothing. Reusable items used on clients known to be infected are tagged accordingly when sent for disinfecting.

Category-specific precautions involve established use of barrier coverings when caring for clients with diseases falling into specific groups (see table). Isolation cards are prepared that identify needed precautions for the specific category.

Disease-specific precautions involve the use of an isolation card identifying required barrier coverings when caring for clients with diseases caused by specific microorganisms that are identified by the mode of disease transmission. Many facilities design isolation cards that identify the necessary precautions (*e.g.*, the use of gloves, gown, masks, goggles, or special disposal of contaminated materials) in a yes/no format. The table includes information found on most cards.

Precautions Used by Health-care Team Members

Isolation/Precaution Systems	Gloves	Gown	Mask	Goggles	Special Handling of Linens/Dishes
Universal precautions (blood/body fluids)	Y	With possible soiling	N	N	Y if contaminated with blood
Body substance isolation	Y	With possible soiling	D	Y with projectile secretions	Basic care with all
Disease-specific	D	D	D	D	D
Category-specific					
Strict	Y	With possible soiling	Y	Y with secretions	Y
Contact	Y	Y	Y	Y with secretions	Y
Enteric	Y	Y	N	N	Y if soiled
Tuberculosis (AFB) isolation	N	Y	Y	Y	Y if soiled
Respiratory	N	N	Y	Y with secretions	Y if soiled

D = depends on disease; N = no, item is not generally required; Y = yes, item is needed in most circumstances (some listed).
Some agencies require double-bagging of soiled materials prior to removal from the room; isolation card should identify these requirements.

Bibliography

Alfaro, R. (1986). *Application of Nursing Process: A Step-by-Step Guide.* Philadelphia: JB Lippincott.

Altersecu, V. (1985). The Ostomy: What Do You Teach the Patient? *American Journal of Nursing.* 85(11) (1250—1253).

Atkinson, L. and Murray, M. (1985). *Fundamentals of Nursing: A Nursing Process Approach.* New York: Macmillan.

Barnes, C. and Kirchhoff, K. (1986). Minimizing Hypoxemia Due to Endotracheal Suctioning: A Literature Review. *Heart & Lung.* 15(2) (164–175).

Bates, B. (1991). *A Guide to Physical Examination and History Taking* (5th ed.). Philadelphia: J.B. Lippincott.

Beeland, K. and Wells, M. (1987). *Clinical Nursing Procedures.* Boston/Monterey: Jones and Bartlett.

Binkley, L. (1984). Keeping Up With Peritoneal Dialysis. *American Journal of Nursing.* 84(6) (729–733).

Birdsall, Carole. (1985). When Is TPN Safe? *American Journal of Nursing.* 85(1) (73).

Boyle, J.S., and Andrews, M.M. (1989). *Transcultural Concepts in Nursing Care.* Boston: Scot Foresman/Little Brown College Division.

Brown, I. (1982). Trach Care? Take Care—Infection's on the Prowl. *Nursing '82.* 82(5) (44–49).

Carnevali, D. (1983). *Nursing Care Planning: Diagnosis and Management* (3rd ed.). Philadelphia: J.B. Lippincott.

Carpenito, L.J. (1987). *Handbook of Nursing Diagnosis* (2nd ed.). Philadelphia: J.B. Lippincott.

Carpenito, L.J. (1992). *Nursing Diagnostic Application to Clinical Practice* (4th ed.). Philadelphia: J.B. Lippincott.

Carroll, P. (1986). Artificial Airways: Real Risks. *Nursing '86.* 86(8) (57–59).

Cline, A. (1989). Streamlined Documentation Through Exceptional Charting. *Nursing Management.* 20 (62–64).

Dick, M., Marce, S., and Gary, J. (1992). How to Boost the Odds of a Painless I.V. Start. *American Journal of Nursing.* 92 (49–50).

Dustin, J. (1990). How Managed Care Can Work for You. *Nursing '90.* 20(10) (56–59).

Ehrhardt, B.S. and Graham, M. (1990). Pulse Oximetry: An Easy Way to Check Oxygen Saturation. *Nursing '90.* 20(3) (50–54).

Erickson, R. (1989). Mastering the Ins and Outs of Chest Drainage, Part 2. *Nursing '89.* 19(6) (47–49).

Eustace, C. (1991). Back Up and Wait. *RN.* 54(6) (49–51).

Ferland, P. (1991). Are You Ready for Ventilator Patients? *Nursing '91.* 91(22) (42–47).

Francis, C.W., Pellegrini, V.D., Jr., Marder, V.J., Totterman, S., Harris, C.M., Gabriel, K.R., Azodo, M.V., and Leibert, K.M. (1992). Comparison of Warfarin and External Pneumatic Compression of Venous Thrombosis After Total Hip Replacement. *Journal of the American Medical Association* 267(21) (2911–2915).

Garner, J. and Simons, B. (1983). CDC Guideline for Isolation Precautions in Hospitals. *Infection Control.* 83(4) (248–325).

Giger, J.N. and Davidhizar, R.E. (1991). *Transcultural Nursing: Assessment and Prevention.* St. Louis: Mosby's Year Book, Inc.

Gonsoulin, S.M. and Broussard, P.C. (1991). Shedding Light on I.V. Therapy. *Nursing '91.* 21(12) (62–64).

Hahn, K. (1990). Brush Up on Your Injection Technique. *Nursing '90.* 20(9) (54–58).

Hamilton, H. and Rose, M. (Eds.) (1983). *Procedures.* Springhouse, PA: Intermed Communications.

Hamilton, H. and Rose, M. (Eds.) (1984). *Assessment.* Springhouse, PA: Springhouse.

Hamilton, H. and Rose, M. (Eds.) (1984). *Diseases.* Springhouse, PA: Springhouse.

Hansen, J.F. (1987). A Timesaving Guide to Better Patient Teaching. *Nursing '87.* 17(11) (129–136).

Hill, M.N. and Grim, C.M. (1991). How to Take a Precise Blood Pressure. *American Journal of Nursing.* 91 (38–42).

Howard, M., Eisenberg, P., and Gianino, M. (1992). Dressing a Central Venous Catheter—A Better Way. *Nursing '92.* 22(3) (60–61).

Iyer, P.W. (1991). New Trends in Charting. *Nursing '91.* 21(1) (48–50).

Iyer, P.W. (1991). Six More Charting Rules. *Nursing '91.* 21(6) (34–39).

Jaffe, M., Skidmore-Roth, L., and Rayman, R. (1986). *Procedure Cards for Clinical Use.* Norwalk: Appleton-Century-Crofts.

Jaffe, M. and Skidmore-Roth, L. (1988). *Home Health Nursing Care Plans.* St. Louis: C.V. Mosby.

Keen, M.F. (1990). Z-track Injections. *Nursing '90.* 20(8) (59).

Luckmann, J. and Sorensen, K. (1987). *Medical-Surgical Nursing* (3rd ed.). Philadelphia: W.B. Saunders.

Malasanos, L., Barkauskas, V., Moss, M., and Stoltenberg-Allen, K. (1986). *Health Assessment* (3rd ed.). St. Louis: C.V. Mosby.

Mandell, M. (1987). Charting: How It Can Keep You Out of Court. *Nursing Life.* 7(5) (46–48).

Marshall, J.C. (1991). Prophylaxis of Deep Venous Thrombosis and Pulmonary Embolism. *Canadian Journal of Surgery.* 34(6) (551–554).

Mathews, J.P. (1991). How to Use an Automated Vital Signs Monitor. *Nursing '91.* 21(2) (60–64).

Mathewson, M. (1986). *Pharmacotherapeutics: A Nursing Approach.* Philadelphia: F.A. Davis.

McConnell, E. (1991). Preventing Postop Complications: Minimizing Respiratory Problems. *Nursing '91.* 91 (November) (33–48)

McGovern, K. (1992). 10 Golden Rules for Administering Drugs Safely. *Nursing '92.* 22(3) (49–55).

McHugh, J. (1987). Perfecting the Three Steps of Chest Physiotherapy. *Nursing '87.* 17(11) (54–57).

McLaughlin-Hagan, M. (1991). Continuous Subcutaneous Infusions. *Nursing '91.* 21(7) (58–59).

Messner, R.L. and Pinkerman, M.L. (1992). Preventing a Peripheral I.V. Infection. *Nursing '92.* 22(6) (34–41).

Metheney, N. (1988). Measures to Test Placement of Nasogastric and Nasointestinal Feeding Tubes: A Review. *Nursing Research.* 37(324).

Millam, D. How to Get Into Hard-to-Stick Veins. *RN Magazine.* 48(4) (34–35).

Millam, D.A. (1992). How to Develop Your Venipuncture Expertise. *Nursing '92.* 22(9) (33–47).

Montanari, J. and Spearing, C. (1986). The Fine Art of Measuring Tracheal Cuff Pressure. *Nursing '86.* 86(7) (46–49).

Morris, L., Kraft, S., Tessem, S., and Reinisch, S. (1988). Nursing the Patient in Traction. *RN.* 51(1). (January) (26–31).

Murphy, T.G. (1992). Low-Tech, High-Touch Perfusion Assessment. *American Journal of Nursing.* 92 (36–45).

National Institute of Health (NIH) Consensus Conference. (1986). Prevention of Venous Thrombosis and Pulmonary Embolism. *Journal of the American Medical Association.* 256(744).

Neeson, J. and May, K. (1986). Comprehensive Maternity Nursing: Nursing Process and the Childbearing Family. Philadelphia: J.B. Lippincott.

Neuberger, G. (1987). Wound Care: What's Clear, What's Not. *Nursing '87.* 17(2) (34–37).

Newton, M., Newton, D., and Fudin, J. (1992). Big Three Injection Routes. *Nursing '92.* 22(2) (34–41).

Norton, B. and Miller, A. (1986). *Skills for Professional Nursing Practice.* Norwalk: Appleton-Century-Crofts.

Nurses' Reference Library. (1984). *Procedures.* Springhouse, PA: Springhouse.

Palau, D. and Jones, S. Test Your Skill at Troubleshooting Chest Tubes. *RN Magazine.* 49(10) (43–45).

Perry, A. and Potter, P. (1986). *Clinical Nursing Skills & Techniques: Basic, Intermediate, & Advanced.* St. Louis: C.V. Mosby.

Persson, A.V., Davis, R.J., and Villavicencio, J.L. (1991). Deep Venous Thrombosis and Pulmonary Embolism. *Surgical Clinics of North America.* 71(6) (1195–1209).

Phipps, W.J., Long, B.C., and Woods, N.F. (1987). *Medical-Surgical Nursing: Concepts and Clinical Practice* (3rd ed.). St. Louis: C.V. Mosby.

Pillitteri, A. (1987). *Child Health Nursing: Care of the Growing Family* (3rd ed.). Boston: Little Brown.

Potter, P. and Perry, A. (1985). *Fundamentals of Nursing: Concepts, Process, and Practice.* St. Louis: C.V. Mosby.

Price, J.L. and Cordell, B. (1984). Patient Education Evaluation: Beyond Intuition. *Nursing Forum.* 21(3) (117–121).

Putterbaugh, S. (1991). Communicating When the Patient Cannot Speak English. *Today's OR Nurse.* 13(1) (31).

Querin, J. and Stahl, L. (1990). 12 Simple Sensible Steps for Successful Blood Transfusion. *Nursing '90.* 20(10) (68–81).

Robertson, R.E. and Kaplan, R.F. (1991). Another Site for the Pulse Oximeter Probe. *Anesthesiology.* 74 (198).

Seidel, H.M., Ball, J.W., Dains, J.E., and Benedict, G.W. (1991). *Mosby's Guide to Physical Examination* (2nd ed.). St. Louis: Mosby Year Book, Inc.

Sheppard, M. and Swearingen, P. Z-Track Injections: A Step-by-step How To for an Unused IM Technique. *American Journal of Nursing.* 84(6) (746–747).

Smith, D. The Ostomy: How Is It Managed? *American Journal of Nursing.* 85(11) (1246–1249).

Smith, D., Nix, K.S., Kemper, J.Y., Liquori, R., Brantly, D.K., Rollins, J.H., Stevens, N.V., and Clutter, L.B. (1991). *Comprehensive Child and Family Nursing Skills.* St. Louis: Mosby Year Book.

Smith, S. and Duell, D. (1992). *Clinical Nursing Skills.* (3rd ed.). Norwalk, CT: Appleton & Lange.

Sonnesso, G. (1991). Are You Ready to Use Pulse Oximetry? *Nursing '91.* 22 (8) (60–64).

Sorenson, K.C. and Luckmann, J. (1986). *Basic Nursing: A Psychophysiologic Approach.* (2nd ed.). Philadelphia: W.B. Saunders.

Speers, A.T. (1989). Patient Education Theory and Practice. *Journal of Nursing Staff Development.* 5(3) (121–126).

Steel, J. (1983). Too Fast or Too Slow—The Erratic IV. *American Journal of Nursing.* 83(6) (898–901).

Steil, C.F. and Deakins, D.A. (1990). Today's Insulins: What You and Your Patient Need to Know. *Nursing '90.* 20(8) (34–39).

Swearingen, P., Sommers, M., and Miller, K. (1988). *Manual of Critical Care : Applying Nursing Diagnosis to Adult Critical Situations.* St. Louis: C.V. Mosby.

Tartaglia, M. (1985). Nursing Diagnosis: Keystone of Your Care Plan. *Nursing '85.* 85(3) (34–38).

Watt, R. (1985). The Ostomy: Why Is It Created? *American Journal of Nursing.* 85(11) (1242–1245).

Weber, J. (1988). *Nurses' Handbook of Health Assessment.* Philadelphia: J.B. Lippincott.

Whaley, L.F. and Wong, D.L. (1987). *Nursing Care of Infants and Children* (3rd ed.). St. Louis: C.V. Mosby.

Wieck, L., King, E., and Dyer, M. (1986). *Illustrated Manual of Nursing Techniques* (3rd ed.). Philadelphia: J.B. Lippincott.

Wong, D., Whaley, L., and Kasprisin, C. *Clinical Handbook of Pediatric Nursing* (2nd ed.). St. Louis: C.V. Mosby.

Young, C. and White, S. (1992). Preparing Patients for Tube Feeding at Home. *American Journal of Nursing.* 92(4) (46–53).

Zori, S. (1984). Bringing the Patient into Focus. *American Journal of Nursing.* 84(11) (1384–1388).

Index